Complementary Health for Women

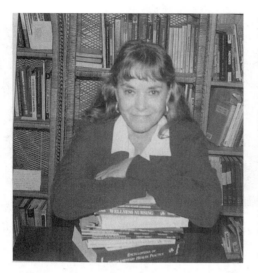

Carolyn Chambers Clark, EdD, ARNP, FAAN, AHN-BC, holds a doctorate from Teachers College, Columbia University. For more than 30 years, she conducted research on wellness self-care, maintained a private practice using complementary and holistic health methods, and provided consultation on complementary health topics. She is a prolific contributor to the literature of wellness and complementary health and is board-certified as an advanced holistic nurse.

Dr. Clark is a faculty member at Walden University in the Health Sciences Department, teaching in both the masters program in nursing and the doctoral program in health services.

Dr. Clark is editor-in-chief of *The Encyclopedia of Complementary Health Practice* (Springer Publishing, 1999), editor of *Health Promotion in Communities: Holistic and Wellness Approaches* (Springer Publishing, 2002), and author of *Wellness Practitioner* (Springer Publishing, 1996), *Integrating Complementary Procedures Into Practice* (Springer Publishing, 2000), *Holistic Assertiveness Skills for Nurses: Empower Yourself and Others!* (2003), and *The Holistic Nursing Approach to Chronic Disease* (2004).

To contact Dr. Clark, subscribe to her free wellness e-newsletter, or find up-to-date wellness research, visit her Web site at www.carolynchambersclark.com.

Complementary Health for Women

A Comprehensive Treatment
Guide for Major Disease and
Common Conditions With

- Evidenced based therapies
- Methods of use
- Dosage and treatment effects
- Cautions
- Handy tips

From Alzheimer's to Stroke

**Carolyn Chambers Clark,
EdD, ARNP, FAAN, AHN-BC**

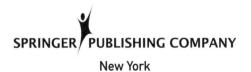

SPRINGER PUBLISHING COMPANY

New York

Springer Publishing Company, Inc.
11 West 42nd Street
New York, NY 10036
www.springerpub.com

Acquisitions Editor: Allan Graubard

Production Editor: Julia Rosen

Cover design: Steven Pisano

Composition: Apex CoVantage

08 09 10 11/ 5 4 3 2 1

Library of Congress Cataloging-in-Publication Data

Clark, Carolyn Chambers.
    Complementary health for women : a comprehensive treatment guide for major disease and common conditions with evidenced based therapies, methods of use, dosage and treatment effects, cautions, handy tips : from Alzheimer's to stroke / Carolyn Chambers Clark.
        p. ; cm.
    Includes bibliographical references and index.
    ISBN 978-0-8261-1087-9 (alk. paper)
    1. Women—Health and hygiene.   2. Women—Diseases—Alternative treatment.
    I. Title.   [DNLM: 1. Complementary Therapies.   2. Women's Health.
3. Evidence Based Medicine.   4. Primary Prevention.   WB 890 C592c 2008]
    RA778.C567 2008
    613'.04244—dc22   2008033652

Printed in the United States of America by Bang Printing.

The author and the publisher of this Work have made every effort to use sources believed to be reliable to provide information that is accurate and compatible with the standards generally accepted at the time of publication. Because medical science is continually advancing, our knowledge base continues to expand. Therefore, as new information becomes available, changes in procedures become necessary. We recommend that the reader always consult current research and specific institutional policies before performing any clinical procedure. The author and publisher shall not be liable for any special, consequential, or exemplary damages resulting, in whole or in part, from the readers' use of, or reliance on, the information contained in this book. The publisher has no responsibility for the persistence or accuracy of URLs for external or third-party Internet Web sites referred to in this publication and does not guarantee that any content on such Web sites is, or will remain, accurate or appropriate.

This book is dedicated to all the women—past, present, and future—who use safe and effective complementary procedures.

Contents

Preface ix

Acknowledgments xi

1   Alzheimer's/Memory 1

2   Anxiety 23

3   Bladder Infections (Cystitis) 37

4   Blood Pressure/Hypertension 45

5   Breast Cancer 65

6   Cervical Cancer 93

7   Colon and Rectal Cancer 105

8   Depression 121

9   Digestion (Constipation, Crohn's, Diarrhea, GERD
    [Heartburn]), IBS/IBD 133

10 Endometrial Cancer 145

11 Falls 157

12 Fatigue 163

13 Fibroids 169

14 Gastric Cancer 173

15 Heart/Blood Vessels 185

16 Incontinence 209

17 Insomnia 215

18 Kidney Conditions 221

19 Liver Conditions 229

20 Lung Conditions 241

21 Menopause 253

22 Migraines 263

23 Osteoporosis/Osteopenia 269

24 Ovarian Cancer 281

25 Overweight/Obesity 287

26 Pain 299

27 Pancreatic Cancer 313

28 PMS 325

29 Polycystic Ovary Syndrome (PCOS) 333

30 Pregnancy/Labor/Delivery 337

31 Stroke 359

Appendix 367

Index 369

Preface

Protocol

Each condition is examined using the following protocol: The alphabetical listing of conditions includes environment, exercise/movement, herbs/essential oils, mindset, nutrition (what to eat, drink, and avoid), stress management, supplements, and touch. If current research-based evidence was not available from a search of www.pubmed.com or a Google search, that element was omitted (e.g., herbs/essential oils or stress management may not appear for certain conditions, even if practitioners do use them). For most conditions, you will find:

a. Actions/expected responses
b. Routes/dosages/frequencies
c. Cautions
d. Assessments
e. Tips on use
f. Other considerations
g. References/other sources

Additional information (standardized assessments, how to apply specific procedures, finding foods containing needed nutrients, etc.) appear as Web addresses within each protocol, which are current as of the date of copyediting the manuscript. If you find a link that is no longer current, please contact me at carolyn@carolynchambersclark.com and I will correct it in the next edition. In the meantime, you can also do a Google search on your computer for whatever the content is and find up-to-date links to guide you.

Research-based references, upon which protocols are based, appear at the end of each condition as References/Other Resources. References provide state-of-the science evidence to support each protocol's information only. For additional research, a Google or www.pubmed.com search is recommended.

A Resource List of Certification and CEU-offering complementary health procedure programs is available in the Appendix (p. 367).

How to Use This Book

This book is meant to be a handy reference that you can carry with you for treatment, self-care, or prevention.

Whenever suggesting any procedures to others (such as meditation, cognitive behavioral approaches, yoga, etc.) that you're not familiar with, it is wise to try them yourself first. This will help you anticipate the questions you might be asked and the reactions others may have to a procedure. Even if you don't wish to try the herbs or supplements, be sure to counsel others to follow the directions on the bottle.

Always encourage others to follow these steps and follow them yourself:

(a) start small and build to the suggested upper limit for supplements or practice,
(b) stop if any negative reaction is observed,
(c) always inform the prescribing health care practitioner(s) about the practices used to make sure no negative interactions occur with prescribed or over-the-counter medications.

All best wishes with this information and do contact me with your reactions and suggestions at carolyn@carolynchambersclark.com. For updated research studies and information as it appears, e-mail me to receive my monthly wellness e-newsletter and/or check updated research on my blog at www.carolynchambersclark.com/id33.html.

In wellness,

Carolyn Chambers Clark
Advanced Registered Nurse Practitioner
Doctorate in Nursing Education
Faculty, Nursing and Health Services, Walden University
Advanced Holistic Nurse, Board-Certified
Fellow, American Academy of Nursing

Acknowledgments

I wish to thank the many women who have asked the important questions about how to use complementary procedures to enhance their health and wellness.

I also wish to thank all the people at Springer Publishing Company involved in the effort to produce this book, especially Allan Graubard who had the vision to realize the importance of my manuscript.

—C. C. C.

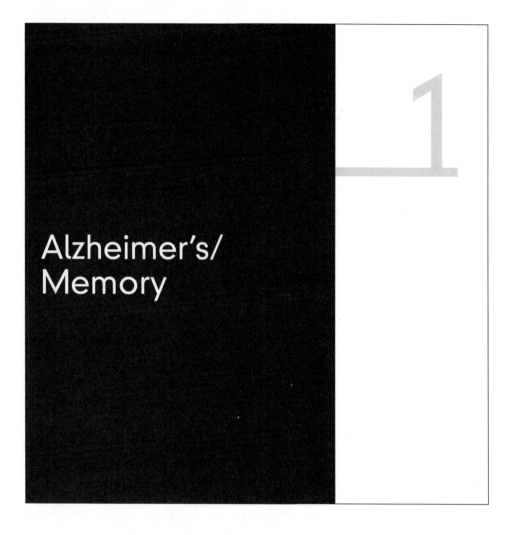

Alzheimer's/ Memory

1

To date, no effective medication has been shown to treat Alzheimer's disease. Recent research has provided evidence of numerous complementary procedures that may either prevent and/or reduce symptoms of the condition.

Environment

1. Aluminum products
   a. *Actions/expected responses:* The combination of fluoride and aluminum has been shown to cause the same pathological changes in the brain tissue that are found in those diagnosed with Alzheimer's.
   b. *Routes/dosages/frequencies:* Avoid antacids, buffered aspirin, aluminum cookware, and underarm antiperspirants.
   c. *Cautions:* Read product labels; some products may contain aluminum salts.
   d. *Assessments:* Take a baseline measure for memory loss and depression and then take a measure after no longer using aluminum-containing products. To assess memory loss, go to: http://www.patient.co.uk/showdoc/40024813

To assess depression, go to: http://www.psychpage.com/learning/library/assess/depression.htm

e. *Tips on use:* Use deodorants instead of antiperspirants; perspiration is the body's natural way of cooling off and ridding the body of toxins and it should not be blocked.

f. *Other considerations:* Eliminate aluminum products from the home and work station.

g. *References/other sources:*

Shcherbatykh, I., & Carpenter, D. O. (2007). The role of metals in the etiology of Alzheimer's disease. *Journal of Alzheimer's Disease, 11*(2), 191–205.

2. Brain toxins from prescribed and over-the-counter medications

a. *Actions/expected responses:* Brain toxins can interfere with clear thinking and memory. For a list of prescribed and over-the-counter medications found to be related to memory loss go to: http://www.worstpills.org/results.cfm?drug_id=0&drugfamily_id=0&disease_id=0&druginduced_id=97&keyword_id=0

b. *Routes/dosages/frequencies:* Avoid prescribed and over-the-counter drugs associated with memory loss.

c. *Cautions:* More than twice as many prescriptions are filled for those 65 and older (23.5 prescriptions per year) than for those younger than 65.

d. *Assessments:* Take a baseline measure for memory loss (see 1d) and then take a measure after medications that lead to memory loss are no longer being used.

e. *Tips on use:* Explore other treatments that are not linked with memory loss with prescribing health care practitioner.

f. *Other considerations:* A medication/memory loss diary can identify which drugs most affect memory.

g. *References/other sources:*

Fogari, R., & Zoppi, A. (2004). Effect of antihypertensive agents on quality of life in the elderly. *Drugs and Aging, 21*(6), 377–393.

Hale, A. S. (1995). Critical flicker fusion threshold and anticholinergic effects of chronic antidepressant treatment in remitted depressives. *British Journal of Clinical Pharmacology, 42,* 239–241.

Kerr, J. S., Powell, J., & Hindmarch, L. (1996). The effects of reboxetine and amitriptyline, with and without alcohol on cognitive function and psychomotor performance. *Journal of Psychopharmacology, 9*(3), 258–266.

Knegtering, H., Eijck, M., & Huijsman, A. (1994). Effects of antidepressants on cognitive functioning of elderly patients: A review. *Drugs and Aging, 5*(3), 192–199.

Moncrieff, J., & Cohen, D. (2005). Rethinking models of psychotropic drug action. *Psychotherapy and Psychosomatics, 74,* 145–153.

Moncrieff, J., & Cohen, D. (2006). Do antidepressants cure or create abnormal brain states? *PloS Med 3*(7). Retrieved July 27, 2008, from http://medicine.plosjournals.org/perlserv/?request=get-document&doi=10.1371/journal.pmed.0030240http://medicine.plosjournals.org/perlserv/?request=get-document&doi=10.1371/journal.pmed.0030240&ct=1

Puustinen, J., Nurminen, J., Kukola, M., Vahlberg, T., Laine, K., & Kivela, S. L. (2007). Associations between use of benzodiazepines or related drugs and health, physical abilities and cognitive function. *Drugs and Aging, 24*(12), 1045–1059.

Van Putten, T., & Marder, S. R. (1987). Behavioral toxicity of antipsychotic drugs. *Journal of Clinical Psychiatry, 48,* 13–19.

3. Fish aquariums
   a. *Actions/expected responses:* Exposing women diagnosed with Alzheimer's to fish aquariums can result in increased nutritional intake and weight, decreased physical aggression, and decreased need for nutritional supplementation, resulting in health care cost savings.
   b. *Routes/dosages/frequencies:* Place an aquarium in the dining area.
   c. *Cautions:* For severe dementia, a specially designed aquarium may be needed to ensure safety.
   d. *Assessments:* Take baseline nutritional data (nutritional intake, weight, need for nutritional supplementation) prior to introducing the aquarium and repeat assessment every 2 weeks for 6 weeks or longer.
   e. *Tips on use:* Encourage women to look at the fish and speak about what they see.
   f. *Other considerations:* Family or caregivers can use aquariums as therapeutic tools to enhance eating behaviors, encourage weight gain, and reduce aggressive behavior.
   g. *References/other sources:*
   Edwards, N. E., & Beck, A. M. (2002). Animal-assisted therapy and nutrition in Alzheimer's disease. *Western Journal of Nursing Research, 24*(6), 697–712.

4. Fluoridated water
   a. *Actions/expected responses:* The combination of fluoride and aluminum has been shown to cause the same pathological changes in the brain tissue that are found in people diagnosed with Alzheimer's.
   b. *Routes/dosages/frequencies:* Drink 8–10 glasses of distilled water daily.
   c. *Cautions:* None.
   d. *Assessments:* Take a baseline measure for memory loss and depression (see 1d) and then take a measure after drinking only distilled water for a week.
   e. *Tips on use:* Distilled water is available at most supermarkets.
   f. *Other considerations:* None.
   g. *References/other sources:*
   Horvath, W., & Isaacson, R. L. (1998). Chronic administration of aluminum-fluoride or sodium-fluoride to rats in drinking water: Alterations in neuronal and cerebrovascular integrity. *Brain Research, 784*(1–2), 284–298.
   Rondeau, V., Commenges, D., Jacqmin-Gadda, H., & Dartigues, J. F. (2000). Relation between aluminum concentrations in drinking water and Alzheimer's disease: An 8-year follow-up study. *American Journal of Epidemiology, 152*(1), 59–66.
   Van der Voet, G. B., Schijns, O., & de Wolff, F. A. (1999). Fluoride enhances the effect of aluminum chloride on interconnections between aggregates of hippocampal neurons. *Archives of Physiological Biochemistry, 107* (1), 15–21.

5. Hydration
   a. *Actions/expected responses:* Low hydration status is related to cognitive functioning, including slowed psychomotor processing speed and poor attention/memory performance in older adults.
   b. *Routes/dosages/frequencies:* Drink 8–10 glasses of water a day.
   c. *Cautions:* Some drinking water may contain toxic substances.

d. *Assessments:* Assess cognitive functioning prior to and after drinking 8–10 glasses of water a day.

e. *Tips on use:* Recommend distilled water.

f. *Other considerations:* As an alternative, women can purchase a reverse osmosis water filter to remove potential toxic substances.

g. *References/other sources:*

Sedman, R. M., Beaumont, J., McDonald, T. A., Reynolds, S., Krowech, G., & Howd, R. (2006). Review of the evidence regarding the carcinogenicity of hexavalent chromium in drinking water. *Journal of Environmental Science and Health Part C, 24,* (1), 155–182.

Suhr, J. A., Hall, J., Patterson, S. M., & Niinisto, R. T. (2004). The relation of hydration to cognitive performance in healthy older adults. *International Journal of Psychophysiology 53*(2), 121–125.

6. Mirror use

a. *Actions/expected responses:* Using a mirror has been shown to raise awareness to needed self-care and can increase communication with caregivers.

b. *Routes/dosages/frequencies:* As tolerated.

c. *Cautions:* At first, feelings of anger or despair may be aroused, but this is quickly followed by relief and calmness.

d. *Assessments:* Take a baseline measure for self-care, anger, and despair prior to using a mirror, and then take a measure after mirror use.

e. *Tips on use:* Gradually expose women to mirror use, encouraging them to look and, if they like, to speak about what they see.

f. *Other considerations:* Family or caregivers can use mirrors as a therapeutic tool to enhance self-care and communication with others.

g. *References/other sources:*

Tabak, N., Bergman, R., & Alpert, R. (1996). The mirror as a therapeutic tool for patients with dementia. *International Journal of Nursing Practice, 2*(3), 155–159.

7. Music

a. *Actions/expected responses:* Aids memory, movement, balance; calms agitation, anxiety, depression; reduces fear-panic; increases appetite.

b. *Routes/dosages/frequencies:* 20-minute sessions.

c. *Cautions:* Stop or change to more soothing music if agitation increases.

d. *Assessments:* Chart changes in memory, thinking, and social function.

e. *Tips on use:* Although not all sources agree, classical music, ballroom dance music, and familiar songs from pleasant situations may be best. According to Campbell (1997), residents from the rural South diagnosed with Alzheimer's could recall the words to songs dramatically better than spoken words or information, when they heard "What a Friend We Have In Jesus," "Amazing Grace," "Psalm 23," "Happy Birthday," and "It's a Small World." Other women may respond well to songs such as "You Made Me Love You" or "Sweet Georgia Brown."

f. *Other considerations:* Memory retention can increase to 75% when asked to sing, hum, or keep time to the beat. Those diagnosed with Alzheimer's who do not talk or interact may sing or dance when music is played.

g. *References/other sources:*

Brotons, M., & Koger, S. (2000). The impact of music therapy on language functioning in dementia. *Journal of Music Therapy, 37*(3), 183–195.

Campbell, D. (1997). *The Mozart effect: Tapping the power of music to heal the body, strengthen the mind and unlock the creative spirit.* New York: Avon.

Clair, A. (2002). The effects of music therapy on engagement in family caregiver and care receiver couples with dementia. *American Journal of Alzheimer's Disease and Other Dementias, 17*(5), 286–290.

Prickett, C. A., & Moore, R. S. (1991). The use of music to aid memory of Alzheimer's patients, *Journal of Music Therapy 28,* 101–110.

Ragneskog, H., Brane, G., Kihlgren, M., Karlsson, I., & Norberg, A. (1996). Dinner music for demented patients: Analysis of video-recorded observations. *Clinical Nursing Research, 5*(3), 262–277.

8. Noise and lighting
   a. *Actions/expected responses:* Noise and lighting conditions can affect food intake at mealtimes.
   b. *Routes/dosages/frequencies:* Reduce noise and increase lighting to enhance food intake.
   c. *Cautions:* None.
   d. *Assessments:* Monitor for noise and lighting and its effect on food intake prior to and after reducing noise and increasing lighting.
   e. *Tips on use:* To start, monitor five days a week at breakfast.
   f. *Other considerations:* None.
   g. *References/other sources:*
      McDaniel, J. H., Hunt, A., Hackes, B., & Pope, J. F. (2001). Impact of dining room environment on nutritional intake of Alzheimer's residents: A case study. *American Journal of Alzheimer's Disease and Other Dementias, 16*(5), 297–302.
9. Power-frequency fields and wireless communications
   a. *Actions/expected responses:* Neurological effects and neurodegenerative diseases, such as Alzheimer's, are associated with modified brain activity due to electromagnetic fields (EMFs).
   b. *Routes/dosages/frequencies:* Current levels of long-term exposure to some kinds of electromagnetic fields are not protective of public health.
   c. *Cautions:* Scientific evidence raises concerns about the health impacts of mobile or cell phone radiation, power lines, interior wiring and grounding of buildings and appliances such as microwaves, wireless technologies, and electric blankets.
   d. *Assessments:* Assess exposure to EMFs listed in item c.
   e. *Tips on use:* Until new public safety limits and limits on further deployment of risky technologies are warranted, avoid exposure to EMFs.
   f. *Other considerations:* An international working group of renowned scientists, researchers, and public health policy professionals (The Bioinitiative Working Group) has released its report on electromagnetic fields and health. It raises serious concerns about the safety of existing public limits that regulate how much EMF is allowable from power lines, cell phones, and many other EMF sources of exposure in daily life.
   g. *References/other sources:*
      Hardell, L., & Sage, C. (2008). Biological effects from electromagnetic field exposure and public exposure standards. *Biomedical Pharmacotherapy, 62*(2), 104–109.
10. Red dishes
    a. *Actions/expected responses:* People with severe Alzheimer's in long-term care can have deficient contrast sensitivity and poor food and liquid

intake. Using high-contrast red or high-contrast blue tableware (as opposed to white tableware) can increase food intake by as much as 35% and liquid intake by as much as 84%.

b. *Routes/dosages/frequencies:* Use red tableware for each meal.

c. *Cautions:* None.

d. *Assessments:* Take a baseline measure for food and liquid intake and then take a measure after change to high-contrast red or blue tableware.

e. *Tips on use:* Try different colored high-contrast tableware to see which works best.

f. *Other considerations:* None.

g. *References/other sources:*

Dunne, T. E., Neargarder, S. A., Cipolloni, P. B., & Cronin-Golumb, A. (2004). Visual contrast enhances food and liquid intake in advanced Alzheimer's disease. *Clinical Nutrition, 23*(4), 533–538.

11. Snoezelen: A multisensory intervention

a. *Actions/expected responses:* Provides statistically significant calming and relaxing of agitation; provides a feeling of dignity, initiative, and freedom of choice. The multisensory environment includes music, light from fiber optic strands, calming image projections, vibrations of bubble tubes, and soothing smells.

b. *Routes/dosages/frequencies:* 30 to 40 minutes.

c. *Cautions:* None reported. Is a pleasant alternative to seclusion or restraints.

d. *Assessments:* Take a baseline measure of agitation prior to and after participating in snoezelen.

e. *Tips on use:* None.

f. *Other considerations:* Snoezelen, a multisensory environmental intervention, has been used successfully in Great Britain and is just beginning to appear in the United States.

g. *References/other sources:*

Chistsey, A. M., Haight, B. K., & Jones, M. M. (2002). Snoezelen: A multisensory environmental intervention. *Journal of Gerontological Nursing, 28*(3), 41–49.

Teitelbaum, A., Volpo, S., Paran, R., Zislin, J., Drumer, D., Raskin, S., et al. (2007). Multisensory environmental intervention (snoezelen) as a preventive alternative to seclusion and restraint in closed psychiatric wards. *Harefuah, 146*(1), 79–80.

Exercise/Movement

1. Rocking in a rocking chair

a. *Actions/expected responses:* Decreases agitation, anxiety, tension, depression, and hyper-responsiveness stress, and indirectly decreases detrimental cortisol levels. Can decrease vocalization/moaning, pacing, and walking. May release pain-relieving brain endorphins, thus increasing quality of life. Can decrease requests for pain medication from one to three fewer requests per week. Balance can also improve.

b. *Routes/dosages/frequencies:* As tolerated from one-half hour to two and a half hours a day. In one study, those who rocked the most improved the most.

    c. *Cautions:* Use only a platform-style rocking chair with a super-stable, immobile base that moves back and forth easily.

    d. *Assessments:* Take a baseline measure for crying, pain medication requests, balance agitation, anxiety, depression, and pacing; then take a measure after treatment.

    e. *Tips on use:* Family members or friends can rock together.

    f. *Other considerations:* Research has shown that rocking can help with agitation, anxiety, depression, falls, and other negative behaviors and that it can increase positive feelings.

    g. *References/other sources:*

        Watson, N., Hauptmann, M., Brink, C., Powers, B., Taillie, E. R., Lash, M., et al. (1998). *As elders rock, emotional burden of dementia eases.* Paper presented to the Eastern Nursing Research Society, April 23–25, Rochester, NY.

2. Walking or other strenuous activity

    a. *Actions/expected responses:* Walking lowers the odds of cognitive decline by 13% and may prevent brain shrinkage in early Alzheimer's.

    b. *Routes/dosages/frequencies:* For every 10 blocks walked by women 65 years or older, there is a drop in risk of cognitive decline.

    c. *Cautions:* If exercise is a new activity, encourage women and their caregivers to start with one block or less and walk at a rate at which easy conversation can be held.

    d. *Assessments:* Take pulse prior to walking and every few minutes when adding this activity. Aerobic activity is not necessary, only walking together at a comfortable, talking-while-walking pace.

    e. *Tips for use:* Suggest caregivers walk with the women if possible, pointing out the sights and observing safety rules.

    f. *Other considerations:* Keep track of number of blocks walked each day and track it versus ability to think clearly and remember. Participating in walking, hiking, bicycling, swimming, weight training, or other strenuous activities for at least 15 minutes three times per week can improve cerebral blood flow and cut dementia risk by one-third.

    g. *References/other sources:*

        American Academy of Neurology. (2008, July 15). Exercise may prevent brain shrinkage in early Alzheimer's disease. *ScienceDaily.* Retrieved July 26, 2008, from http://www.sciencedaily.com/releases/2008/07/080714162632.htm

        Larsson, E. G., Wang, L., Bowen, J. D., McCormick, W. C., Teri, L., Crane, P., et al. (2006). Exercise is associated with reduced risk for incident dementia among persons 65 years of age and older. *Annals of Internal Medicine, 144,* 73–81.

        Yaffe, E., Barnes, D., & Nevitt, M. (2001). A prospective study of physical activity and cognitive decline in elderly women: Women who walk. *Archives of Internal Medicine, 161,* 1703–1708.

Herbs/Essential Oils

1. Ginkgo biloba

    a. *Actions/expected responses:* Speeds up working memory and information processing, improves social functioning, improves blood flow to the brain.

Is equally effective as cholinesterase inhibitors in the treatment of mild to moderate Alzheimer's dementia.

b. *Routes/dosages/frequencies:* 24% standardized extract/capsules of 60–80 mg and take one to three times a day, following dosage on bottle.

c. *Cautions:* Ginkgo must be carefully coordinated with medications because it can interact with aspirin and antiplatelet drugs, increasing clotting time. Avoid using concurrently with anticonvulsants, buspirone, trazadone, St. John's wort, MAOIs or fluoexetine, and never exceed suggested dosage. Not to be used during pregnancy, given to children, or used by those with coagulation or platelet disorders, hemophilia, seizures, or hypersensitivity to this herb. Adverse reactions could include transient headache, anxiety, restlessness, vomiting, lack of appetite, diarrhea, flatulence, or rash, but a meta-analysis of unconfounded, randomized, double-blind controlled studies found no significant differences between ginkgo and placebo in the proportion of participants experiencing adverse events.

d. *Assessments:* Chart changes in memory, thinking, and social function prior to and after taking ginkgo.

e. *Tips on use:* Follow bottle directions.

f. *Other considerations:* Discuss use with a certified or expert herbalist for best results. Ginkgo may take from 1–6 months to achieve full effectiveness.

g. *References/other sources:*

Birks, J., Grimley, E. V., & Van Dongen, M. (2002). Ginkgo biloba for cognitive impairment and dementia. *Cochrane Database System Review 4,* CD0031230.

Itil, T., & Martorano, D., (1995). Natural substances in psychiatry (ginkgo biloba) in dementia. *Psychopharmacology Bulletin, 31*(1), 147–158.

LeBars, P. L., Katz, M., & Berman, N. (1997). A placebo-controlled, double-blind randomized trial of an extract of gingko biloba for dementia. *Journal of the American Medical Association, 278,* 1327–1332.

Skidmore-Roth, L. (2006). *Mosby's handbook of herbs and natural supplements* (3rd ed.). St. Louis, MO: ElsevierMosby.

Stough, C., Clarke, J., Lloyd, J., & Nathan, P. J. (2001). Neuropsychological changes after 30-day gingko biloba administration in healthy participants. *International Journal of Neuropsychopharmacology, 4*(2), 131–134.

Weitstein, A. (2000). Cholinesterase inhibitors and gingko extracts—Are they comparable in the treatment of dementia? Comparison of published placebo-controlled efficacy studies of at least six months' duration. *Phytomedicine, 6*(6), 393–401.

2. Lemon balm

a. *Actions/expected responses:* It is memory-enhancing, calming, and can improve cognitive performance.

b. *Routes/dosages/frequencies:* Drink as a tea, starting with one cup a day and work up to no more than three cups a day. To keep the tea for up to one year, it should be stored in a sealed container away from heat and moisture. Lemon balm can also be taken as a standardized extract 60 drops per day.

c. *Cautions:* The herb is not to be used during pregnancy or lactation or given to children, nor should it be used by persons diagnosed with hypothyroidism or by those hypersensitive to it. Adverse reactions may include nausea, anorexia, and hypersensitivity reactions. Lemon balm may potentiate the sedative effects of barbiturates and central nervous system depressants, and it may decrease the absorption of iron salts, so separate intake of the herb from any medications or drugs by two hours.

  d. *Assessments:* Assess for hypersensitivity reactions, use of barbiturates, other central nervous system depressants or iron salts. Take a baseline for memory and calmness and then chart changes in memory and increased calmness with use of the herb.

  e. *Tips on use:* Pour boiling water over tea leaves or bags and allow it to set for 10 minutes; strain if necessary. For standardized extract, follow directions on the bottle.

  f. *Other considerations:* Discuss use with a certified or expert herbalist for best results. Lemon balm may take from 1–6 months to achieve effectiveness.

  g. *References/other sources:*

Blumenthal, M. (1998). *The complete German Commission E monographs and therapeutic guide to herbal medicines.* Austin, TX: American Botanical Council.

Kennedy, D. O., Wake, G., Savelev, S., Tildesley, N. T., Perry, E. K., Wesnes, K. A., et al. (2003). Modulation of mood and cognitive performance following acute administration of single doses of Melissa officinalis (lemon balm) with human CNS nicotinic and muscarine receptor-binding properties. *Neuropsychopharmacology, 28*(10), 1871–1881.

Mindset

1. Bingo versus daily physical activity
  a. *Actions/expected responses:* Bingo-enhanced performance on the Boston Naming Test and a Word List Recognition Task while engaging in physical activity did not reach statistical significance.
  b. *Routes/dosages/frequencies:* As tolerated.
  c. *Cautions:* None.
  d. *Assessments:* Take a baseline measure for short-term memory, concentration, word retrieval, and word recognition, and then take a measure after increasing bingo play.
  e. *Tips on use:* Playing bingo every day if possible is recommended.
  f. *Other considerations:* Past research has shown that pharmacological measures can enhance functional capacities for those with Alzheimer's but may result in unacceptable side effects.
  g. *References/other sources:*

Sobel, B. P. (2001). Bingo vs. physical intervention in stimulating short-term cognition in Alzheimer's disease patients. *American Journal of Alzheimer's Disease and Other Dementias, 16*(2), 115–120.

2. Reading, solving crossword puzzles, playing musical instruments, playing board games, visiting museums, and dancing
  a. *Actions/expected responses:* Reduced risk of Alzheimer's and memory impairment.
  b. *Routes/dosages/frequencies:* Frequent participation in cognitively stimulating activities is associated with reduced risk of Alzheimer's.
  c. *Cautions:* None.

    d. *Assessments:* Take a baseline measure of participation in activities. Chart changes in memory, thinking, and social function as activities increase.

    e. *Tips on use:* Encourage family participation.

    f. *Other considerations:* See "Routes/Dosages/Frequencies."

    g. *References/other sources:*

        Verghese, J., Lipton, R. B., Katz, M. J., Hall, C. B., Derby, C. A., Kuslansky, G., et al. (2003). Leisure activities and the risk of dementia in the elderly. *New England Journal of Medicine, 348*(25), 2508–2516.

        Wilson, R. S., de Leon, M., Barnes, L. L., Schneider, J. A., Bienias, J. L., et al. (2002). Participation in cognitively stimulating activities and risk of incident Alzheimer disease. *Journal of American Medical Association, 287*(6), 742–748.

3. Talking

    a. *Actions/expected responses:* Spending 10 minutes talking to another person can improve memory and performance. Talking about a social issue can be as effective as engaging in intellectual activities such as doing crossword puzzles.

    b. *Routes/dosages/frequencies:* Daily.

    c. *Cautions:* None.

    d. *Assessments:* Take a baseline measure of memory and performance using a Mini Mental Examination (see http://www.bami.us/MiniMental.htm).

    e. *Tips on use:* Take a baseline on how often the person engages in social talk and then chart changes in improved cognition as activities increase. If possible, family members should participate in talking to the woman daily for at least 10 minutes.

    f. *Other considerations:* Instruct women/caregivers that visiting with a friend or neighbor is also useful and can decrease social isolation.

    g. *References/other sources:*

        University of Michigan. (2007, November 1). Ten minutes of talking improves memory and test performance. *ScienceDaily.* Retrieved November 12, 2007, from http://www.sciencedaily.com/releases/2007/10/071029172856.htm

Nutrition

1. Apples/apple juice

    a. *Actions/expected responses:* Apples improve memory and learning and may protect against Alzheimer's by increasing the production in the brain of the essential neurotransmitter acetylcholine, which can slow mental decline in women already diagnosed with the condition.

    b. *Routes/dosages:* Two 8-ounce glasses of apple juice or two to three apples a day (preferred).

    c. *Cautions:* None unless allergic to apples.

    d. *Assessments:* Monitor for which form is most easily used and which produces the best effects.

    e. *Tips on use:* Choose juice that contains no added sugar and that includes apple skins; choose organic apples when possible to eliminate toxic effects of spraying.

f. *Other considerations:* For food-mind information go to http://www.mind.org.uk/Information/Booklets/Mind+guide+to/Mindguidetofoodandmood.htm

g. *References/other sources:*

Chan, A., Groves, V., & Shea, T. B. (2006). Apple juice concentrate maintains acetylcholine levels following dietary compromises. *International Journal of Alzheimer's Disease, 9*(3), 287–291.

Tchantchoa, F., Graves, M., Ortiz, D., Rogers, E., & Shea, T. B. (2004). Dietary supplementation with apple juice concentrate alleviates the compensatory increase in glutathione synthase transcription and activity that accompanies dietary and genetically induced oxidative stress. *Journal of Nutrition Health and Aging, 8,* 92–97.

2. Blueberries

a. *Actions/expected responses:* Blueberries protect against age-related oxidative stress; they improve learning, balance, memory, and coordination.

b. *Routes/dosages/frequencies:* 1 cup of fresh or frozen berries daily.

c. *Cautions:* None unless allergic to the berries.

d. *Assessments:* Monitor for allergies; keep track of learning, balance, memory, and coordination after starting daily blueberries.

e. *Tips on use:* Keep frozen berries in freezer and take out 15–30 minutes prior to eating.

f. *Other considerations:* None.

g. *References/other sources:*

Goyarzu, P., Lau, F. C., Kaufmann, J., Jennings, R., Taglialatela, G., Joseph, J., et al. (2003). *Age-related increase in brain NF-B is attenuated by blueberry-enriched antioxidant diet.* Program No. 98.3. Abstract. Washington DC: Society for Neuroscience.

Joseph, J. A., Shukitt-Hale, B., Denisova, N. A., Bielinski, D., Martin, A., McEwen, J. J., et al. (1999). Reversals of age-related declines in neuronal signal transduction, cognitive, and motor behavioral deficits with blueberry, spinach, or strawberry dietary supplementation. *Journal of Neuroscience, 19*(18), 8114–8121.

Spangler, E. L., Duffy, K., Devan, B., Guo, Z., Bowker, J., Shukitt-Hale, B., et al. (2003). *Rats fed a blueberry-enriched diet exhibit greater protection against a kainate-induced learning impairment.* Program No. 735.10. Abstract. Washington DC: Society for Neuroscience.

3. Curry

a. *Actions/expected responses:* Older women (ages 60–93) who consumed curry occasionally often or very often had significantly better scores on the Mini-Mental State Examination (MMSE) than those who never or rarely consumed curry.

b. *Routes/dosages/frequencies:* Curcumin, from the curry spice turmeric, possesses potent antioxidant and anti-inflammatory properties and can reduce B-amyloid and plaque burden in the brain.

c. *Cautions:* The herb is safe in food doses and up to 12 grams a day. In larger quantities it can have strong activity in the common bile duct that might aggravate the passage of gallstones in women currently suffering from the condition.

d. *Assessments:* Take a baseline measure using the MMSE prior to and after curry consumption.

e. *Tips on use:* Counsel caregivers to serve curry or food seasoned with curcumin at least once a week; doing so more often may produce better results.

f. *Other considerations:* None.

g. *References/other sources:*

Anand, P., Kunnumakkara, A. B., Newman, R. A., & Aggarwal, B. B. (2007). Bioavailability of curcumin: Problems and promises. *Molecular Pharmacology, 4*(6), 807–818.

Ng, T-P., Chiam, P-C., Lee, T., Chua, H-C., Lim, L., & Kua, E-H. (2006). Curry consumption and cognitive function in the elderly. *American Journal of Epidemiology, 164*(9), 898–906.

4. Fish oil

a. *Actions/expected responses:* Deficiencies in essential, mainly omega-3 and omega-6 long chain polyunsaturated fatty acids (LC-PUFA) results in visual and cognitive impairment and disturbances in mental functions in animals and could be the main reason for the increasing incidence of mental disorders in humans. DNA microassays found that fish oil diets altered the expression of several genes involved in modulating protein aggregation.

b. *Routes/dosages/frequencies:* Serve fish 3–4 times/week or provide fish oil caplets (available at health food stores) and follow the direction on bottle.

c. *Cautions:* None unless there are allergies to fish.

d. *Assessments:* Take a baseline measure for clear thinking and memory, and then take a measure after fish meals or fish oil supplements have been implemented.

e. *Tips on use:* Keep oil caplets in the refrigerator so they don't become rancid.

f. *Other considerations:* None.

g. *References/other sources:*

American Academy of Neurology. (2007, November 13). Eating fish, omega-3 oils, fruits and veggies lowers risk of memory problems. *ScienceDaily.* Retrieved November 15, 2007, from http://www.sciencedaily.com/releases/2007/11/071112163630.htm

Puskas, L. G., & Kitajka, K. (2006). Nutrigenomic approaches to study the effects of n-3 PUFA diet in the central nervous system. *Nutrition and Health, 18*(3), 227–232.

5. Flavonoids in fruits and vegetables

a. *Actions/expected responses:* The intake of antioxidant flavonoids in tea, fruits, and vegetables is inversely related to the risk of dementia. Apples, bananas, and oranges protect against neurodegenerative diseases including Alzheimer's.

b. *Routes/dosages/frequencies:* 5–10 servings (1/2 cup) daily.

c. *Cautions:* None unless there are allergies to specific fruits or vegetables.

d. *Assessments:* Take a baseline measure for fruits, vegetables, and tea daily, and then take a measure after these foods are increased in the diet.

e. *Tips on use:* Fresh or frozen fruits and vegetables contain the most nutrients and the least salt and sugar.

f. *Other considerations:* None.

g. *References/other sources:*

Engelhart, M. J., Geerlings, M. I., Ruitenberg, A., van Swieten, J. C., Hofman, A., Witteman, J. C., et al. (2002). Dietary intake of antioxidants and risk of Alzheimer's disease. *Journal of American Medical Association, 287*(24), 3223–3229.

Heo, H. J., Choi, S. J., Choi, S-G., Shin, D.-H., Lee, J. M., & Lee, C. Y. (2008). Effects of banana, orange, and apple on oxidative stress-induced neurotoxicity in PC12 cells. *Journal of Food Science, 73*(2), H28–H32.

6. Garlic

a. *Actions/expected responses:* Oxidative damage is a major factor in dementia. Aged garlic extract (AGE) has been shown to prevent Alzheimer's progression by scavenging oxidants, increasing superoxide dismutase, catalase glutathione peroxidase, and glutathione levels, and inhibits lipid peroxidation and inflammatory prostaglandins.

b. *Routes/dosages/frequencies:* Two capsules with meals twice a day.

c. *Cautions:* AGE may interact with antiplatelet or anticoagulant drugs, but it appears safe for warfarin therapy.

d. *Assessments:* Assess women for use of antiplatelet or anticoagulant drugs. Assess memory prior to and after taking garlic.

e. *Tips on use:* Keep bottle in a cool, dry place.

f. *Other considerations:* The methyl allyl trisulfide in garlic dilates blood vessel walls and may be responsible for better circulation to the brain.

g. *References/other sources:*

Borek, C. (2006). Garlic reduces dementia and heart-disease risk. *Journal of Nutrition, 136*(3 Suppl.), 810S–812S.

Chauhan, N. B., & Sandoval, J. (2007). Amelioration of early cognitive deficits by aged garlic extract in Alzheimer's transgenic mice. *Phytotherapy Research, 21*(7), 629–640.

Macan, H., Uykimpang, R., Alconcel, M., Takasu, J., Razon, R., Amagase, H., et al. (2006). Aged garlic extract may be safe for patients on warfarin therapy. *Journal of Nutrition 136*(3 Suppl.), 793S–795S.

7. Green and black tea

a. *Actions/expected responses:* Tea protects against the build-up of plaque from amyloid deposits associated with an increase in brain cell damage and death from oxidative stress. Green tea polyphenols might explain the observed association with improved cognitive function. Women who drank more than two cups of green tea a day had a 50% lower chance of having cognitive impairment, compared to those who drank less than three cups a week. Black tea can also protect against the build up of amyloid proteins.

b. *Routes/dosages/frequencies:* Two to three cups of green or black tea a day.

c. *Cautions:* Caffeine may increase restlessness and talkativeness; decaffeinated green or black tea is preferable.

d. *Assessments:* Assess for allergies or sensitivity to the tea. Assess cognitive impairment prior to and after drinking green or black tea.

e. *Tips for use:* Steep teabags in boiling water for 10 minutes; let cool and drink.

f. *Other considerations:* None.

g. *References/other sources:*

Bastinetto, S., Brouillette, J., & Quirion, R. (2007). Neuroprotective effects of natural products: Interaction with intracellular, amyloid peptides and a possible role for transthyretin. *Neurochemical Research, 32*(10), 1720–1725.

Rezai-Zadeh, K., Shytle, D., Sun, N., Takashi, M., Hou, H., Jeanniton, D., et al. (2005). Green tea epigallocatechin-e-gallate (EGCG) modulates amyloid precursos protein cleavage and reduces cerebral amyloidosis in Alzyeimer transgenic mice. *Journal of Neuroscience, 25*(38), 8807–8814.

8. High-fat diet (avoid)

   a. *Actions/expected responses:* A high-fat diet may increase risk of Alzheimer's, especially in those with the APOE e4 allele marker. In one study, women who consumed the highest-fat diets had a sevenfold higher risk of developing Alzheimer's than those who ate lower-fat diets. Participants age 20–39 who carried the genetic marker and ate a diet in which more than 40% of calories were from fat had an almost 23-fold higher risk of Alzheimer's than those who didn't carry the marker and followed high-fat diets. These control subjects also ate more dietary antioxidants (fruits and vegetables).

   b. *Routes/dosages/frequencies:* Lower fat intake, especially saturated animal fats (meats, dairy products) and eat increased amounts of fruits and vegetables.

   c. *Cautions:* High-fat consumption at a relatively early age can portend development of Alzheimer's.

   d. *Assessments:* Assess women for high-fat consumption.

   e. *Tips for use:* Increase vegetable and fruit intake and reduce intake of meat and dairy products.

   f. *Other considerations:* None.

   g. *References/other sources:*
      Petot, G. (2000). *Alzheimer's disease risk increases with high-fat diet.* Presented at World Alzheimer's Conference, July 9–18, Washington, DC.

9. Onion

   a. *Actions/expected responses:* Antioxidant effect of onions leads to enhanced memory.

   b. *Routes/dosages/frequencies:* Encourage caregivers to serve onions as often as possible.

   c. *Cautions:* None unless allergic or sensitive to onions.

   d. *Assessments:* Assess for allergies or sensitivity. Assess for memory prior to and after eating onions for several weeks.

   e. *Tips for use:* If onion breath is a problem for women, cook the onions rather than eating them raw in salads or sandwiches.

   f. *Other considerations:* None.

   g. *References/other sources:*
      Nishimura, H., Higuchi, O., Tateshita, K., Tomobe, K., Okuma, Y., & Nomura, Y. (2006). Antioxidative activity and ameliorative effects of memory impairment of sulfur-containing compounds in allium species. *Biofactors, 26*(2), 135–146.

10. Sugary sodas (avoid)

    a. *Actions/expected responses:* Excess drinking of sugary beverages like soda may increase the risk of Alzheimer's.

    b. *Routes/dosages/frequencies:* Five (and possibly fewer cans of soda) a day.

c. *Cautions:* Sugar is associated with an increase in Alzheimer's progression.

d. *Assessments:* Assess daily intake of soda.

e. *Tips on use:* Suggest women wean themselves off soda and replace it with green tea, filtered water with lemon or frozen berries, or diluted (unsweetened) apple juice.

f. *Other considerations:* High sugar intake is also associated with higher cholesterol levels, insulin resistance, learning deficits, and memory loss. Mice fed on a sugar diet had twice as many amyloid plaque deposits, an anatomical hallmark of Alzheimer's.

g. *References/other sources:*

American Society for Biochemistry and Molecular Biology. (2007). Sugary beverages may increase Alzheimer's risk. *ScienceDaily*. Retrieved December 16, 2007, from http://www.sciencedaily.com/releases/2007/12/0712814299.htm

11. Thiamine (vitamin B1)

a. *Actions/expected responses:* A significant proportion of women diagnosed with Alzheimer's may have a thiamine deficiency, which may have an impact on cognitive function.

b. *Routes/dosages/frequencies:* Eating thiamine-rich foods may help improve cognitive function.

c. *Cautions:* None.

d. *Assessments:* Assess cognitive function before and after eating thiamine-rich foods.

e. *Tips on use:* For thiamine-rich foods, direct women and caregivers to http://www.feinberg.northwestern.edu/nutrition/factsheets/thiamin.pdf

f. *Other considerations:* Counsel caregivers to choose the healthier thiamine-rich foods, such as sunflower seeds, wheat germ, soy milk, and baked or black beans.

g. *References/other sources:*

Gold, M., Chen, M. F., & Johnson, K. (1995). Plasma and red blood cell thiamine deficiency with dementia of the Alzheimer's type. *Archives of Neurology, 51*(11), 1081–1086.

12. Vitamin B3

a. *Actions/expected responses:* Vitamin B3 (niacin) restores memory loss associated with Alzheimer's.

b. *Routes/dosages/frequencies:* Foods containing niacin should be eaten daily.

c. *Cautions:* Avoid meat sources.

d. *Assessments:* Assess for memory loss before and after eating additional niacin-containing foods.

e. *Tips on use:* Counsel caregivers to offer women foods high in niacin as listed at www.feinberg.northwestern.edu/nutrition/factsheets/vitamin-b3.html

f. *Other considerations:* Suggest caregivers provide the healthiest sources of niacin—for example, chunk tuna from U.S. waters, organic peanut butter, and wild (not farmed) salmon.

g. *References/other sources:*

Morris, M. C., Evans, D. A., Bienias, J. L., Scherr, P. A., Tangney, C. C., Hebert, L. E., et al. (2004). Dietary niacin and the risk of incident Alzheimer's disease and of cognitive decline. *Journal of Neurology Neurosurgery and Psychiatry, 75*, 1093–1099.

13. Vitamin B12 and folate
    a. *Actions/expected responses:* Vitamin B12 is involved in synthesizing carbohydrates, fats, and protein; a deficiency can manifest as pernicious anemia, as degeneration of the axon and nerves in the head, as depression, or as dementia. Women with low levels of B12 or folate may have twice the risk of developing Alzheimer's as do those with higher levels of these two nutrients. Taking folic acid and vitamin B12 can reduce homocysteine blood levels; homocysteine compromises brain function by damaging the lining of blood vessels in the brain. Drinking five or more cups of coffee a day raises homocysteine significantly and should be avoided.
    b. *Routes/dosages/frequencies:* Vegetarians and vegans (who avoid fish, dairy products, and eggs) are especially at risk for folate deficiency. Folic acid (the synthetic form of folate) is metabolized in the liver, while folate is metabolized in the gut, an easily saturated system. Fortification can lead to significant unmetabolized folic acid entering the blood stream, with the potential to cause a number of health problems. Undigested folic acid accelerates cognitive decline in older adults with low vitamin B12 status. For sources of folate go to http://ohioline.osu.edu/hyg-fact/5000/5553.html
    c. *Cautions:* Avoid foods fortified with folic acid and eat foods high in folate instead.
    d. *Assessments:* Take a baseline measure for dementia and depression and then take a measure after increasing vitamin B12 and folate.
    e. *Tips on use:* Calcium supplementation can improve B12 absorption. Teach caregivers good sources of vitamin B12 and folate, how to include them in daily menus, and how to reduce coffee intake below five cups a day by serving half caffeinated coffee with one-half decaffeinated coffee/cup or serving tea half the time.
    f. *Other considerations:* The following medications can lead to B12 deficiencies and a need for more foods high in folate: H2 blockers (such as ranitidine), proton pump inhibitors (e.g., omeprazole), colchicines, zicovudine, nitrous oxide anesthesia, metformin, phenformin, and potassium supplements.
    g. *References/other sources:*

    Herrmann, W. (2006). Significance of hyperhomocysteinemia. *Clinical Laboratory, 52*(7–8), 367–374.

    Kruman, I. I., Kumaravel, T. S., Lohani, A., Pedersen, W. A., Cutler R. G., Kruman, Y., et al. (2002). Folic acid deficiency and homocysteine impair DNA repair in hippocampal neurons and sensitize them to amyloid toxicity in experimental models of Alzheimer's disease. *Journal of Neuroscience, 22*(5), 1752–1762.

    Luchsinger, A., Tang, M-X., Miller, J., Green, R., & Mayeux, R., (2007). Relation of higher folate intake to lower risk of Alzheimer disease in the elderly. *Archives of Neurology, 64,* 12–14.

    Pettit, J. L. (2002). Vitamin B12. *Clinicians Review, 12*(7), 64, 66.

    Seshadri, S., Beiser, A., Sellub, J., Jacques, P. F., Rosenberg, I. H., D'Agostino, R. B., et al. (2002). Plasma homocysteine as a risk factor for dementia and Alzheimer's disease. *New England Journal of Medicine, 346,* 476–483.

    Wright, J., Dainty, J., & Fingles, P. (2007). Folic acid metabolism in human subjects: Potential implications for proposed mandatory folic acid fortification in the UK. *British Journal of Nutrition, 98,* 667–675.

14. Weight loss (avoid)
   a. *Actions/expected responses:* Weight loss is a common problem, is a predictive factor of mortality and decreases quality of life for both women and caregivers. A nutrition education program can prevent weight loss and have a significant effect on cognitive function.
   b. *Routes/dosages/frequencies:* One approach that has proved successful is the Mediterranean diet, which includes a high intake of vegetables, legumes, fruits, whole grain cereals, fish, and unsaturated fatty acids such as olive oil; low intake of saturated fatty acids, dairy products, meat, and poultry; and low to moderate intake of alcohol. For more information, go to http://www.mayoclinic.com/health/mediteraneandiet/CL00011
   c. *Cautions:* Drink no more than one 5-ounce glass of red wine a day; drinking more has been linked with health problems including cancers.
   d. *Assessments:* Evaluate weight, nutritional state, cognitive function, mood, and behavior disorders prior to and after switching to a Mediterranean food plan.
   e. *Tips on use:* Hispanic women may be more likely to adhere to the Mediterranean food plan than are African Americans and may show a 20%–40% reduction in risk of Alzheimer's after being on the food plan.
   f. *Other considerations:* None.
   g. *References/other sources:*
      Riviere, S., Gillette-Guyonnet, S., Voisin, T., Reynish, E., Andrieu, S., Lauque, S., et al. (2001). A nutritional education program could prevent weight loss and slow cognitive decline in Alzheimer's disease. *Journal of Nutritional Health and Aging, 5*(4), 295–299.
      Scarmeas, N., Stern, Y., Mayeux, R., & Luchsinger, J. A. (2006). Mediterranean diet, Alzheimer's disease and vascular mediation. *Archives of Neurology, 63,* 1709–1717.
15. Western diet: Sugar, refined carbohydrates, and animal products (avoid)
   a. *Actions/expected responses:* Excessive dietary intake of sugar, refined carbohydrates, and animal products (meat and dairy products with high content of saturated fat), also known as a traditional Western diet, is linked with Alzheimer's.
   b. *Routes/dosages/frequencies:* Avoiding meat, dairy products, sugar and refined carbohydrates (cakes, pies, candy, etc.) and increasing fish and/or fish oils, vegetables, whole grain cereals, legumes, and soy products can reduce Alzheimer's symptoms.
   c. *Cautions:* Evaluate allergies to specific fruits or vegetables.
   d. *Assessments:* Take a baseline measure for Alzheimer's symptoms with the Western diet and then take a measure after instituting nutritional substances that can reduce symptoms of dementia.
   e. *Tips on use:* Encourage caregivers to move away from a Western diet when planning menus.
   f. *Other considerations:* For menus to share with caregivers, go to: http://www.prevention.com/cda/categorypage.do?channel=nutrition.recipes&category=recipes
   g. *References/other sources:*
      Berrino, F. (2002). Western diet and Alzheimer's disease. *Epidemiology and Prevention, 26*(3), 107–115.

Whitmer, R., Gunderson, E. P., Barrett-Connor, E., Quesenberry, P., Jr., & Yaffe, K. (2005). Obesity in middle age and future risk of dementia: A 27 year longitudinal population based study. *British Medical Journal, 330,* 1360–1364.

Stress Management

1. Imagery
    a. *Actions/expected responses:* Repeatedly picturing oneself completing a cognitive task is as effective at managing stress as practicing the task.
    b. *Routes/dosages/frequencies:* Coach women to use imagery up to 45 minutes a day. Ask them to make a vivid image of what they want to remember.
    c. *Cautions:* None.
    d. *Assessments:* Take a baseline measure for memory prior to women using imagery and then take a measure after treatment.
    e. *Tips on use:* Teach caregivers and clients how to use imagery and that daily practice improves results.
    f. *Other considerations:* For more information on using imagery to improve memory go to: http://www.helpguide.org/life/improving_memory.htm,
    g. *References/other sources:*
    Wright, C. J., & Smith, D. K. (2007). The effect of a short-term PETTLEP imagery intervention on a cognitive task. *Journal of Imagery Research in Sport and Physical Activity, 2*(1). Retrieved August 30, 2008 from http://www.bepress.com/jirspa/vol2/iss1/sty1
2. Meditation
    a. *Actions/expected responses:* Meditation decreases the chronic stress that can lead to Alzheimer's and especially memory loss. Women with memory loss reported their thinking was clearer and their memory better after meditating. All wanted to continue the practice.
    b. *Routes/dosages/frequencies:* Practice meditation 12 minutes a day.
    c. *Cautions:* Not all women will be able to focus on traditional meditation approaches.
    d. *Assessments:* Take a baseline measure for memory prior to meditation and then take a measure after treatment.
    e. *Tips on use:* Use simple meditation approaches like focusing on breathing in and out or counting while walking. For more ideas, go to http://www.imcleveland.org/meditation/
    f. *Other considerations:* Teach caretakers how to do meditation if possible.
    g. *References/other sources:*
    Khalsa, D. S. (2007). *Stress reduction and Alzheimer's prevention: Two studies using SPECT.* Presentation at 6th World Congress on Stress, October 11–13, Vienna, Austria.
    Peavy, G. M., Lange, K. L., Salmon, D. P., Patterson, T. L., Goldman, S., Gamst, A. C., et al. (2007). The effects of prolonged stress and APOE genotype on memory and cortisol in older adults. *Biological Psychiatry, 62*(5), 472–478.

Supplements

1. Lecithin
   a. *Actions/expected responses:* Lecithin increases acetylcholine at receptor sites in the nervous system, improving memory. One of the chemical components of lecithin is phosphatidylcholine, a precursor to acetylcholine. Memory may increases significantly after taking lecithin for 4–6 weeks.
   b. *Routes/dosages/frequencies:* Use lecithin capsules at 20–45 grams a day, starting at the lower dosage and increasing gradually as needed.
   c. *Cautions:* Lecithin is not to be taken by pregnant or lactating women or by children.
   d. *Assessments:* Monitor for allergies; keep track of memory changes.
   e. *Tips on use:* Keep bottle in cool dry place.
   f. *Other considerations:* Lecithin is also found in peanuts, beef liver, and egg yolks; the lecithin in the yolk protects against the cholesterol in eggs.
   g. *References/other sources:*
      Higgins, J. P., & Flicker, L. (2003). Lecithin for dementia and cognitive impairment. *Cochrane Database System Reviews, 3,* CD001015.
      Kansas State University. (2001). Eggs have a lipid that lowers cholesterol absorption. ScienceDaily. Retrieved July 27, 2008, from http://www.sciencedaily.com/releases/2001/10/011029073601.htm

2. Pycnogenol
   a. *Actions/expected responses:* Pycnogenol protects against senile plaques characteristic of Alzheimer's.
   b. *Routes/dosages/frequencies:* By mouth, 100–150 mg daily.
   c. *Cautions:* Not to be used by pregnant or lactating women or by children.
   d. *Assessments:* Monitor for allergies; keep track of learning, balance, memory, and coordination after starting daily pycnogenol.
   e. *Tips on use:* Start at lowest dose and gradually increase if necessary.
   f. *Other considerations:* Be sure to remind women/caregivers to consult with prescribing health care practitioner.
   g. *References/other sources:*
      Liu, F., Lau, B. H., Peng, Q., & Shah, V. (2000). Pycnogenol protects vascular endothelial cells from beta-amyloid-induced injury. *Biological Pharmaceutical Bulletin, 23*(6), 735–737.
      Skidmore-Roth, L. (2006). Pycnogenol. In *Handbook of herbs and natural supplements* (pp. 868–869). St. Louis, MO: ElsevierMosby.

3. Selenium
   a. *Actions/expected responses:* Increasing evidence suggests a role for oxidative stress in several neurodegenerative diseases, including Alzheimer's, and that selenium compounds may function as protective antioxidants.
   b. *Routes/dosages/frequencies:* By mouth, no more than 400 mcg per day.
   c. *Cautions/adverse reactions:* Rare, but do not exceed suggested dosage. For more information on how to find selenium in foods, go to http://ods.od.nih.gov/factsheets/selenium.asp
   d. *Assessments:* Evaluate symptoms prior to and after increasing dietary selenium.

   e. *Tips on use:* If a selenium supplement is taken, factor in the intake of these foods to keep the dosage of selenium under 400 mcg. The highest level of selenium is found in Brazil nuts (275 mcg/3–4 nuts), fish (20–68 mcg/3 ounces), and whole wheat spaghetti (36 mcg/cup).

   f. *Other considerations:* None.

   g. *References/other sources:*

     Schrauzer, G. N. (2001). Nutritional selenium supplements: Product types, quality and safety. *Journal of American College of Nutrition, 20*(1), 1–4.

     Xiong, S., Markesbery, W. R., Shao, C., & Lovell, M. A. (2007). Seleno-L-methionine protects against beta-amyloid and iron/hydrogen peroxide-mediated neuron death. *Antioxidants and Redox Signaling, 9*(4), 457–467.

4. Vitamins and trace elements

   a. *Actions/expected responses:* Cognitive functions improve after supplementation with modest amounts of vitamins and trace elements.

   b. *Routes/dosages/frequencies:* A daily multivitamin pill taken with a meal.

   c. *Cautions:* None.

   d. *Assessments:* Take a baseline measure for immediate and long-term memory, abstract thinking, problem-solving ability, and attention.

   e. *Tips on use:* Examine multivitamin information on the bottle to make sure there are no fillers, dyes, starches, or other unnecessary substances contained in the tablets or capsules.

   f. *Other considerations*: Older women should take these vitamins as a way to significantly improve cognition and thus quality of life and the ability to perform activities of daily living. Such a nutritional approach may delay the onset of Alzheimer's.

   g. *References/other sources:*

     Chandra, R. K. (2001). Effect of vitamin and trace-element supplementation on cognitive function in elderly subjects. *Nutrition, 17*(9), 709–712.

5. Vitamins C and E

   a. *Actions/expected responses:* Evidence shows that vitamin C, which is water soluble, might serve to recharge the antioxidate capacity of vitamin E. Taken together, these two vitamins can slow the progression of Alzheimer's. When compared to a cholinesterase inhibitor, women who took vitamin E alone were 26 percent less likely to die than women who didn't take vitamin E.

   b. *Routes/dosages/frequencies:* 2,000 IU vitamin E and 2,000 mg vitamin C daily.

   c. *Cautions:* None noted in the study, however vitamin E is a blood thinner and vitamin C should be taken with a full glass of water. Use ester C form if ascorbic acid form is irritating to gastrointestinal tract.

   d. *Assessments:* Take a baseline measure for Alzheimer's symptoms and then take a measure after taking vitamins E and C.

   e. *Tips on use:* For vitamin E, start at 400 IU and gradually build up to 2,000 IU while monitoring blood pressure.

   f. *Other considerations:* Discuss the use of vitamins E and C with prescribing health care practitioner.

   g. *References/other sources:*

     American Academy of Neurology (2008, April 17). Vitamin E may help Alzheimer's patients live longer, study suggests. *ScienceDaily*. Retrieved

May 14, 2008, from http://www.sciencedaily.com/releases/2008/04/080415194438.htm

Engelhart, M. J., Geerlings, M. I. K., Ruitenberg, A., van Swieten, J. C., Hofman, A., Witteman, J. C., et al. (2002). Dietary intake of antioxidants and risk of Alzheimer's disease. *Journal of American Medical Association, 287*(24), 3223–3229.

Exposito, E., Rotilio, D., DiMatteo, V., DiGiulio, C., Cacchio, M., & Algeri, S. (2002). A review of specific dietary antioxidants and the effects on biochemical mechanisms related to neurodegenerative processes. *Neurobiology and Aging, 23*(5), 719–735.

Zandi, P. P. (2004). Using vitamin E and C supplements together may reduce risk of Alzheimer's disease. *Archives of Neurology, 61*, 82–88.

Touch

1. Foot acupressure and massage
   a. *Actions/expected responses:* Decreases agitation and a hyper-responsiveness to stress, and indirectly decreases detrimental cortisol levels. Can decrease yelling, pacing, and walking, and can help with quiet time, pulse, and respiration, sleep quality,
   b. *Routes/dosages/frequencies:* Massage the feet for 10–15 minutes daily.
   c. *Cautions:* Contraindications may include venous stasis, phlebitis, and traumatic and deep tissue injuries.
   d. *Assessments:* Take a baseline measure for vocalizations, pacing, and/or walking prior to administering foot acupressure and massage and then take a measure after treatment.
   e. *Tips on use:* Specific acupressure points to use include the (a) the middle of the bottom of the feet, about 2 inches down from the toes, (b) around the ankles, and (c) the front webbing about 1 inch down between the first and second toes. For more on foot massage, go to http://www.eclecticenergies.com.
   f. *Other considerations:* Teach caregivers how to do foot massage whenever possible.
   g. *References/other sources:*
      Sutherland, J., Peakes, J., & Bridges, C. (1999). Foot acupressure and massage for patients with Alzheimer's disease and related dementias. *Image, Journal of Nursing Scholarship, 31*(4), 347–348.
      Yang, M. H., Wu, S. C., Lin, J. G., & Lin, L. C. (2007). The efficacy of acupressure for decreasing agitated behaviour in dementia: A pilot study. *Journal of Clinical Nursing, 16*(2), 308–315.
2. Hand aromatherapy and massage
   a. *Actions/expected responses:* Decreases negative emotion and agitation significantly.
   b. *Routes/dosages/frequencies:* Lavender aromatherapy hand massage daily for 2 weeks.
   c. *Cautions:* None.
   d. *Assessments:* Take a baseline measure for agitation and negative emotion and then take a measure of both after treatment.

e. *Tips on use:* Place a few drops of lavender oil in an ounce or two of olive or castor oil and then mix. (Practice this sequence on yourself first.) Place a few drops of mixed oil in the palm of the woman's left hand and hold that hand in yours. Massage the woman's palm with your thumb, working out in circles. Work down each finger and use the thumbnail to stimulate the ends of the women's fingers. Work up and down the thumb (correlates to the head of the woman) with the pad of your thumb, using a very firm stroke. Stroke down the hand and up the forearm using thumb and fingers. Compare the two hands for tone, color, and temperature. Repeat with other hand.

f. *Other considerations:* For more massage specifics go to http://www.cool nurse.com/massage.htm

g. *References/other sources:*

Lee, S. Y. (2005). The effect of lavender aromatherapy on cognitive function, emotion and aggressive behavior of elderly with dementia. *Taehan Kanho Hakhoe Chi, 35*(2), 303–312.

3. Therapeutic touch (TT)

a. *Actions/expected responses:* Decreases agitation and a hyper-responsiveness to stress, and indirectly decreases detrimental cortisol levels. Can decrease vocalization and pacing and walking.

b. *Routes/dosages/frequencies:* Apply therapeutic touch for 5–7 minutes, two times a day.

c. *Cautions:* The aged, extremely ill, or dying should be given a gentle treatment by an experienced practitioner.

d. *Assessments:* Take a baseline measure for vocalizations, pacing, and/or walking prior to administering therapeutic touch and then take a measure after treatment.

e. *Tips on use:* Center and calm yourself by closing your eyes and focusing on breathing in your abdomen. When relaxed, rub your hands together and feel the tingling sensation as you slowly pull your hands apart. When able to feel the energies balancing between the hands, hold the intent to balance the other person's energy. Start above the head and keep an inch or so away from the body, bring your hands slowly down, sweeping down the body slowly, ending a few inches past the feet. For more information, go to http://www.healgrief.com/Site/Heal_Grief_in_Your_Body.html (retrieved July 27, 2008).

f. *Other considerations:* Regular TT treatments may enhance the effect achieved.

g. *References/other sources:*

Woods, D. L., & Dimond, M. (2002). The effect of therapeutic touch on agitated behavior and cortisol in persons with Alzheimer's disease. *Biological Research in Nursing, 4*(2), 104–114.

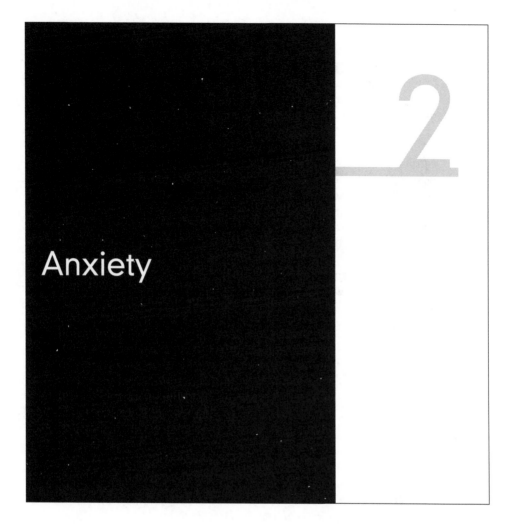

Anxiety

Worry about an unknown event, or anxiety, is often treated by antianxiety drugs that can have numerous negative consequences. Recent research provides evidence for complementary procedures that are safe and effective.

Environment

1. Music
   a. *Actions/expected responses:* Significantly less anxiety can occur in women who listen to sedative music compared to those who received either scheduled rest or treatment as usual.
   b. *Routes/dosages/frequencies:* 30-minute sessions.
   c. *Cautions:* Stop or change the music if agitation increases.
   d. *Assessments:* Assess anxiety on a scale from 1 (calm) to 10 (extreme anxiety) before and after listening to calming music.
   e. *Tips on use:* Investigate healing music such as that listed at http://www.healingmusic.org

    f. *Other considerations:* Play segments of available CDs, DVDs, or tapes containing calming music and see to which produce the most favorable response.

    g. *References/other sources:*

       Evans, D. (2002). The effectiveness of music as an intervention for hospital patients: A systematic review. *Journal of Advanced Nursing, 37,* 8–18.

       Galaal, K. A., Deane, K., Sangal, S., & Lopes, A. D. (2007). Interventions for reducing anxiety in women undergoing colposcopy. *Cochrane Database of Systematic Reviews 3.* Retrieved July 27, 2008, from http://www.cochrane.org/reviews/en/ab006013.html

       Voss, J., Good, M., Yates, B., Baun, M., Thompson, A., & Hertzog, M. (2004). Sedative music reduces anxiety and pain during chair rest after open-heart surgery. *Pain, 112*(1–2), 197–203.

2. Smoking cessation

    a. *Actions/expected responses:* Panic attacks (a symptom of high anxiety) are strongly associated with smoking and nicotine dependence.

    b. *Routes/dosages/frequencies:* Both occasional and regular smoking increase the risk of panic attacks.

    c. *Cautions:* None.

    d. *Assessments:* Assess active and passive smoking behaviors. Women who smoke should keep a smoking/mood diary to chart their reactions to cigarettes.

    e. *Tips on use:* Investigate smoking cessation programs such as http://www.helpguide.org/mental/quit_smoking_cessation.htm

    f. *Other considerations:* Develop individualized smoking cessation programs based on lifestyle and preferences.

    g. *References/other sources:*

       Isensee, B., Wittchen, H. U., Stein, M. B., Hofler, M., & Lieb, R. (2003). Smoking increases the risk of panic: Findings from a prospective community. *Archives of General Psychiatry, 60*(7), 692–700.

Exercise/Movement

1. Dance

    a. *Actions/expected responses:* Dance (modern and otherwise) can significantly reduce anxiety.

    b. *Routes/dosages/frequencies:* 50–60 minutes a day or as tolerated.

    c. *Cautions:* Wear appropriate clothes and shoes and only dance on safe surfaces.

    d. *Assessments:* Assess vital signs and balance and consult with primary caregiver prior to undertaking an exercise program.

    e. *Tips on use:* Complete warm-up prior to dancing and cool-downs afterward. For suggestions, go to http://library.thinkquest.org/12819/text/warmupcooldown.html

    f. *Other considerations:* Exercise may be especially useful to decrease painful joints.

    g. *References/other sources:*

       Leslie, A., & Rust, J. (1984). Effects of dance on anxiety. *Perceptual Motor Skills 58*(3), 767–772.

Noreau, L., Martineau, H., Roy, L., & Belzile, M. A. (1995). Effects of a modified dance-based exercise on cardiorespiratory fitness, psychological state and health status of persons with rheumatoid arthritis. *Physical Medicine & Rehabilitation, 74*(1), 19–27.

2. Housework
   a. *Actions/expected responses:* Any physical activity, including housework, is enough to boost mental health and reduce anxiety.
   b. *Routes/dosages/frequencies*: 20 minutes a day.
   c. *Cautions:* Go to http://exercise.lifetips.com.
   d. *Assessments:* Assess amount of daily physical activity.
   e. *Tips on use:* Go to http://exercise.lifetips.com.
   f. *Other considerations:* Gardening and sports also lower risk of distress; participating in sports lowered distress by 33%.
   g. *References/other sources:*
      British Medical Journal. (2008, April 10). Just 20 minutes of weekly housework boosts mental health. *ScienceDaily.* Retrieved April 20, 2008, from http://www.sciencedaily.com/releases/2008/04/080409205840.htm

3. Rocking chair use
   a. *Actions/expected responses:* Decreases agitation, anxiety, tension, and a hyper-responsiveness stress, and indirectly decreases detrimental cortisol levels.
   b. *Routes/dosages/frequencies:* As tolerated from one-half hour to two and a half hours a day. Those who rock the most often improve the most.
   c. *Cautions:* Use only a platform-style rocking chair with a super-stable, immobile base that moves back and forth easily.
   d. *Assessments:* Take a baseline measure of agitation and anxiety, and then take a measure after treatment.
   e. *Tips on use:* Rocking together with a family member or friend may encourage rocking.
   f. *Other considerations:* Research has shown rocking can help with agitation and anxiety, and can increase positive feelings.
   g. *References/other sources:*
      Watson, N. (1998). Rocking chair therapy for dementia patients: Its effect on psychosocial well-being and balance. *American Journal of Alzheimer's Disease and Other Dementias, 13*(6), 296–308.
      Watson, N., Hauptmann, M., Brink, C., Powers, B., Taillie, E.R., Lash, M., et al. (1998). *As elders rock, emotional burden of dementia eases.* Presented to the Eastern Nursing Research Society, April 23–25, Rochester, NY.

4. Walking
   a. *Actions/expected responses:* Significantly lowers anxiety level.
   b. *Routes/dosages/frequencies:* As tolerated, walking at the fastest pace possible while still able to carry on a conversation.
   c. *Cautions:* Clear any exercise program with primary care practitioner.
   d. *Assessments:* Take a baseline measure of agitation and anxiety, and then take a measure after exercise. Optional: Use the Six-Minute Walk Test. See the next item.
   e. *Tips on use:* Assessments are available at six-minute walk test: http://www.pulmonaryrehab.com/au/index.asp?page=19, Hospital and Anxiety

Scale: http://www.nfer-nelson.co.uk or email information@nfer-nelson.co.uk, Respiratory Questionnaire: http://libbyasbestos.org/docs/StGeorgesQuestionnaire.pdf

f. *Other considerations:* Wear appropriate clothes and shoes and carry sufficient water (preferably distilled or reverse-osmosis filtered) to remain hydrated (1 cup of water every 15 minutes of exercise).

g. *References/other sources:*

Berk, M. (2007). Should we be targeting exercise as a routine mental health intervention? *Act Neuropsychiatrica 19*(3), 217–218.

De Moor, M. H. M., Beem, A. L., Stubbe, J. H., Boomsma, D. I., & De Geus, E. J. C. A. (2006). Regular exercise, anxiety, depression & personality: A population based study. *Preventive Medicine, 42*(4), 273–279.

5. Yoga

a. *Actions/expected responses:* Stress can significantly decrease after completing a yoga program.

b. *Routes/dosages/frequencies:* 60-minute sessions.

c. *Cautions:* Go to http://yoga.lifetips.com/cat/56770/yoga-cautions/

d. *Assessments:* None.

e. *Tips on use:* Because yoga exerts pressure on internal organs, women should wait at least 2 hours after a meal and 30 minutes to 1 hour after a snack to practice. For more information about yoga, go to http://www.mothernature.com/Library/Bookshelf/Books/21/54.cfm

f. *Other considerations:* To avoid knee injury when doing yoga, keep the knees straight (especially in standing poses). The knees should be forward in line with the ankle and foot, and you should not allow them to twist inward or outward.

g. *References/other sources:*

McCaffrey, R., Ruknui, P., Hatthakit, U., & Kasetsomboon, P. (2005). The effects of yoga on hypertensive persons in Thailand. *Holistic Nursing Practice, 19*(4), 173–180.

Herbs/Essential Oils

1. Ginkgo biloba

a. *Actions/expected responses:* Ginkgo stabilizes mood and reduces anxiety.

b. *Routes/dosages/frequencies:* Special extract EGb 761, 240 mg (reduced global rating of anxiety by 12.1 points)–460 mg/day (reduced global rating of anxiety by 14.3 on the Hamilton Rating Scale for Anxiety [HAMA]).

c. *Cautions:* Ginkgo should not be used during pregnancy or lactation or given to children. The herb is safe and well-tolerated and may be of particular value in older adults with anxiety related to cognitive decline. Adverse reactions may include transient headache, nausea, anorexia, diarrhea, flatulence, and rash. Should not be taken concurrently with anticoagulants or platelet inhibitors because of ginkgo's blood-thinning ability. Ginkgo may also decrease the activity of anticonvulsants. May cause hypomania if given with buspirone, fluoxetine, or St. John's wort. MAOI action may be increased if taken concurrently. Coma may result if taken with trazadone.

    d. *Assessments:* Assess for hypersensitivity reactions. If present, discontinue use of this herb. Use HAMA prior to and after taking ginkgo for 4 weeks. See http://www.anxietyhelp.org/information/hama.html

    e. *Tips on use:* Ginkgo takes 1–6 months for full effect.

    f. *Other considerations:* Do not use ginkgo with anticoagulants, platelet inhibitors, trazadone, or MAOIs.

    g. *References/other sources:*

        Arnoldt, K. H., Kieser, M., & Schwabe, W. (2007). Ginkgo biloba special extract EGb 761 in generalized anxiety disorder and adjustment disorder with anxious mood: A randomized, double-blind, placebo-controlled trial. *Journal of Psychiatric Research, 41*(6), 472–480.

        Skidmore-Roth, L. (2006). Gingko. In *Mosby's handbook of herbs and natural supplements* (pp. 487–492). St. Louis, MO: ElsevierMosby.

2. Lavender and rosemary essential oils

    a. *Actions/expected responses:* Protects the body from oxidative stress by decreasing the stress hormone cortisol.

    b. *Routes/dosages/frequencies:* Sniff aroma of essential oils for 5 minutes.

    c. *Cautions:* None known.

    d. *Assessments:* Assess for hypersensitivity (skin reactions, nausea, or anorexia).

    e. *Tips on use:* Keep aromatherapy products away from heat and moisture in a sealed container.

    f. *Other considerations:* Can use one or the other essential oil as both protect against oxidative stress.

    g. *References/other sources:*

        Atsumi, T., & Tonosaki, K. (2007). Smelling lavender and rosemary increases free radical scavenging activity and decreases cortisol level in saliva. *Psychiatry Research, 150*(1), 89–96.

3. Lemon balm

    a. *Actions/expected responses:* Has a sedative effect, reducing anxiety.

    b. *Routes/dosages/frequencies:* Tea infusion. Pour boiling water over 1.5–4.6 grams of the herb or one tea bag and let steep for 10 minutes and cool prior to sipping.

    c. *Cautions:* Not to be used during pregnancy or lactation or by individuals with hypothyroidism or who are sensitive to the herb.

    d. *Assessments:* Assess for hypersensitivity (skin reactions), nausea, or anorexia.

    e. *Tips on use:* Keep lemon balm products away from heat and moisture in a sealed container; can be kept for up to one year.

    f. *Other considerations:* Avoid using lemon balm if taking barbiturates, other central nervous system depressants, or iron salts.

    g. *References/other sources:*

        Skidmore-Roth, L. (2006). Lemon balm. In *Mosby's handbook of herbs and natural supplements* (pp. 649–652). St. Louis, MO: ElsevierMosby.

4. Peppermint tea

    a. *Actions/expected responses:* Analgesic and anesthetic effects in the central and peripheral nervous system.

    b. *Routes/dosages/frequencies:* Place 1 tbsp of leaves in 2 cups boiling water and steep 15 minutes; take two or three times a day.

    c. *Cautions:* Adverse reactions to peppermint tea have not been reported. Until more information is available, counsel pregnant or lactating women and their children not to drink peppermint tea.

    d. *Assessments:* Assess for sensitivity to peppermint tea and avoid if sensitive. Assess anxiety level prior to and after drinking one to two cups of peppermint tea.

    e. *Tips on use*: Store peppermint tea in a cool, dry place.

    f. *Other considerations:* Animal studies demonstrate a relaxation effect on gastrointestinal (GI) tissues, analgesic and anesthetic effects in the central and peripheral nervous system, immunomodulating actions, and chemopreventive potential.

    g. *References/other sources:*

        McKay, D. L., & Blumberg, J. B. (2006). A review of the bioactivity and potential health benefits of peppermint tea. *Phytotherapy Research, 20*(8), 619–633.

5. Sage

    a. *Actions/expected responses:* Increased alertness, calmness, and contentedness are associated with taking the herb.

    b. *Routes/dosages/frequencies:* 600 mg dried sage leaf.

    c. *Cautions:* Because sage is a uterine stimulant, it should not be used during pregnancy or lactation or given to children. Persons with sensitivity to sage should not use it. Sage can decrease the action of anticonvulsants; avoid concurrent use. Sage can increase the action of antidiabetic agents and central nervous system depressants. The herb may decrease the absorption of iron salt; separate doses by at least 2 hours.

    d. *Assessments:* Assess mood predose and at 1 and 4 hours postdose using a 10-point scale from 0 = no anxiety to 10 = extremely high anxiety.

    e. *Tips on use:* Monitor for diabetes mellitus and seizure disorders closely.

    f. *Other considerations:* Store sage in a sealed container away from heat and moisture. Sage essential oil is safer and can be used in a diffuser, sniffed, or placed in a warm bath (5–10 drops depending on the size of tub).

    g. *References/other sources:*

        Kennedy, D. O., Pace, S., Haskell, C., Okello, E. J., Milne, A., Scholey, A. B., et al. (2006). Effects of cholinesterase inhibiting sage (Salvia officinalis) on mood, anxiety and performance on a psychological stressor battery. *Neuropsychopharmacology, 31*(4), 845–852.

        Skidmore-Roth, L. (2006). Sage. In *Mosby's handbook of herbs and natural supplements* (pp. 908–911). St. Louis, MO: ElsevierMosby.

Mindset

1. Affirmations

    a. *Actions/expected responses:* Self-affirmation of personal values and beliefs buffers neuroendocrine and psychological stress.

    b. *Routes/dosages/frequencies:* Repeat aloud or write positive affirmations up to 20 times a day such as "I am safe and protected," "I love and approve of myself," and "I trust the process of life."

    c. *Cautions:* Ensure that affirmations are positive and acceptable.

d. *Assessments:* Assess anxiety prior to and after completing affirmations for a week.

e. *Tips on use*: Write favorite affirmations on 3 by 5 cards and put them in places where they will be read frequently.

f. *Other considerations:* Find more affirmation information at http://www. successconsciousness.com/index_00000a.htm

g. *References/other sources:*

Hay, L. (2000). *Heal your body.* Carlsbad, CA: Hay House.

Schwarzer, R., Babler, J., Kwiatek, P., Schroder, K., & Zang, J. W. (1997). The assessment of optimistic self-beliefs: Assessment of general perceived self-efficacy in thirteen cultures. *World Psychology, 3*(1–2), 177–190.

2. Cognitive-behavioral therapy (CBT)

a. *Actions/expected responses:* Helps uncover and alter distortions of thought or perception that increase their anxiety. Individuals with persistent panic attacks are encouraged to test out beliefs they have related to such attacks, such as specific fears related to bodily sensations, and to develop realistic responses to such beliefs.

b. *Routes/dosages/frequencies:* Keep a daily log of thought and perception problems that lead to anxiety, such as believing external events cause anxiety and fear, that people are helpless and fragile and have no control over what they experience or feel, that there is a perfect love and relationship, that anger is bad and destructive, that the past determines the present, that adults must have love and approval to survive, that worth is determined by achievement, that it's possible to be perfect and competent at all times, and that it's important to always please other people and never go after what you want. Read *How to Stubbornly Refuse to Make Yourself Miserable About Anything* by Albert Ellis.

c. *Cautions:* Women with acute stress disorder may not find this approach helpful.

d. *Assessments:* Assess anxiety prior to and after cognitive behavioral work.

e. *Tips on use:* Question any beliefs that lead to anxiety.

f. *Other considerations:* See CBT information at http://www.mind.org.uk/ Information/Booklets/Making+sense/MakingSenseCBT.htm

g. *References/other sources:*

Bryant, R. A., Sackville, T., Dang, S. T., Moulds, M., & Guthrie, R. (1999). On treating acute stress disorder: Evaluation of cognitive behavior therapy and supportive counseling techniques. *American Journal of Psychiatry 156*(11), 1780–1786.

Nutrition

1. Coffee/caffeine (avoid)

a. *Actions/expected responses:* Anxiety attacks, including panic, sweating, and trembling have been related to consuming large amounts of caffeine daily in the form of coffee, tea, chocolate, sodas, and over-the-counter pain medications (Anacin, Excedrin, Midol, NoDoz).

b. *Routes/dosages/frequencies:* Depending on the person, one or more cups of coffee or caffeinated foods, beverages, or pain medications can increase anxiety symptoms.

    c. *Cautions:* Caffeine inhibits the absorption of adenosine, a body hormone that is calming. This can lead to sleep problems. Dehydration is one of the main concerns, as is the loss of calcium, which can accelerate bone loss.

    d. *Assessments:* Keep a caffeine diary for a week and jot down number of cups of coffee, tea, sodas, coffee ice cream or yogurt, over-the-counter pain meds, and NoDoz, and to assess their anxiety, panic, and trembling.

    e. *Tips on use:* Withdrawal symptoms, including headache, sleepiness, and irritability, usually occur. A good way to avoid withdrawal from caffeine is to drink one-half cup of coffee and one-half cup of hot water or decaffeinated coffee and over the course of a week slowly eliminate caffeinated coffee.

    f. *Other considerations:* Studies have shown that 200 mg or more of caffeine daily increases anxiety ratings and can induce panic attacks. For caffeine sources, go to http://www.cspinet.org/new/cafchart.htm

    g. *References/other sources:*

        Johns Hopkins Medical Center. (2007). *Caffeine dependence.* Retrieved November 13, 2007, from http://www.caffeinedependence.org/caffeine_dependence.html

        Kendall, P. (2003). *The effects of caffeine on hydration and bone loss.* Retrieved December 3, 2007, from http://www.ext.colostate.edu/pubs/columnn/nn031103.html

2. Vitamin B6

    a. *Actions/expected responses:* Lack of vitamin B6 is related to increases in anxiety. Vitamin B6 is a building block for serotonin; decreased levels of serotonin have been associated with increased stress and anxiety.

    b. *Routes/dosages/frequencies:* 1.6 mg/day for most women. Pregnant women require an additional 0.1 mg per day, and those who are lactating require an additional 0.7–0.8 mg daily. For food sources of vitamin B6, go to http://dietary-supplements.info.nih.gov/factsheets/vitaminb6.asp#h2 or http://lpi.oregonstate.edu/infocenter/vitamins/vitaminB6

    c. *Cautions:* If taken as a supplement, vitamin B6 can cause neurological disorders, such as loss of sensation in legs and imbalance, when taken in high doses (200 mg or more per day) over a long period of time. Vitamin B6 toxicity can damage sensory nerves, leading to numbness in the hands and feet as well as difficulty walking, which recedes when the vitamin supplement is withdrawn.

    d. *Assessments:* On a scale from 0 (no anxiety) to 10 (extreme anxiety), assess anxiety prior to and at 1 and 4 hours after eating more vitamin B6-rich foods.

    e. *Tips on use:* It is safer to take a multivitamin and even safer to eat foods rich in vitamin B6. This vitamin is sensitive to ultraviolet light and heat, so large amounts of this nutrient are lost during the cooking process. Raw fruits and vegetables are preferable. If women take multivitamins counsel them to store the bottles in a cool dry place and keep their covers tightly closed.

    f. *Other considerations:* Several surveys have found that more than half of all women over age 60 consume less than the current recommended daily allowance of vitamin B6 (1.5 mg/day).

    g. *References/other sources:*

    University of Miami School of Medicine. (1995). Researchers at UM School of Medicine link vitamin B6 deficiency to stress. *Vital Signs,* 19.

3. Vitamin C

    a. *Actions/expected responses:* The equivalent of 2 grams a day of vitamin C has been shown to reduce the level of stress hormones circulating in the blood and reduce other typical indicators of physical and emotional stress.

    b. *Routes/dosages/frequencies:* Ester C is less irritating to the stomach and bladder mucosa than other forms of vitamin C. Eating a diet rich in vitamin C—including green peppers, citrus fruits and juices, strawberries, tomatoes, broccoli, turnip greens and other leafy greens, sweet and white potatoes, and cantaloupe—is a healthy alternative to taking a vitamin pill. Other excellent sources include papaya, mango, watermelon, Brussels sprouts, cauliflower, cabbage, winter squash, red peppers, raspberries, blueberries, cranberries, and pineapples.

    c. *Cautions:* Avoid taking vitamin C supplements after eating a meal containing fat. High levels of vitamin C can produce diarrhea and GI upset. Drink a full glass of water or juice when taking a vitamin pill. Whenever possible, focus instead on eating more vitamin C-rich fruits and vegetables.

    d. *Assessments:* Assess for weight loss, frequent infections, and anxiety prior to and after increasing vitamin C intake.

    e. *Tips on use:* Vitamin C is not stored or manufactured in the body, so it is needed daily.

    f. *Other considerations:* Some experts recommend taking a sharper look at the present recommended daily allowance and remembering that our prehistoric ancestors probably consumed large amounts of vitamin C in a diet rich in fruits.

    g. *References/other sources:*

    American Chemical Society. (1999). Vitamin C may alleviate the body's response to stress. *ScienceDaily.* Retrieved November 11, 2007, from www.sciencedaily.com/releases/1999/08/990823072615.htm

4. Whole grains

    a. *Actions/expected responses:* Higher whole-grain intake is associated with a reduced risk of hypertension in middle-aged and older women.

    b. *Routes/dosages/frequencies:* Daily intake of four servings of whole grain breads, cereals, or pasta.

    c. *Cautions:* Refined grains (found in foods made from white flour, such as white bread, refined cereals in boxes, cakes, pies, cookies, or white spaghetti and macaroni) do not lower the risk of hypertension.

    d. *Assessments:* Assess women's intake of whole grains.

    e. *Tips on use:* Counsel women to read labels carefully and eat only whole grains.

    f. *Other considerations:* Increased whole grain intake may also prevent hypertension.

    g. *References/other sources:*

    Wang, L., Gaziano, J. M., Liu, S., Manson, J. E., Buring, J. E. R., & Sesso, H. D. (2007). Whole- and refined-grain intake and the risk of hypertension in women. *American Journal of Clinical Nutrition, 86*(2), 472–479.

Stress Management

1. Autogenic training
   a. *Actions/expected responses:* Autogenic training is a relaxation technique consisting of six mental exercises that used calming statements or thoughts and is aimed at relieving tension, anger, and stress. It has been shown to produce a statistically significantly greater reduction in both state (temporary) and trait (long-term) anxiety as compared to laughter therapy or a control group receiving no intervention.
   b. *Routes/dosages/frequencies:* Can be used effectively with individuals or groups. Ninety-second sessions five to eight times a day, either sitting or lying down. It may take up to 10 months to master the series.
   c. *Cautions:* Focus on the solar plexus is not used for women who have ulcers, diabetes, or any condition involving bleeding from the abdominal region.
   d. *Assessments:* Take a baseline measure for anxiety prior to completing the series of exercises and then take one after completing them.
   e. *Tips on use:* Focus on a different series of body/mind statements or thoughts each week, starting with the arms for 3 minutes four to seven times a day. Weeks 1–3 focus on bringing heaviness to arms and legs. Weeks 4–7 focus on bringing warmth and heaviness to the arms and legs. Week 8 focuses on calming and steadying the heartbeat, week 9 on easy breathing, week 10 on solar plexus (unless the women has ulcers, diabetes or any abdominal bleeding). Week 11 focuses on cooling the forehead, and week 12 on individualized themes such as being quiet, still, at ease, or relaxed.
   f. *Other considerations:* For more information on the procedure, go to http://www.guidetopsychology.com/autogen.htm
   g. *References/other sources:*
      Kanji, N., White, A., & Ernst, E. (2006). Autogenic training to reduce anxiety in nursing students: Randomized controlled trial. *Journal of Advanced Nursing, 53*(6), 729–735.
      Sakai, M. (1997). Application of autogenic training for anxiety disorders: A clinical study in a psychiatric setting. *Fukuoka Igaku Zasshi, 88*(3), 56–64.
2. Breathing retraining
   a. *Actions/expected responses:* Breathing retraining, with or without physical exercise, can reduce breathing frequency, a frequent cause of anxiety.
   b. *Routes/dosages/frequencies:* 30 minutes a day for 6–12 weeks can retrain fast, shallow breathing to slower, *less* frequent breathing.
   c. *Cautions:* None. Abdominal breathing is preferable to shallow chest breathing.
   d. *Assessments:* Assess anxiety level prior to and after breathing retraining.
   e. *Tips on use:* Focus on letting breathing slowly move down toward the abdomen.
   f. *Other considerations:* For more information go to http://www.citytech.cuny.edu/files/students/counseling/stresshb.pdf
   g. *References/other sources:*
      Han, J. N., Stegen, K., De Valck, C., Clement, J., & Van de Woestijne, K. P. (1996). Influence of breathing therapy on complaints, anxiety and

breathing pattern in patients with hyperventilation syndrome and anxiety disorders. *Journal of Psychosomatic Research, 41*(5), 481–493.

Kim, S., & Kim, H. A. (2005). Effects of relaxation breathing exercises on anxiety, depression and leukocytes in hemopoietic stem cell transplantation patients. *Cancer Nursing, 28*(1), 79–83.

3. Mindfulness meditation
   a. *Actions/expected responses:* Anxiety showed statistically significant improvements in subjective and objective symptoms in both short-term and long-term treatment after using mindfulness meditation.
   b. *Routes/dosages/frequencies:* 8-week group stress reduction intervention.
   c. *Cautions:* May not be congruent with the following diagnoses: antisocial personality disorder, borderline personality disorder, current major depressive disorder, physical impairment that precludes attending class, posttraumatic stress disorder, psychosis, social anxiety (if it interferes with participation in class), substance abuse or addiction (current or recovery within the past year), suicidal intent or plan, or unstable medical diagnosis.
   d. *Assessments:* Rate anxiety from 0 (no anxiety) to 10 (extreme anxiety) prior to and after participating in mindfulness sessions.
   e. *Tips on use:* For more information go to http://www.stjohn.org/innerpage. aspx?PageID=1779
   f. *Other considerations:* Other Web sites that may be useful are http://www. mindfulnessmeditationcentre.org/breathingGathas.htm or http://www. meditationcenter.com
   g. *References/other sources:*
      Kabat-Zinn, J. (1990). *Full catastrophe living: The program of the stress reduction.* Clinic of the University of Massachusetts Medical Center. New York: Delta.
      Miller, J. J., Fletcher, K., & Kabat-Zinn, J. (1995). Three-year follow-up and clinical implications of a mindfulness meditation-based stress reduction intervention in the treatment of anxiety disorders. *General Hospital Psychiatry, 17*(3), 192–200.
      Pass, J. E. (2005). Mindfulness-based stress reduction: Applications for nurse practitioners. *The American Journal for Nurse Practitioners, 9*(7–8), 9–18.

4. Relaxation therapy
   a. *Actions/expected responses:* Relaxation therapy produces a calming effect by stilling the body and is now supported by strong evidence for the treatment of anxiety.
   b. *Routes/dosages/frequencies:* 20 minutes a day.
   c. *Cautions:* In a relaxed state, lower levels of medication, especially insulin, may be needed. Complete relaxation may result in a hypotensive state.
   d. *Assessments:* Assess level of anxiety before and after relaxation.
   e. *Tips on use:* Avoid holding the breath and picture breathing in and out of the abdomen. For more information go to http://www.webmd.com/ migraines-headaches/guide/relaxation-techniques
   f. *Other considerations:* Taking blood pressure at the conclusion of a relaxation training session may help identify individuals prone to hypotensive states.

g. *References/other sources:*
   Ernst, E., Pittler, M. H., Wider, B., & Boddy, K. (2007). Mind-body therapies: Are the trial data getting stronger? *Alternative Therapies in Health and Medicine, 13*(5), 62–64.

   Scogin, F., Rickard, H. C., Keither, S., Wilson, J., & McElreath, L. (1992). Progressive and imaginal relaxation training for elderly persons with subjective anxiety. *Psychology and Aging, 7*(3), 419–424.

   Winter, J. C. (1988). *Relationship between research and practice: Nurses' attitudes about relaxation therapy.* Doctoral dissertation, Columbia University, New York.

Supplements

1. Vitamin D
   a. *Actions/expected responses:* Vitamin D deficiency is associated with anxiety.
   b. *Routes/dosages/frequencies:* Vitamin D3 is produced in light-skinned women by 4–10 minutes of exposure of face, arms, or back to the noonday sun, and by 60–80 minutes of exposure for darker-skinned women. Individuals living at latitudes north of 35 degrees or who may not receive exposure to the sun or who are older than 49 years may need to take a tablespoon of cod liver oil daily.
   c. *Cautions:* Taking amounts over 100,000 IU of vitamin D per day as a supplement may be toxic: signs of toxicity include anorexia, nausea/vomiting, polyuria, polydipsia, weakness, nervousness, and pruritus. Vitamin D supplements can suppress the proper operation of the immune system.
   d. *Assessments:* Assess level of anxiety before and after exposure to sun and/or ingesting cod liver oil.
   e. *Tips on use:* The vitamin D2 that is added to so-called fortified foods and many multivitamins, and is usually written in prescriptions, is inefficiently metabolized in humans; only 20%–40% is metabolized into biologically active vitamin D3.
   f. *Other considerations:* Women using corticosteroids may require additional vitamin D.
   g. *References/other sources:*
   Armstrong, D. J., Meenagh, G. K., Bickle, I., Lee, A. S., Curran, E. S., & Finch, M. B. (2007). Vitamin D deficiency is associated with anxiety and depression in fibromyalgia. *Clinical Rheumatology, 26*(4), 551–554.

   Autoimmunity Research Foundation. (2008, January 27). Vitamin D deficiency study raises new questions about disease and supplements. *ScienceDaily.* Retrieved February 13, 2008, from http://www.science daily.com/releases/2008/01/080125223302.htm

   Jockers, B. S. (2007). Vitamin D sufficiency: An approach to disease prevention. *The American Journal for Nurse Practitioners, 11*(10), 43–50.

   Lansdowne, A. T., & Provost, S. C. (1998). Vitamin D_3 enhances mood in healthy subjects during winter. *Psychopharmacology, 135*(4), 319–323.

Touch

1. Acupressure
   a. *Actions/expected responses:* Acupressure at specific relaxation points has been shown to be an effective treatment for anxiety.
   b. *Routes/dosages/frequencies:* 10 to 15 minutes daily. *Foot acupressure:* on the sole of the foot about one third down below the second and third toes (solar plexus), right below the ankle bone on the outside of the foot, and on top of the foot between the tendons of the big toe and second toe about an inch down from the toes. *Hand acupressure:* center of the palm where middle finger touches the palm when it is gently bent forward, in the middle of the wrist crease between the tendons on the inside of the arm, and level with the little finger (works well for palpitations and irritability).
   c. *Cautions:* Foot acupressure should not be applied to individuals with venous stasis, phlebitis, and traumatic and deep tissue injuries. Acupressure of any kind is not advised for premature infants who can withstand only limited physical contact.
   d. *Assessments:* Use a visual analogue scale of 0 to 100 mm to rate anxiety. If this is impossible, rate changes in behavior after treatment begins.
   e. *Tips on use:* Use tip of thumb to press and knead points for 1–2 minutes. Practice these movements to find the points and the amount of pressure that is healing and does not tickle or is too painful.
   f. *Other considerations:* Find more specific directions and photographs of foot massage at http://www.chinese-holistic-health-exercises.com/foot-massage-techniques.html
   g. *References/other sources:*

   Mora, B., Iannuzzi, M., Lang, T., Steinlechner, B., Barker, R., Dobrovits, M., et al. (2007). Auricular acupressure as a treatment for anxiety before extracorporeal shock wave lithotripsy in the elderly. *The Journal of Urology 178*(1), 160–164.

   Sutherland, J., Peaks, J., & Bridges, C. (1999). Foot acupressure and massage for patients with Alzheimer's disease and related dementias. *Image, Journal of Nursing Scholarship, 31*(4), 147–148.

   Tsay, S. L., Wang, J. C., Lin, K. C., & Chung, U. L. (2005). Effects of acupressure therapy for patients having prolonged mechanical ventilation support. *Journal of Advanced Nursing, 52*(2), 142–150.

2. Massage with aromatherapy
   a. *Actions/expected responses:* Aromatherapy massage (lavender, chamomile, rosemary, and lemon) exerts significant positive effects on anxiety.
   b. *Routes/dosages/frequencies:* 20 minutes sessions three times a week for 6 weeks.
   c. *Cautions:* The aged, extremely ill, or dying individuals may require a gentle massage. The head is also a sensitive area; only gentle sweeping motions are used and energy is not concentrated in that area.
   d. *Assessments:* Ask women to chart behavior mood prior to and after massage.
   e. *Tips on use:* Go to http://www.ehow.com/how_12801_aromatherapy-with-bodywork.html
   f. *Other considerations:* Avoid concentrating energy in any area where cancer may reside.

    g. *References/other sources:*

Rho, K. H., Han, S. H., Kim, K. S., & Lee, M. S. (2006). Effects of aromatherapy massage on anxiety and self-esteem in Korean elderly women: A pilot study. *International Journal of Neuroscience, 116*(12), 1447–1555.

3. Reflexology

    a. *Actions/expected responses:* Women who self-applied foot reflexology reduced their stress responses.

    b. *Routes/dosages/frequencies:* Daily for 6 weeks, 15–60 minutes.

    c. *Cautions:* Pregnant women should avoid foot reflexology because certain manipulations can lead to premature labor. Those with foot problems, gout, arthritis, and vascular conditions such as varicose veins should be careful using this procedure.

    d. *Assessments:* Assess anxiety/stress on a scale of 1 (none) to 10 (extremely anxious) prior to and after foot reflexology sessions.

    e. *Tips on use:* For foot charts, see http://groups.msn.com/Alternatives ToPainandDisease/reflexologyinstructionspg1.msnw

    f. *Other considerations:* http://groups.msn.com/AlternativesToPainand Disease/reflexologyinstructionspg2.msnw

    g. *References/other sources:*

Kesselring, A. (1994). Foot reflex zone massage. *Schweizerische Medizinische Wochenschrift, 62,* 88–93.

Lee, Y. M. (2006). Effect of self-foot reflexology massage on depression, stress response and immune functions of middle aged women. *Taehan Kanho Hakkoe Chi, 36*(1), 179–188.

4. Therapeutic touch

    a. *Actions/expected responses:* Therapeutic touch (TT) includes centering, assessing, unruffling the field, and transfer of energy.

    b. *Routes/dosages/frequencies:* The hands are used to assess the energy field and transfer energy.

    c. *Cautions:* In general, the body will accept the amount of energy needed. Aged, extremely ill, or dying women may require a gentle energy input. The head is also a sensitive area; only gentle sweeping motions are used and energy is not concentrated in that area or in an area where cancer resides.

    d. *Assessments:* The hands are used to assess energy levels and note disordered energy patterns.

    e. *Tips on use:* The techniques of TT can be learned in a short period of time, perhaps hours, but knowing when and how to use the techniques requires practice. To start, go to http://www.healgrief.com/Site/Heal_Grief_in_Your_ Body.html

    f. *Other considerations:* Specific healing colors may be pictured and used in the healing process.

    g. *References/other sources:*

Gagne, D., & Toye, R. C. (1994). The effects of therapeutic touch and relaxation therapy in reducing anxiety. *Archives of Psychiatric Nursing, 8*(3), 184–189.

Simington, J. A., & Laing, G. P. (1993). Effects of therapeutic touch on anxiety in the institutionalized elderly. *Clinical Nursing Research, 2*(4), 438–450.

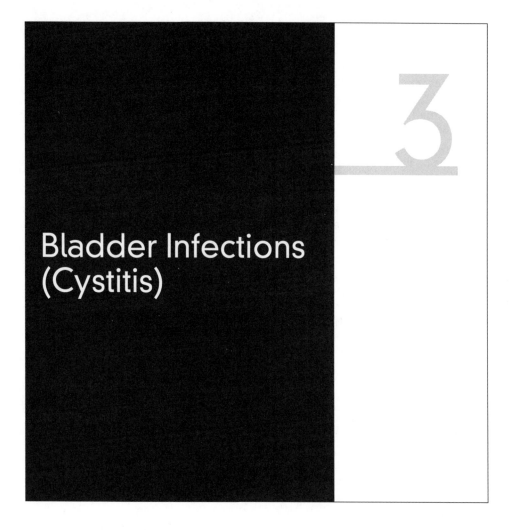

Bladder Infections (Cystitis)

Bladder symptoms can often be assuaged by nutritional, exercise, and relaxation approaches. These complementary procedures work well in concert with traditional medical approaches.

Environment

1. Good bladder hygiene for urinary symptoms
   a. *Actions/expected responses:* Emptying the bladder, soaking in a warm tub, wiping from front to back, wearing a diaphragm that isn't too large, using nonallergenic menstrual pads, changing tampons each urination, drinking six to eight glasses of fluid a day, urinating prior to and after intercourse, and making sure the angle of the penis matches the angle of the vagina so abrasions do not occur are actions that can reduce or even eliminate bladder inflammation or infections.
   b. *Routes/dosages/frequencies:* Complete all the actions in "Actions/Expected Responses" for best results.

c. *Cautions:* Chemical contamination from spermicidal barrier methods of contraception, regular douching, deodorant sanitary napkins or tampons, and frequent or vigorous sexual activity while using a condom are predisposing factors.

d. *Assessments:* Keep a daily diary of bladder hygiene and urinary symptoms to see what foods, supplements, medications, and situations affect cystitis.

e. *Tips on use:* Devise a bladder action card (that lists helpful actions) to post in the bathroom.

f. *Other considerations:* None.

g. *References/other sources:*

Foxman, B., Geiger, A. M., Palin, K., Gillespie, B., & Koopman, J. S. (1995). First-time urinary tract infection and sexual behavior. *Epidemiology 6*(2), 162–168.

Hooten, T. M., Scholes, D., Stapleton, A. E., Roberts, P. I., Winter, C., Gupta, K., et al. (2000). A prospective study of asymptomatic bacteriuria in sexually active young women. *The New England Journal of Medicine, 343*(14), 992–997.

Khalsa, S. (2006). Living without cystitis. *Health Counselor, 6*(2), 15–17.

Exercise/Movement

1. Exercises that avoid excessive motion in the lower abdomen
   a. *Actions/expected responses:* Swimming, walking in water, or upper and lower body aerobics performed while sitting or standing in place are best because they do not use excessive abdominal motion.
   b. *Routes/dosages/frequencies:* 60-minute sessions.
   c. *Cautions:* Counsel women to stop any exercise that increases bladder discomfort.
   d. *Assessments:* Assess bladder discomfort prior to and after completing exercise.
   e. *Tips on use:* Wait at least 1 hour after a meal and 30 minutes to 1 hour after a snack to exercise.
   f. *Other considerations:* Suggest women exercise with a buddy or friend who can provide support and encouragement.
   g. *References/other sources:*
      Crutchfield, N. S., & Wilen, S. B. (1998). Interstitial cystitis, a diagnostic and therapeutic dilemma. *Advance for Nurse Practitioners, 1*(9), 54–56.

2. Hatha yoga
   a. *Actions/expected responses:* Yoga may reduce pain of interstitial cystitis.
   b. *Routes/dosages/frequencies:* Participate in yoga class or use a yoga tape (do a Google search for yoga tapes) at home in 30–60-minute sessions.
   c. *Cautions:* Go to http://yoga.lifetips.com/cat/56770/yoga-cautions/
   d. *Assessments:* Assess for heavy menstrual flow, pregnancy, knee problems, and conditions that may affect yoga practice.
   e. *Tips on use:* Because yoga exerts pressure on internal organs, wait at least 2 hours after a meal and 30 minutes to 1 hour after a snack to practice. For more information about yoga, go to http://www.mothernature.com/Library/

Bookshelf/Books/21/54.cfm and http://www.santosha.com/asanas/asana.html

f. *Other considerations:* To avoid knee injury when doing yoga, keep the knees straight (especially in standing poses). The knees should be forward in line with the ankle and foot and should not twist inward or outward.

g. *References/other sources:*

Ripoll, E., & Mahowald, D. (2002). Hatha yoga therapy management of urologic disorders. *World Journal of Urology, 20*(5), 306–309.

Herbs/Essential Oils

1. Peppermint, menthol, rosemary, and clove essential oils
   a. *Actions/expected responses:* The four oils all have antimicrobial actions.
   b. *Routes/dosages/frequencies:* Fill a bathtub until the hips are covered. Place 5–10 drops of either peppermint, menthol, rosemary, or clove essential oil in the water and swirl it around to disperse it, and then soak for 15–20 minutes.
   c. *Cautions:* Avoid using essential oils anywhere near the eyes.
   d. *Assessments:* Evaluate number of bladder infections/distress prior to and after using essential oil in a sitz bath (that soaks only the hips and buttocks).
   e. *Tips on use:* Only use essential oils; other oils do not have the same healing qualities.
   f. *Other considerations:* Experiment with different oils and see which one is most soothing. Clove and rosemary have been shown to possess synergistic activity.
   g. *References/other sources:*

Fu, Y., Zu, Y., Chen, L., Shi, W., Wang, Z., Sun, S., et al. (2007). Antimicrobial activity of clove and rosemary essential oils alone and in combination. *Phytotherapy Research, 21*(10), 989–994.

Luqman, S., Dwivedi, G. R., Darokar, M. P., Kalra, A., & Khanuja, S. P. (2007). Potential of rosemary oil to be used in drug-resistant infections. *Alternative Therapies in Health and Medicine, 13*(5), 54–59.

Schelz, Z., Molnar, J., & Hohmann, J. (2006). Antimicrobial and antiplasmid activities of essential oils. *Fitoterapia, 77*(4), 279–285.

Mindset

1. Affirmations
   a. *Actions/expected responses:* Self-affirmation of personal values and beliefs buffers neuroendocrine and psychological stress.
   b. *Routes/dosages/frequencies:* Repeat aloud or write positive affirmations up to 20 times a day, such as "I easily release the old and welcome change in my life" and "I let go of all anger and cover myself with hope and love."
   c. *Cautions:* Wait until panic or high anxiety has lessened before trying affirmations.

    d. *Assessments:* Assess reaction to doing affirmations and see "Stress Management" section for other approaches if necessary.

    e. *Tips on use:* Assess beliefs about their infection/inflammation and use them to develop positive affirmations—for example, "My bladder is healthy" or "I let go of ideas that upset me."

    f. *Other considerations:* For more information go to http://www.successconsciousness.com/index_00000a.htm

    g. *References/other sources:*

        Creswell, J. D., Welch, W. T., Taylor, S. E., Sherman, D. R., Gruenwald, T. L., & Hay, L. (2000). *Heal your body.* Carlsbad, CA: Hay House.

        Kolea, S. L., & van Knippenberg, A. (2006). Controlling your mind without ironic consequences: Self-affirmation eliminates rebound effects after thought suppression. *Journal of Experimental Social Psychology, 43*(4), 671–677.

        Mann, T. (2005). Affirmation of personal values buffers neuroendocrine and psychological stress responses. *Psychological Science, 16,* 946–851.

        Schwarzer, R., Babler, J., Kwiatek, P., Schroder, K., & Zang, J. W. (1997). The assessment of optimistic self-beliefs: Assessment of general perceived self-efficacy in thirteen cultures. *World Psychology, 3*(1–2), 177–190.

Nutrition

1. Berry juices

    a. *Actions/expected responses:* Fresh juices, especially cranberry and blueberry juice, are associated with a decreased risk of recurrence of urinary tract infections.

    b. *Routes/dosages/frequencies:* Drink one-half pint of unsweetened cranberry or blueberry juice daily.

    c. *Cautions:* Fresh juice may be more effective at eliminating existing infections than warding off new ones for some women and vice versa for others.

    d. *Assessments:* Chart the effect of drinking fresh berry juices versus urinary symptoms.

    e. *Tips on use:* Avoid juices containing high levels of high fructose corn syrup.

    f. *Other considerations:* Use only 100% natural fruit juice. Corn syrup is correlated with high blood sugar, the buildup of fat cells, and obesity.

    g. *References/other sources:*

        Kontiokari, T., Laitinen, J., Jarvi, L., Pokka, T., Sundqvist, K., & Uhari, M. (2003). Dietary factors protecting women from urinary tract infections. *American Journal of Clinical Nutrition, 77*(3), 600–604.

        University of Michigan Health System. (2007, September 6). The power of fruit juice. *ScienceDaily.* Retrieved November 20, 2007, from http://www.sciencedaily.com/releasese/2007/09/070905175237.htm

2. Fermented milk products

    a. *Actions/expected responses:* Fermented milk products containing probiotic bacteria are associated with a decreased risk of recurrence of urinary tract infections.

b. *Routes/dosages/frequencies:* Ingest acidophilus soured milk, berry and fruit cultured milk, kefir, or yogurt three times per week.

c. *Cautions:* None unless allergic to the product.

d. *Assessments:* Assess allergies to cultured milk.

e. *Tips on use:* Not all yogurts contain live organisms, so it's important to read labels prior to buying a product.

f. *Other considerations:* None.

g. *References/other sources:*

> Kontiokari, T., Laitinen, J., Jarvi, L., Pokka, T., Sundqvist, K., & Uhari, M. (2003). Dietary factors protecting women from urinary tract infections. *American Journal of Clinical Nutrition, 77*(3), 600–604.

> Zarate, G., & Nader-Macias, M. E. (2006). Influence of probiotic vaginal lactobacilli on in vitro adhesion of urogenital pathogens to vaginal epithelial cells. *Letters in Applied Microbiology, 43*(2), 174–180.

3. Tea and garlic

a. *Actions/expected responses:* Tea and garlic juice were shown to have strong antibacterial activity on a broad spectrum of pathogens including resistant strains such as methicillin- and ciprofloxacin-resistant staphylococci, vancomycin-resistant enterococci, and ciprofloxacin-resistant Pseudomonas aeruginosa.

b. *Routes/dosages/frequencies:* As tolerated.

c. *Cautions:* Garlic may interact with some antiplatelet medications but may be safe while taking warfarin.

d. *Assessments:* Ask women to rate bladder infection symptoms prior to and after ingesting garlic juice or tea.

e. *Tips on use:* Tea can be sipped throughout the day and used in sitz baths. Garlic juice can be added to cooked foods.

f. *Other considerations:* None.

g. *References/other sources:*

> Lee, Y. L., Cesario, T., Wang, Y., Shanbrom, E., & Thrupp, L. (2003). Antibacterial activity of vegetables and juices. *Nutrition, 19*(11–12), 904–906.

> Macan, H., Uykimpang, R., Clconcel, M., Takasu, J., Razon, R., Amagase, H., et al. (2006). Aged garlic extract may be safe for patients on warfarin therapy. *Journal of Nutrition, 136*(3 Suppl.), 793S–795S.

4. Triggering foods (avoid)

a. *Actions/expected responses:* Avoid alcohol, apples, artificial sweeteners, avocados, bananas, beans (fava and lima), brewer's yeast, canned figs, cantaloupes, carbonated drinks, cheese (aged), citrus, chocolate, chicken livers, corned beef, grapes, guavas, mayonnaise, nuts, onions, peaches, pickled herring, pineapples, plums, prunes, raisins, rye bread, soy sauce, spicy foods, strawberries, tomatoes, vinegar, sour cream, yogurt, vitamins buffered with aspartate, and caffeine. They are considered bladder irritants.

b. *Routes/dosages/frequencies:* Avoid bladder-irritating foods at all times.

c. *Cautions:* Not all individuals react to all bladder irritants.

d. *Assessments:* Complete a food diary by recording everything consumed, and then eliminating possible irritants for several weeks, and especially 2 hours prior to sleep.

e. *Tips on use:* Once potential irritants have been eliminated, counsel women to slowly add back the foods one at a time over several weeks until bladder irritants are identified.

f. *Other considerations:* Irritating symptoms can often be relieved by drinking a glass of water with one teaspoon of baking soda stirred in.

g. *References/other sources:*

Crutchfield, N. S., & Wilen, S. B. (1998). Interstitial cystitis, a diagnostic and therapeutic dilemma. *Advance for Nurse Practitioners, 5*(9), 54–56.

Stress Management

1. Relaxation therapy

a. *Actions/expected responses:* Relaxation therapy produces a calming effect by stilling the body and enhancing circulation.

b. *Routes/dosages/frequencies:* 20 minutes a day.

c. *Cautions:* In a relaxed state, lower levels of medication, especially insulin, may be needed. Complete relaxation may result in a hypotensive state.

d. *Assessments:* Assess level of anxiety before and after relaxation.

e. *Tips on use:* Avoid holding the breath while breathing in and out of the abdomen. For more information go to http://www.webmd.com/migraines headaches/guide/relaxation-techniques

f. *Other considerations:* Taking blood pressure at the conclusion of a relaxation training session may help identify inclination for hypotensive states.

g. *References/other sources:*

Ernst, E., Pittler, M. H., Wider, B., & Boddy, K. (2007). Mind-body therapies: Are the trial data getting stronger? *Alternative Therapies in Health and Medicine, 13*(5), 62–64.

Supplements

1. Vitamins A, B6, B12, C, D, E and folic acid, and trace elements of iron, zinc, copper, and selenium

a. *Actions/expected responses:* These supplements work in synergy to contribute to the body's natural defense, cellular immunity, and antibody production. Inadequate intake and status of these vitamins and trace elements may lead to suppressed immunity, which predisposes to infections.

b. *Routes/dosages/frequencies:* All are taken by mouth.

c. *Cautions:* Follow suggested dosage on bottles.

d. *Assessments:* Assess frequency and intensity of bladder infections prior to and after taking supplements.

e. *Tips on use:* Tell women to keep supplements in a dry, cool place.

f. *Other considerations:* Stop taking any supplement if a negative reaction occurs.

g. *References/other sources:*

Maggini, S., Wintergerst, E. S., Beveridge, S., & Hornig, D. H. (2007). Selected vitamins and trace elements support immune function by strengthening epithelial barriers and cellular and humoral immune responses. *British Journal of Nutrition, 1*(Suppl.), S29–S35.

Touch

1. Foot reflexology
   a. *Actions/expected responses:* A meta-analysis of studies on foot reflexology concluded this procedure enhances urination and bladder tonus.
   b. *Routes/dosages/frequencies:* 45–60 minute sessions, as tolerated.
   c. *Cautions:* Pregnant women should avoid foot reflexology because certain manipulations can lead to premature labor. Those with foot problems, gout, arthritis, and vascular conditions such as varicose veins should be careful using this procedure.
   d. *Assessments:* Evaluate bladder sensations prior to and after foot reflexology sessions.
   e. *Tips on use:* Focus on massaging bladder and kidneys. For foot charts, see http://groups.msn.com/AlternativesToPainandDisease/reflexologyinstructionspg1.msnw
   f. *Other considerations:* See http://groups.msn.com/AlternativesToPainandDisease/reflexologyinstructionspg2.msnw
   g. *References/other sources:*
      Kesselring, A. (1994). Foot reflex zone massage. *Schweizerische Medizinische Wochenschrift, 62,* 88–93.

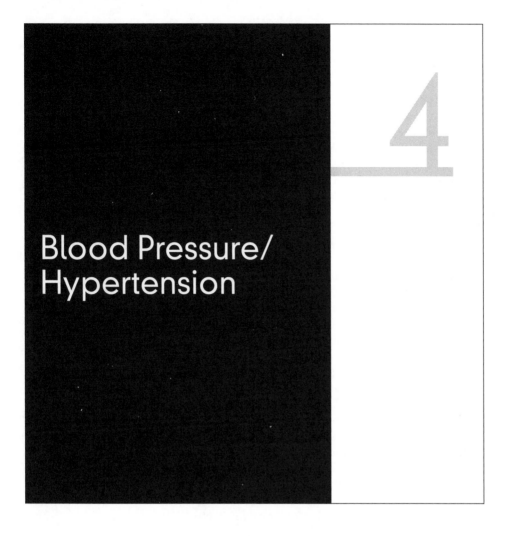

Blood Pressure/ Hypertension

Blood pressure can be lowered through nutrition, exercise, and relaxation approaches. These complementary procedures work well in concert with traditional medical approaches.

Environment

1. Alcohol and smoking
   a. *Actions/expected responses:* Drinking alcohol and smoking both increase diastolic blood pressure.
   b. *Routes/dosages/frequencies:* Goal is to eliminate use of alcohol and cigarettes.
   c. *Cautions:* Alcohol and cigarettes are also associated with other conditions, including heart disease and cancer.
   d. *Assessments:* Determine a baseline by assessing number of drinks per day and number of cigarettes smoked.
   e. *Tips on use:* For information on tobacco and alcohol cessation, go to http://www.cdc.gov/tobacco/quit_smoking/index.htm and http://www.eckerd.edu/health/links/index.php

    f. *Other considerations:* Using nondrug therapy, and strictly adhering to it, cases of prehypertension can be prevented from progressing to a hypertension stage, and medications in grade 1 (mild) hypertension can be reduced or stopped.

    g. *References/other sources:*

        Dickey, R. A., & Janick, J. J. (2001). Lifestyle modifications in the prevention and treatment of hypertension. *Endocrine Practice, 7*(5), 392–399.

        Sainani, G. S. (2003). Non-drug therapy in prevention and control of hypertension. *Journal of Association of Physicians in India, 51,* 1001–1006.

2. Drug links

    a. *Actions/expected responses:* A number of prescription and nonprescription drugs can cause transient or sustained increase in blood pressure.

    b. *Routes/dosages/frequencies:* Zero use if possible.

    c. *Cautions:* NSAIDS (COX-1 and COX-2), amphetamines, decongestants, anorectics, oral contraceptives, adrenal steroid hormones, cyclosporine and tacrolimus, erythropoietin, licorice, chewing tobacco, ephedra, ma huang, and bitter orange can raise blood pressure.

    d. *Assessments:* Assess use of listed drugs.

    e. *Tips on use:* Reduce or stop taking the listed drugs by discussing the topic with prescribing health care provider to find alternatives.

    f. *Other considerations:* Monitor blood pressure and discuss reducing blood pressure–elevating medication use with the prescribing health care practitioner.

    g. *References/other sources:*

        Chobanian, A. V., Bakris, G. L., & Black, H. R. (2003). The seventh report of the Joint Committee on the Prevention, Detection, Evaluation and Treatment of High Blood Pressure: The JNC 7 report. *Journal of the American Medical Association, 289,* 2560–2572.

3. Music

    a. *Actions/expected responses:* Self-selected music decreased perceived blood pressure and perceived stress, and enhanced sense of personal control and well-being to levels not seen in women who did not listen to the music.

    b. *Routes/dosages/frequencies:* Play soothing music during or prior to stressful situations.

    c. *Cautions:* Avoid choosing rock music; it can raise heart rate.

    d. *Assessments:* Assess blood pressure prior to and after listening to music.

    e. *Tips on use:* Classical music, ballroom dance music, and familiar songs may be best for lowering blood pressure.

    f. *Other considerations:* None.

    g. *References/other sources:*

        Allen, K., Golden, L. H., Izzo, J. L., Ching, M. I., Forrest, A., Niles, C. R., et al. (2001). Normalization of hypertensive responses during ambulatory surgical stress by perioperative music. *Psychosomatic Medicine, 63*(3), 487–492.

        Campbell, D. (1997). *The Mozart effect: Tapping the power of music to heal the body, strengthen the mind, and unlock the creative spirit.* New York: Avon Books.

4. Sunlight
   a. *Actions/expected responses:* Studies show a strong correlation between high vitamin D consumption and lower blood pressure.
   b. *Routes/dosages/frequencies:* For light-skinned women, 10–15 minutes of direct midday sun at least twice a week on the face, arms, hands, or back is sufficient, according to the National Institutes of Health. Darker-skinned women may require three to six times as much exposure.
   c. *Cautions:* More frequent exposure could result in skin cancer. Insufficient exposure to the sun can result in improper absorption of calcium and phosphorus, leading to imperfect skeletal formation as well as bone disorders. Vitamin D supplements can suppress the immune system.
   d. *Assessments:* Assess the amount of time women spend in direct sunlight.
   e. *Tips on use:* Develop a plan for obtaining sufficient sunlight, depending on lifestyle. Eating lunch outside when weather permits could be one solution. In colder climes, taking a tablespoon of cod liver oil daily, eating fatty fish and fish oils, and egg yolks may work. Supplements of Vitamin D3 (calciferol) may be necessary in certain cases.
   f. *Other considerations:* Vitamin D2, found in fortified foods, especially breads and cereals, is poorly metabolized by the body. Certain drugs can interfere with vitamin D metabolism, including corticosteroids, phenytoin, heparin, cimetidine, isoniazid, rifampin, phenobarbital, and primidone. Find alternate medications whenever possible to enhance vitamin D3 absorption.
   g. *References/other sources:*
      Demgrow, M. (2007, June). High vitamin D: Treatment for cancer prevention? *The Clinical Advisor, 54,* 57.
      Jockers, B. S. (2007). Vitamin D sufficiency: An approach to disease prevention. *The American Journal for Nurse Practitioners, 11*(10), 43–50.
5. Water
   a. *Actions/expected responses:* Water replaces lost fluids while caffeinated beverages and alcohol increase fluid output, leeching out needed liquids, minerals, and vitamins. Dehydration can lead to hypertension, while hydration is a treatment for high blood pressure.
   b. *Routes/dosages/frequencies:* At least 8–10 glasses a day.
   c. *Cautions:* Tap water and even bottled water can contain parasites, weed killers, nitrates (correlated with spontaneous miscarriage and so-called blue-baby syndrome), salmonella, E. coli, chlorine, fluoride and other potentially dangerous substances.
   d. *Assessments:* Assess type and quantity of water drunk.
   e. *Tips on use:* Counsel women to drink (and cook with) only distilled water or reverse-osmosis filtered water.
   f. *Other considerations:* Fluid intake is probably adequate when thirst is rarely experienced and when urine is colorless or slightly yellow. With age, women experience less thirst. Drink water before thirst sets in because by that time, dehydration may already have taken over.
   g. *References/other sources:*
      Doull, J., Boekelheide, K., Farishian, B. G., Isaacson, R. L., Klotz, J. B., Limeback, H., et al. (2006). *Committee on Fluoride in Drinking Water Board on Environmental Studies and Toxicology, Division of Earth and Life Sciences, National Research Council of the National Academies.*

Fluoride in drinking water: A scientific review of EPA's standards. Washington, DC: National Academies Press.

Manz, F. (2007). Hydration and disease. *Journal of American College of Nutrition, 26*(5 Suppl.), 535S–541S.

Exercise/Movement

1. T'ai chi
   a. *Actions/expected responses:* T'ai chi lowered blood pressure in women nearly as much as moderate-intensity aerobic exercise.
   b. *Routes/dosages/frequencies:* 12-week program lowered systolic blood pressure an average of 8.4 mm of mercury for the aerobic exercise group and 7 mm Hg in the t'ai chi group.
   c. *Cautions:* Older women who tend to fall or become dizzy should be closely monitored.
   d. *Assessments:* Assess blood pressure and suggest hypertensive women find a t'ai chi exercise group.
   e. *Tips on use:* Find a t'ai chi group to join by looking in the newspaper in the health section or searching the Yellow Pages.
   f. *Other considerations:* None.
   g. *References/other sources:*
      American Heart Association. (1998, March 20). T'ai chi lowers blood pressure for older adults. *ScienceDaily.* Retrieved November 23, 2007, from http://www.sciencedaily.com/releases/1998/03/980320075947.htm
2. Walking, jogging, ergometric cycling, or swimming
   a. *Actions/expected responses:* Even modest amount of weekly exercise can significantly improve blood pressure levels in hypertensive women.
   b. *Routes/dosages/frequencies:* Exercising 61–90 minutes a week significantly reduces systolic BP (11.7 mm Hg), with a 6.9 mm Hg average reduction for women who exercised 30 to 60 minutes a week, compared to nonexercising women whose BP remained constant.
   c. *Cautions:* Exclusion criteria include antihypertensive medication use and cardiovascular disease. Discuss exercise plans with prescribing health care practitioner.
   d. *Assessments:* Assess blood pressure prior to and at rest after completing exercise for several weeks.
   e. *Tips on use:* Complete warm-up and cool-down stretches prior to exercising.
   f. *Other considerations:* Exercising more than 90 minutes may not significantly lower blood pressure. Older women may benefit most from moderate to high-intensity interval walking.
   g. *References/other sources:*
      British Medical Journal. (2007, August 20). Even low levels of weekly exercise drive down blood pressure. *ScienceDaily.* Retrieved November 23, 2007, from http://www.sciencedaily.com/releases/2007/08/070813192701.htm
      Ishikawa-Takata, K., Ohta, F., & Tanaka, H. (2003). Just one hour of weekly exercise may lower BP. *American Journal of Hypertension, 16,* 629–633.

Mayo Clinic. (2007, July 13). When it comes to walking, it's all good, says Mayo Clinic researcher. *ScienceDaily*. Retrieved November 23, 2007, from http://www.sciencedaily.com/releases/2007/07/070711134426.htm

Herbs/Essential Oils

1. Aromatherapy
   a. *Actions/expected responses:* A blending of lavender, ylang-ylang, and bergamot essential oils reduced blood pressure in women with essential hypertension, as compared to a placebo group and a control group.
   b. *Routes/dosages/frequencies:* The blended oils are inhaled once daily for 4 weeks.
   c. *Cautions:* None known.
   d. *Assessments:* Assess blood pressure prior to and after inhaling essential oils.
   e. *Tips on use:* Either of the following methods can be used: (a) Add 20 drops of blended oil to 1/2 ounce carrier oil (peanut, castor, olive) and mix well; (b) place 3 drops in palm, rub hands together and inhale for 1 minute.
   f. *Other considerations:* Essential oils are for external use only unless supervised by a qualified aromatherapist. Keep out of reach of children. Avoid while pregnant. Do not expose to mucous membranes or eyes.
   g. *References/other sources:*
      Hwang, J. H. (2006). The effects of the inhalation method using essential oils on blood pressure and stress responses of women with essential hypertension. *Taehan Kanho Hakhoe Chi, 36*(7), 1123–1124.

Mindset

1. Affirmations
   a. *Actions/expected responses:* Self-affirmation of personal values and beliefs buffers neuroendocrine and psychological stress that can raise blood pressure.
   b. *Routes/dosages/frequencies:* Repeat aloud or write positive affirmations up to 20 times a day such as "I am at peace. I joyously release the past."
   c. *Cautions:* None known.
   d. *Assessments:* Monitor blood pressure prior to and after women use affirmations for several weeks.
   e. *Tips on use:* Choose affirmations that seem agreeable and possible.
   f. *Other considerations:* See affirmations information at http://www.success consciousness.com/index_00000a.htm
   g. *References/other sources:*
      Creswell, J. D., Welch, W. T., Taylor, S. E., Sherman, D. R., Gruenwald, T. L., & Hay, L. (2000). *Heal your body*. Carlsbad, CA: Hay House.
      Kolea, S. L., & van Knippenberg, A. (2006). Controlling your mind without ironic consequences: Self-affirmation eliminates rebound effects after thought suppression. *Journal of Experimental Social Psychology, 43*(4), 671–677.
      Mann, T. (2005). Affirmation of personal values buffers neuroendocrine and psychological stress responses. *Psychological Science, 16*, 946–851.

Schwarzer, R., Babler, J., Kwiatek, P., Schroder, K., & Zang, J. W. (1997). The assessment of optimistic self-beliefs: Assessment of general perceived self-efficacy in thirteen cultures. *World Psychology, 3*(1–2), 177–190.

2. Cognitive-behavioral therapy (CBT)

   a. *Actions/expected responses:* CBT can result in less of the exaggeration and generalization of negative thinking that can raise blood pressure. Indications for use are hyperreactivity to stress, high levels of occupational stress, and difficulty tolerating or complying with antihypertensive drugs.

   b. *Routes/dosages/frequencies:* Daily to weekly. Includes homework that helps examine how thoughts set off negative feelings that can affect blood pressure.

   c. *Cautions:* If not ready to examine thoughts and feelings, consider yoga, qigong, visualization and breathing exercises, autogenic training, or progressive muscle relaxation, all of which can help reduce blood pressure.

   d. *Assessments:* Assess view of life situations. See http://www.healthatoz. com/healthatoz/Atoz/common/standard/transform.jsp?requestURI=/ healthatoz/Atoz/ency/cognitive-behavioral_therapy.jsp

   e. *Tips on use:* To turn irrational thinking into rational thought, write down specifics about: (a) a recent interchange between you and one other person who upset you; (b) rational observations of the other person (e.g., she is new to the job and under a lot of pressure); (c) irrational ideas (e.g., I can't stand being humiliated in public, I'm falling apart); (d) the main feelings evoked (e.g., anger, rage, humiliation); (e) refuting the irrational ideas (e.g., I'm not really falling apart; it's not pleasant, but I can handle it); (f) the worst thing that could happen (e.g., I could retaliate and lose my job); (g) good things that could occur as a result of the incident (e.g., I can learn to deal with difficult situations); (h) alternate thoughts (e.g., I'm okay and it's okay to feel anger and know I can still function and learn to handle this kind of situation); and (i) alternate emotions (e.g., I feel less angry now and calmer). For more information see http://www.mind.org.uk/Informa tion/Booklets/Making+sense/MakingSenseCBT.html

   f. *Other considerations:* Keep using the cognitive-behavioral model with emerging situations. Make positive statements about your efforts and point out ongoing irrational thoughts. Remember that cognitive behavioral therapy has been shown to reduce blood pressure. If necessary, make an appointment to consult with a cognitive-behavioral therapist.

   g. *References/other sources:*

Granath, J., Ingvarsson, S., von Thiele, U., & Lundberg, U. (2006). Stress management: A randomized study of cognitive behavioural therapy and yoga. *Cognitive Behavioural Therapy, 35*(1), 3–10.

Schwickert, M., Langhorst, J., Paul, A., Michalsen, A., & Dobos, G. J. (2006). Stress management in the treatment of essential arterial hypertension. *Fortschritte der Medizin, 148*(47), 40–42.

Nutrition

1. Apples, berries, and onions

   a. *Actions/expected responses:* Apples, berries and onions contain quercetin, an antioxidant flavonol associated with reduced blood pressure.

b. *Routes/dosages/frequencies:* Eat as many apples, berries, and onions as possible every day.

c. *Cautions:* Avoid any produce that brings on unwanted reactions.

d. *Assessments:* Assess blood pressure prior to and after eating apples, berries and onions daily for a month.

e. *Tips on use:* Eat the skins of apples whenever possible; they contain the most antioxidants.

f. *Other considerations:* None.

g. *References/other sources:*

Edwards, R. L., Lyon, T., Litwin, S. E., Rabovsky, A. L., Symons, J. D., & Jalili, T. (2007). Quercetin reduces blood pressure in hypertensive subjects. *The Journal of Nutrition, 137*(11), 2405–2411.

2. Beet juice

a. *Actions/expected responses:* Beetroot juice can significantly reduce blood pressure.

b. *Routes/dosages/frequencies:* Drink a glass of beetroot juice a day.

c. *Cautions:* None known unless hypersensitive to beets.

d. *Assessments:* Assess blood pressure 1, 4, and 24 hours after ingestion of beetroot juice.

e. *Tips on use:* Combine 1 cup of beetroot juice with 1/2 cup of juice from green, leafy vegetables, for an added decrease in blood pressure.

f. *Other considerations:* Juicers are available at health food stores or online.

g. *References/other sources:*

Queen Mary, University of London. (2008, February 6). Daily glass of beet juice can beat high blood pressure, study shows. *ScienceDaily.* Retrieved February 28, 2008, from http://www.sciencedaily.com/releases/2008/02/080205123825.htm

3. Calcium

a. *Actions/expected responses:* Calcium reduces the risk of high blood pressure and preeclampsia in pregnant women.

b. *Routes/dosages/frequencies:* 1,200–1,500 mg for pregnant women daily. For dairy and nondairy sources of calcium, go to www.health.gov/dietary guidelines/dga2005/document/html/appendixB.htm

c. *Cautions:* None except sensitivities to dairy foods. In this case, suggest nondairy sources of calcium.

d. *Assessments:* Assess blood pressure prior to and after ingesting 1,200 to 1,500 mg of calcium.

e. *Tips on use:* Calcium from nondairy sources is more readily absorbed. A high-protein and high-phosphorus diet (soda, milk) make calcium absorption more difficult.

f. *Other considerations:* Vitamin D is needed for calcium to be absorbed.

g. *References/other sources:*

Bucher, H. C., Gayatt, G. H., Cook., R. J., Hotala, R., Cook, D. J., Lang, J. D., et al. (1996). Effect of calcium supplementation on pregnancy-induced hypertension and preeclampsia—A meta-analysis of randomized controlled trials. *Journal of the American Medical Association, 275*(13), 1113–1117.

4. Coffee (avoid)

a. *Actions/expected responses:* Coffee consumption is associated with increased blood pressure and plasma homocysteine.

    b. *Routes/dosages/frequencies:* Eliminate coffee to reduce blood pressure.

    c. *Cautions:* Cutting out coffee without slowly reducing its effects can result in a withdrawal syndrome. Cut coffee with 1/2 cup of decaffeinated beverage and slowly withdraw over a week to reduce withdrawal.

    d. *Assessments:* Assess blood pressure prior to and after eliminating coffee from use.

    e. *Tips on use:* Eliminate coffee completely to maintain lowered blood pressure.

    f. *Other considerations:* Older women may be more vulnerable to the adverse effects of caffeine.

    g. *References/other sources:*

        Higdon, J. V., & Frei, B. (2006). Coffee and health: A review of recent human research. *Critical Reviews of Food Science and Nutrition, 46*(2), 101–123.

5. Cola beverages (avoid)

    a. *Actions/expected responses:* Consumption of sugared or diet cola is associated with an increased risk of hypertension.

    b. *Routes/dosages/frequencies:* By mouth.

    c. *Cautions:* The risk of hypertension rises with number of cans of sugared cola or sugar-free cola drunk daily.

    d. *Assessments:* Assess amount of cola drunk.

    e. *Tips on use:* Use water with lemon or frozen berries as an alternative to colas. Use stevia as a sweetener; it has been shown to repair DNA.

    f. *Other considerations:* Some as yet unidentified ingredient other than the caffeine may be responsible for the increased hypertension risk.

    g. *References/other sources:*

        Ghanta, S., Banerjee, A., Poddar, A., & Chattopadhyay, S. (2007). Oxidative DNA damage preventive activity and antioxidant potential of Stevia rebaudiana (Bertoni) Bertoni, a natural sweetener. *Journal of Agriculture and Food Chemistry, 55*(26), 10962–10967.

        Winkelmayer, W. C., Stampfer, M. J., Willett, W. C., & Curhan, G. C. (2005). Habitual caffeine intake and the risk of hypertension in women. *Journal of the American Medical Association, 294*(18), 2330–2335.

6. CoQ10

    a. *Actions/expected responses:* Coenzyme Q10 (CoQ10) is an endogenous cofactor required for mitochondrial energy production and has been shown to lower systolic blood pressure by up to 17 mm Hg and diastolic blood pressure by up to 10 mm Hg without significant side effects.

    b. *Routes/dosages/frequencies:* Food sources of CoQ10 include mackerel, salmon, sardines, organ meats, boiled peanuts, and raw spinach.

    c. *Cautions:* Eat only Spanish mackerel and Alaskan salmon for best results and least contamination.

    d. *Assessments:* Assess blood pressure prior to and three weeks after increasing CoQ10 in the menu.

    e. *Tips on use:* Eat several foods rich in CoQ10 daily to help lower blood pressure.

    f. *Other considerations:* For other food sources, go to www.extension.iastate.edu/nutrition/supplements/coenzyme_q10.php

    g. CoQ10 is also available as a capsule if additional amounts of the cofactor are required.

h. *References/other sources:*

Rosenfeldt, F. L., Has, S. J., Krum, H., Hadj, A., Ng, K., Leong, J. Y., et al. (2007). Coenzyme Q10 in the treatment of hypertension: A meta-analysis of the clinical trials. *Journal of Human Hypertension, 21*(4), 297–306.

Sha, S. A., Sander, S., Cios, D., Lipeika, J., Kluger, J., & White, C. M. (2007). Electrocardiographic and hemodynamic effects of coenzyme Q10 in healthy individuals: A double-blind, randomized controlled trial. *Annals of Pharmacotherapy, 41*(3), 420–425.

7. DASH diet

a. *Actions/expected responses:* DASH (dietary approaches to stop hypertension) diet lowers blood pressure.

b. *Routes/dosages/frequencies:* Daily meals high in fruits, vegetables (total of 10 servings or 1/2 cup daily of each), low-fat dairy products, whole grains, poultry, fish, and nuts and reduced in fat, red meat, and refined sugars lowers blood pressure.

c. *Cautions:* None.

d. *Assessments:* Assess blood pressure prior to and after using the DASH regimen.

e. *Tips on use:* Slowly begin to switch meal plans away from fat, red meat, and refined sugars and to the DASH diet by increasing the use of chicken and fish and eating more fresh fruit. Use stevia as a sweetener. It has no calories or side effects and has been shown to repair DNA.

f. *Other considerations:* Simple diet advice from health care practitioners can have a positive influence on motivation to make lifestyle change.

g. *References/other sources:*

Bhatt, S. P., Luqman-Arafath, T. K., & Guleria, R. (2007). Non-pharmacological management of hypertension. *Indian Journal of Medical Science, 61*(11), 616–624.

Ghanta, S., Banerjee, A., Poddar, A., & Chattopadhyay, S. (2007). Oxidative DNA damage preventive activity and antioxidant potential of Stevia rebaudiana (Bertoni) Bertoni, a natural sweetener. *Journal of Agriculture and Food Chemistry, 55*(26), 10962–10967.

Svetky, L. P., Simons-Morton, D., & Vollmer, W. M. (1999). Effects of dietary patterns on blood pressure: Subgroup analysis of the dietary approaches to stop hypertension (DASH) randomized clinical trial. *Archives of Internal Medicine, 159,* 285.

8. Dietary fiber

a. *Actions/expected responses:* A diet high in fiber can lower blood pressure according to a meta-analysis of 24 trials.

b. *Routes/dosages/frequencies:* Eating a bowl of oatmeal (not instant, which is highly processed; preferably steel cut), at least four pieces of whole grain bread (or dried beans such as black, pinto, or kidney), and four to six fresh fruits and vegetables daily can help lower blood pressure.

c. *Cautions:* Drink sufficient water (8–10 glasses a day) to process the fiber.

d. *Assessments:* Fewer than half of Americans eat the recommended levels of fibrous foods. Keep a record of foods eaten for several days and point out any lack of dietary fiber. Assess favored fibrous foods.

e. *Tips on use:* Set a goal to eat more favored fibrous foods in the upcoming weeks.

    f. *Other considerations:* Dietary fiber also improves mineral absorption in the GI system, which may indirectly modulate blood pressure.

    g. *References/other sources:*

        Dietary fiber helps control BP. (2005, March). *The Clinical Advisor,* 12.

        Myers, V. H. (2007). Nutritional effects on blood pressure. *Current Opinion in Lipidology, 18*(1), 20–24.

9. Fish

    a. *Actions/expected responses:* Salmon, sardines, and tuna are rich sources of omega-3 fatty acids used to treat hypertension.

    b. *Routes/dosages/frequencies:* The American Heart Association recommends consumption of two servings of fish per week and foods high in alpha-linolenic acid (tofu and other forms of soybeans, canola, and walnut and flaxseed and their oils, which can be converted to omega-3 in the body) for women who have no history of coronary heart disease and more for those with known coronary heart disease.

    c. *Cautions:* Eat fish at least twice a week, to use chunk white tuna and salmon caught off the coast of the United States (to reduce chances of mercury exposure and farm-fed fish), and eat more soybeans, canola, walnut, and flaxseeds and their oils.

    d. *Assessments:* Assess weekly intake of fish. Take blood pressure prior to and every month after increasing fish intake.

    e. *Tips on use:* Find fish recipes that are appealing at http://allrecipes.com/Recipes/Seafood/Fish/Main.aspx

    f. *Other considerations:* The authors of one large randomized clinical trial concluded that individuals who are overweight and hypertensive who change their eating habits to incorporate more fish and protein may be able to decrease or potentially discontinue their antihypertensive medication.

    g. *References/other sources:*

        American Heart Association. (2002). Fish and omega-3 recommendations. Retrieved July 27, 2008, from http://www.americanheart.org/presenter.jhtml?identifier=4632

        Bao, D. Q., Mori, T. A., Burke, V., Puddey, I. B., & Bewilin, L. J. (1998). Effects of dietary fish and weight reduction on ambulatory blood pressure in overweight hypertensives. *Hypertension, 32*(4), 710–717.

        Covington, M. B. (2004). Omega-3 fatty acids. *American Family Physician, 70*(1), 133–140.

        Norwegian School of Veterinary Science. (2008, February 28). Farmed fish fed cheap food may be less nutritious for humans. *ScienceDaily.* Retrieved March 9, 2008, from http://www.sciencedaily.com/releases/2008/02/080226164105.htm

10. Folate

    a. *Actions/expected responses:* Folate has important beneficial effects on endothelial function. High folate intake was associated with a decreased risk of hypertension, particularly in younger women. Because national surveys revealed most women did not consume adequate folate, a grain fortification program is in place.

    b. *Routes/dosages/frequencies:* Leafy green vegetables (like spinach and turnip greens), fruits (citrus fruits and juices), and dried beans and peas are all natural sources of folate that can help meet the suggested amount of 1,000 micrograms (mcg) per day. Women on diets who do not eat breads, cereals or pasta, who abuse alcohol, or who take medications that interfere with folate absorption may not receive sufficient amounts of the nutrient and may need additional amounts.

   c. *Cautions:* Medications and medical conditions that increase the need for folate or result in an increased excretion of folate include: anticonvulsant medications, metformin, sulfasalazine, triamterene, methotrexate, barbiturates, pregnancy and lactation, alcohol abuse, malabsorption, kidney dialysis, liver disease, and certain anemias. Because folate is a water-soluble B-vitamin, unneeded amounts will be eliminated in the urine.

   d. *Assessments:* Assess for signs of folate deficiency: anemia, diarrhea, loss of appetite, weight loss, weakness, sore tongue, headaches, heart palpitations, irritability, forgetfulness, behavioral disorders, and an elevated level of homocysteine.

   e. *Tips on use:* Avoid flour-fortified foods as a source of folic acid; new research has shown the introduction of flour fortified with folic acid into common foods has been linked to colon cancer.

   f. *Other considerations:* Exceeding 1,000 micrograms (mcg) per day of folate may trigger vitamin B12 deficiency. To compensate, women can take a multivitamin that contains B12 or eat at least one food daily that contains B12: nutritional yeast (unless susceptible to candida), clams, eggs, herring, kidney, liver, mackerel, seafood, milk, or dairy products.

   g. *References/other sources:*

Blackwell Publishing Ltd. (2007, November 5). Folic acid linked to increased cancer rate, historical review suggests. *ScienceDaily.* Retrieved November 29, 2007, from http://www.sciencedaily.com/releases/2007/11/07/071102111956.htm

Office of Dietary Supplements. (2005). Dietary supplement fact sheet: *Folate.* NIH Clinical Center. National Institutes of Health. Bethesda, MD. Retrieved July 27, 2008, from Office of Dietary Supplements. Folate fact sheet. http://ods.od.nih.gov/factsheets/folate.asp

11. Fruits and vegetables

   a. *Actions/expected responses:* Fruits and vegetables contain potassium, magnesium, and calcium which can improve blood pressure levels and reduce coronary heart disease and stroke.

   b. *Routes/dosages/frequencies:* Eat 10 fruits and/or vegetables a day to help reduce high blood pressure.

   c. *Cautions:* None unless specific sensitivity to fruits or vegetables exists.

   d. *Assessments:* Assess for sensitivity to fruits and vegetables.

   e. *Tips on use:* Buy in-season fresh or frozen fruits and vegetables.

   f. *Other considerations:* Avoid microwaving vegetables and fruits; microwaving broccoli resulted in a loss of 97%, 74%, and 87% of its three major antioxidant compounds, respectively; steaming for 5 minutes resulted in a loss of only 11%, 0%, and 8%, respectively, of the same antioxidants.

   g. *References/other sources:*

Houston, M.C., and Harper, K.J. (2005). Potassium, magnesium, and calcium: Their role in the treatment of hypertension. *Journal of Clinical Hypertension, 19*(7) (Supplement 2), 3–11.

12. Garlic
   a. *Actions/expected responses:* Garlic has antioxidant properties that can help lower blood pressure.
   b. *Routes/dosages/frequencies:* Two capsules daily of aged garlic extract (AGE) can reduce blood pressure. Garlic can also be used in cooking.
   c. *Cautions:* Assess for allergy to garlic and use of antiplatelet drugs.
   d. *Assessments:* Assess blood pressure prior to and after taking garlic.
   e. *Tips on use:* Take AGE with meals. Keep container in a dry, cool place.
   f. *Other considerations:* Garlic may be safe while taking warfarin.
   g. *References/other sources:*
   > Macan, H., Uykimpang, R., Clconcel, M., Takasu, J., Razon, R., Amagase, H., et al. (2006). Aged garlic extract may be safe for patients on warfarin therapy. *Journal of Nutrition, 136*(3 Suppl.), 793S–795S.
   > Sener, G., Sakarcan, A., & Yegen, B. C. (2007). Role of garlic in the prevention of ischemia-reperfusion injury. *Molecular Nutrition and Food Research, 51*(11), 1345–1352.

13. Green tea
   a. *Actions/expected responses:* Hypertension decreased by 35% in women who drank 120 to 599 ml per day of green tea, and was further reduced by 65% for those who drank three cups or more.
   b. *Routes/dosages/frequencies:* By mouth, daily. Available in capsules, extract, or tea.
   c. *Cautions:* Should not be used by women with hypersensitivity to green tea or by those with kidney inflammation, gastrointestinal ulcers, insomnia, cardiovascular disease, or increased intraocular pressure. High doses of green tea can result in palpitations and irregular heartbeat, anxiety, nervousness, insomnia, nausea, heartburn, and increased stomach acid. The decaffeinated form may be a better choice for these reasons.
   d. *Assessments:* Assess for hypersensitivity and take blood pressure prior to and after drinking green tea.
   e. *Tips on use:* Store green tea in a cool, dry place.
   f. *Other considerations:* Antacids may decrease the therapeutic effects of green tea, and green tea may interact with anticoagulants/antiplatelets, increasing risk of bleeding. Avoid drinking green tea while taking MAOIs or bronchodilators.
   g. *References/other sources:*
   > Skidmore-Roth, L. (2006). Green tea. In *Mosby's handbook of herbs and natural supplements* (3rd ed., pp. 535–539). St. Louis, MO: Elsevier-Mosby.
   > Yang, Y. C., Lu, F. H., Wu, J. S., Wu, C. H., & Cheng, C. J. (2004). The protective effect of habitual tea consumption on hypertension. *Archives of Internal Medicine, 164*(14), 1534–1540.

14. Magnesium
   a. *Actions/expected responses:* Women who eat foods containing magnesium are least likely to have hypertension.
   b. *Routes/dosages/frequencies:* To find foods highest in magnesium go to http://www.health.gov/dietaryguidelines/dga2005/document/html/appendixB.htm and scroll down.

c. *Cautions:* Magnesium absorption can be reduced by diuretics, antibiotics, and antineoplastic medications. Women who substitute alcohol for food, have poorly controlled diabetes or malabsorptive problems, or who are older are at risk for magnesium deficiency. Women who take magnesium-containing antacids and laxatives may have excessive magnesium consumption.

d. *Assessments:* Assess magnesium intake and whether magnesium-containing antacids and laxatives are used.

e. *Tips on use:* Eat whole grain breads and cereals and other magnesium-rich foods daily.

f. *Other considerations:* A woman should have 320 mg of magnesium a day unless she's pregnant, then 360 mg. Women with kidney or GI conditions may not be able to limit excretion of dietary magnesium and may require supplementation.

g. *References/other sources:*

Song, Y., Sesso, H. D., Manson, J. E., Cook, N. R., Buring, J. E., & Liu, S. (2006). Dietary magnesium intake and risk of incident hypertension among middle-aged and older US women in a 10-year follow-up study. *American Journal of a Cardiology, 98*(12), 1616–1621.

15. Pomegranate juice

a. *Actions/expected responses:* Consumption of pomegranate juice by hypertensive women resulted in a 5% reduction in systolic blood pressure.

b. *Routes/dosages/frequencies:* 2 ounces of pomegranate juice per day.

c. *Cautions:* None, unless hypersensitive to the juice.

d. *Assessments:* Assess use of pomegranate juice.

e. *Tips on use:* Serve pomegranate juice without ice to guarantee easier absorption.

f. *References/other sources:*

Aviram, M., & Dornfield, L. (2001). Pomegranate juice consumption inhibits serum angiotensin converting enzyme activity and reduces systolic blood pressure. *Atherosclerosis, 158,* 195–198.

16. Salt (avoid)

a. *Actions/expected responses:* A meta-analysis of available studies lead to the conclusion that restricting sodium intake to levels below 6 grams per day (as most international guidelines such as those of the U.S. Dietary Guideline Committee and the Scientific Advisory Committee on Nutrition recommend) clearly reduces blood pressure and may reduce the need for antihypertensives by as much as 30%.

b. *Routes/dosages/frequencies:* Reduce intake of salt, aiming for 6 grams (about a teaspoon) a day.

c. *Cautions:* Reducing intake of salt is important because hypertension is associated with stroke in salt-sensitive women.

d. *Assessments:* Assess blood pressure prior to and after restricting high sodium foods for a month.

e. *Tips on use:* It is not necessary to totally restrict salty foods, but it is important to reduce their use. Read labels and choose low-salt or no salt alternatives. Use herbs, lemon juice, and garlic to enhance food taste. Throw away salt shakers.

f. *Other considerations:* Women taking antihypertensive medication who restrict salty foods in the diet can reduce the need for medication by as much as 30%.

g. *References/other sources:*

Cappuccio, F. P., Markandu, N. D., Carney, C., Sagnella, G. A., & MacGregor, G. A. (1997). Double-blind randomized trial of modest salt restriction in older people. *Lancet, 350*(9081), 850–854.

Walter, J., Mackenzie, A. D., Dunning, J. (2007). Does reducing your salt intake make you live longer? *Interactions in Cardiovascular Thoracic Surgery, 6*(6), 793–798.

17. Sesame oil

a. *Actions/expected responses:* When used as the sole cooking oil, sesame oil can reduce blood pressure to normal in hypertensive women (with a blood pressure reading of 166/101 on the average) who are already taking the calcium channel blocker nifedipine.

b. *Routes/dosages/frequencies:* Cook daily with sesame oil.

c. *Cautions:* Monitor for allergic reaction to sesame oil.

d. *Assessments:* Take blood pressure prior to and after using sesame oil for cooking every 15 days and on day 60.

e. *Tips on use:* This oil is made from pressed sesame seeds and comes in two varieties: light (made with untoasted seeds) and dark (made with toasted seeds). Light sesame oil has a nutty flavor and is especially good for cooking. Dark sesame oil (Asian) has a stronger flavor and should only be used in small quantities for flavoring foods—not cooking. Both varieties are high in polyunsaturated fat.

f. *Other considerations:* The effect of the oil on blood pressure may be due to polyunsaturated fatty acids (PUFA) and the compound sesamin—a lignan present in sesame oil. Both compounds have been shown to reduce blood pressure.

g. *References/other sources:*

Pugalendi, K. V., Sambandam, G., & Rao, M. R. (2003). *Sesame oil helps reduce blood pressure-lowering medicine.* Presented to the 15th Scientific Meeting of the Inter-American Society of Hypertension. San Antonio, TX, April, 28. Retrieved December 12, 2007, from http://www.americanheart.org/presenter.jhtml?identified=3011334

18. Soy nuts

a. *Actions/expected responses:* Substituting soy nuts for other protein sources in a healthy diet appears to lower blood pressure in postmenopausal women.

b. *Routes/dosages/frequencies:* 1/2 cup of unsalted soy nuts for 8 weeks.

c. *Cautions:* None.

d. *Assessments:* Assess blood pressure prior to and after eating soy nuts.

e. *Tips on use:* Include soy nuts in a healthy diet consisting of two meals of fatty fish (such as salmon or tuna) per week.

f. *Other considerations:* Use unsalted soy nuts to help reduce blood pressure.

g. *References/other sources:*

JAMA and Archives Journals. (2007, May 29). Soy nuts may improve blood pressure in postmenopausal women. *ScienceDaily*. Retrieved November 25, 2007, from http://www.sciencedaily.com/releases/2007/051070528160754.htm

19. Tomatoes
    a. *Actions/expected responses:* Natural antioxidants from tomato reduce blood pressure in women.
    b. *Routes/dosages/frequencies:* By mouth daily.
    c. *Cautions:* None unless sensitive to tomatoes.
    d. *Assessments:* Assess sensitivity to tomatoes.
    e. *Tips on use:* Encourage women not sensitive to tomatoes to eat tomatoes to reduce their blood pressure.
    f. *Other considerations:* None.
    g. *References/other sources:*
       Englehard, Y. N., Gazer, B., & Paran, E. (2006). Natural antioxidants from tomato extract reduce blood pressure in patients with grade-1 hypertension. *American Heart Journal, 151*(1), 100.

Stress Management

1. Autogenic training (AT)
    a. *Actions/expected responses:* Autogenic training is a relaxation technique consisting of six mental exercises and is aimed at relieving tension, anger, and stress. The exercises produce a statistically significantly greater reduction in both systolic and diastolic blood pressure as compared to laughter therapy or a control group receiving no intervention.
    b. *Routes/dosages/frequencies:* AT can be used effectively with individuals or groups. Ninety-second sessions five to eight times a day, either sitting or lying down, are recommended. It may take up to 10 months to master the series.
    c. *Cautions:* The solar plexus theme or statement is not used for individuals who have ulcers, diabetes, or any condition involving bleeding from the abdominal region.
    d. *Assessments:* Take a baseline blood pressure measure prior to beginning autogenic training, after completing the exercises for several weeks, and again at the end of the series.
    e. *Tips on use:* For more information go to http://www.guidetopsychology.com/autogen.htm
    f. *Other considerations:* Although statistically significant, findings only relate to short-term effects with AT.
    g. *References/other sources:*
       Kanji, N., White, A., & Ernst, E. (2006). Autogenic training to reduce anxiety in nursing students: Randomized controlled trial. *Journal of Advanced Nursing, 53*(6), 729–735.
       Watanabe, Y., Halberg, F., Carnelissen, G., Saito, Y., Fukuda, K., Otsujka, K., et al. (1996). Chronobiometric assessment of autogenic training effects upon blood pressure and heart rate. *Perceptual Motor Skills, 83*(3, Pt. 2), 1395–1410.
2. Transcendental meditation
    a. *Actions/expected responses:* A meta-analysis of studies showed that transcendental meditation technique produces a statistically significant reduction in high blood pressure that is at least as great as the changes

found with major changes in diet or exercise. The changes due to meditation are associated with at least a 15% reduction in rates of heart attack and stroke.

b. *Routes/dosages/frequencies:* 1 hour is often recommended for the best results.

c. *Cautions:* Avoid trying to force something to happen or make the mind blank or put too much emphasis on doing it right.

d. *Assessments:* Assess blood pressure prior to meditating and after several weeks of practice.

e. *Tips on use:* It's not necessary or advisable to meditate on an empty stomach. It is permissible to eat lightly prior to meditating.

f. *Other considerations:* Meditation is best accomplished in a quiet, comfortable place. Women can be counseled to sit in a comfortable chair, on the bed, on the floor, or anywhere that is comfortable. The legs can be kept in whatever position that is comfortable. For specific kinds of meditation go to http://www.meditationcenter.com/info/index.html

g. *References/other sources:*

University of Kentucky. (2007, December 5). Transcendental meditation effective in reducing high blood pressure, study shows. *ScienceDaily.* Retrieved December 10, 2007, from http://www.sciencedaily.com/re leases/2007/12/071204121953.htm

3. Yoga

a. *Actions/expected responses:* Women who practiced yoga showed significant improvement in blood pressure.

b. *Routes/dosages/frequencies:* 60-minute sessions for 10 weeks.

c. *Cautions:* Go to http://yoga.lifetips.com/cat/56770/yoga-cautions/

d. *Assessments:* Assess blood pressure prior to and after completing 1 month of yoga practice.

e. *Tips on use:* Because yoga exerts pressure on internal organs, wait at least 2 hours after a meal and 30 minutes to 1 hour after a snack to practice. For more information about yoga, go to http://www.mothernature.com/Li brary/Bookshelf/Books/21/54.cfm. For more information on various asanas go to http://www.santosha.com/asanas/asana.html

f. *Other considerations:* To avoid knee injury when doing yoga, keep the knees straight (especially in standing poses). The knees should be forward in line with the ankle and foot and should not twist inward or outward.

g. *References/other sources:*

Ernst, E. (2005). Complementary/alternative medicine for hypertension: A mini-review. *Wiener Medizinische Wochenschrift, 155*(17–18), 386–391.

Sivasankaran, S., Pollard-Quintner, S., Sachdeva, R., Pugeda, J., Hoq, S. W., Granath, J., et al. (2006). Stress management: A randomized study of cognitive behavioural therapy and yoga. *Cognitive Behavioural Therapy, 35*(1), 3–10.

Zarich, S. W. (2006). The effect of a six-week program of yoga and meditation on brachial artery reactivity: Do psychosocial interventions affect vascular tone? *Clinical Cardiology, 29*(9), 393–398.

Supplements

1. Potassium
   a. *Actions/expected responses:* Potassium supplementation significantly reduces blood pressure in African Americans, a population at high risk for hypertension because they may have difficulty reducing their sodium intake. Potassium is also useful in reducing blood pressure in young healthy volunteers.
   b. *Routes/dosages/frequencies:* 1,600 mg per day in tablet form.
   c. *Cautions:* In general, potassium supplements are well-tolerated, but watch for complaints of eructation (belching), abdominal pain, and flatulence, which were noted in two studies, and a third documented adverse effect such as stomach pain, bright-red blood in the stools, diarrhea, nausea, and vomiting. Only one individual dropped out of a study because of gastric discomfort.
   d. *Assessments:* Assess blood pressure prior to and after taking potassium supplements.
   e. *Tips on use:* Keep potassium supplements in a cool, dry place.
   f. *Other considerations:* Women without salt-related hypertension may achieve similar results from eating potassium-rich foods.
   g. *References/other sources:*
   Brancati, F. L., Appel, L. J., Seidler, A. J., & Whelton, P. K. (1996). Effect of potassium supplementation on blood pressure in African Americans consuming a low-potassium diet. *Archives of Internal Medicine, 156*(1), 61–67.
   Braschi, A., & Naismith, D. J. (2008). The effect of dietary supplement of potassium chloride or potassium citrate on blood pressure in predominantly normotensive volunteers. *British Journal of Nutrition 99(6)*, 1284-1292.
   Whelton, P. K., He, J., Culter, J. A., Brausatu, F. L., Appel, L. J., Fallmanny, D., et al. (1997). Effects of oral potassium on blood pressure. Meta analysis of randomized controlled clinical trials. *Journal of the American Medical Association, 277*(201), 1624–1632.
2. Pycnogenol
   a. *Actions/expected responses:*Pycnogenol, an extract of bark from the French maritime pine, contains the bioflavonoids catechin and taxifolin as well as phenolcarbonic acids. Antioxidants, such as bioflavonoids, enhance blood vessel function.
   b. *Routes/dosages/frequencies:* 180 mgm a day.
   c. *Cautions:* Until more research is completed, pregnant and lactating women should not use this supplement, nor should it be given to children.
   d. *Assessments:* Assess reaction to pycnogenol and any blood pressure changes.
   e. *Tips on use:* Store supplement in a cool, dry place.
   f. *Other considerations:* Pycnogenol has also been found useful in preventing venous thrombosis, thrombophlebitis, gingival bleeding and plaque, inflammatory bowel disease, venous insufficiency, digestive conditions, and menopause symptoms.

g. *References/other sources:*

Nishioka, K., Hidaka, T., Nakamura, S., Umemura, T., Jitsuiki, D., Soga, J., et al. (2007). Pycnogenol, French maritime pine bark extract, augments endothelium-dependent vasodilation in humans. *Hypertension Research, 30*(9), 775–780.

3. Vitamins C and E

   a. *Actions/expected responses:* The enhancement of antioxidant status by vitamins C and E supplementation is essential for hypertensive women and is associated with lower blood pressure.

   b. *Routes/dosages/frequencies:* 1,000 mg vitamin C and 400 IU vitamin E a day were shown to reduce blood pressure significantly.

   c. *Cautions:* Monitor for signs of reduced blood pressure. Vitamin E is a blood thinner and can reduce the amount of prescribed blood thinners needed.

   d. *Assessments:* Assess blood pressure prior to and after 8 weeks of taking the two vitamins.

   e. *Tips on use:* Keep bottles in a cool, dry place.

   f. *Other considerations:* Oxidative stress is involved in the pathogenesis of essential hypertension. Vitamins A and C are antioxidants.

   g. *References/other sources:*

   Rodrigo, R., Prat, H., Passalacqua, W., Araya, J., & Bachler, J. P. (2008). Diminution of oxidative stress through vitamins C and E supplementation associated with blood pressure reduction in essential hypertension. *Clinical Science (Lond), 114*(10), 625–634.

Touch

1. Acupuncture

   a. *Actions/expected responses:* Acupuncture proved effective and safe for the treatment of mild to moderate hypertension in a randomized, single-blind clinical trial.

   b. *Routes/dosages/frequencies:* 22 sessions of 30 minutes duration for a period of 6 weeks.

   c. *Cautions:* Two women dropped out of the study because they said that acupuncture was too painful. No other side effects were reported.

   d. *Assessments:* Take blood pressure prior to and after acupuncture.

   e. *Tips on use:* Acupuncture sessions must be repeated at least once every 3 months or blood pressure may return to pretreatment levels.

   f. *Other considerations:* Specific acupoints trigger neurons in the hypothalamus, midbrain, and medulla to release chemicals that reduce excitatory responses in the cardiovascular system that lower blood pressure.

   g. *References/other sources:*

   Hur, M. H., Oh, H., Lee, M. S., Kim, C., Choi, A. N., & Shin, G. R. (2007, April). Acupuncture provides short-term drop in high blood pressure. *Clinical Psychiatry News,* 72.

   Li, P., Longhurst, J., & Dodge, L. K. (2007). *Acupuncture works in lowering blood pressure in hypertensive patients.* Presented at the Society for

Neuroscience Conference, San Diego Convention Center Halls B-H. November 5, San Diego, CA.

2. Biofeedback

a. *Actions/expected responses:* Women who participated in biofeedback sessions with a machine reduced their blood pressure as compared to a control group who self-monitored their systolic and diastolic pressure.

b. *Routes/dosages/frequencies:* Once a week treatment for four sessions.

c. *Cautions:* Prepare women for what to expect if they choose to have biofeedback.

d. *Assessments:* Assess blood pressure prior to and after treatment program.

e. *Tips on use:* For more information see http://psychotherapy.com/bio.html

f. *Other considerations:* Biofeedback can be simple, like reading a scale, or more complex, like using a biofeedback machine to feed back information about the body.

g. *References/other sources:*

Nakso, M., Nomura, S., Shimosawa, T., Yashiuchi, K., Kumano, H., Kuboki, T., et al. (1997). Clinical effects of blood pressure biofeedback treatment on hypertension by auto-shaping. *Psychosomatic Medicine, 59*(3), 331–338.

3. Foot reflexology

a. *Actions/expected responses:* Administered foot reflexology significantly decreased systolic blood pressure; self-administered foot reflexology proved just as good for decreasing diastolic blood pressure.

b. *Routes/dosages/frequencies:* Twice a week for 4–6 weeks.

c. *Cautions:* See http://www.wikihow.com/Give-a-Foot-Massage

d. *Assessments:* Take blood pressure prior to and after foot reflexology.

e. *Tips on use:* See Web site under "Cautions."

f. *Other considerations:* None unless there are leg or foot injuries or disease.

g. *References/other sources:*

Park, H. S., & Cho, G. Y. (2004). Effects of foot reflexology on essential hypertension patients. *Taehan Kanho Hakkoe Chi, 34*(5), 739–750.

4. Massage therapy

a. *Actions/expected responses:* Significant differences in systolic and diastolic blood pressures of 58 climacteric women were observed after massage therapy was performed once weekly for two 8-week periods. Aromatherapy massage using lavender, rose geranium, rose, and jasmine essential oils was given to the experimental group only.

b. *Routes/dosages/frequencies:* 30 minute massage weekly with self-administered abdominal daily massage at home.

c. *Cautions:* The aged, extremely ill, or dying individuals may require a gentle massage. The head is also a sensitive area; only gentle sweeping motions are used, and energy is not concentrated in that area or in an area where cancer resides.

d. *Assessments:* Assess blood pressure prior to and after massage.

e. *Tips on use:* Go to http://www.ehow.com/how_12801_aromatherapy-with-bodywork.html

f. *Other considerations:* Practice will improve massage skills.

g. *References/other sources:*

Hur, M. H., Oh, H., Lee, M. S., Kim, C., Choi, A. N., & Shin, G. R. (2007). Effects of aromatherapy massage on blood pressure and lipid profile in Korean climacteric women. *International Journal of Neuroscience, 117*(9), 1281–1287.

Sharpe, P. A., Williams, H. G., Granner, M. I., & Hussey, J. R. (2007). A randomized study of the effects of massage therapy compared to guided relaxation on well-being and stress perception among older adults. *Complementary Therapies in Medicine, 15*(3), 157–163.

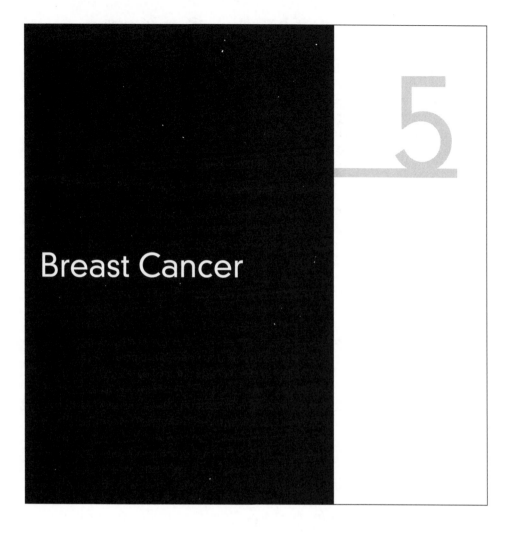

5

Breast Cancer

Medical treatment for breast cancer includes chemotherapy, surgery, and radiation. Recent research provides evidence for complementary procedures that may prevent and/or help treat breast cancer.

Environment

1. Acrylamide
   a. *Actions/expected responses:* Acrylamide is a carcinogen linked to breast cancer in humans.
   b. *Routes/dosages/frequencies:* This cancer-causing substance is formed when frying, baking, or grilling carbohydrate-rich foods at temperatures above 120° C, including bread, French fries, and biscuits.
   c. *Cautions:* The longer the cooking time and the lower the water content, the higher the acrylamide content in the heat-processed food.
   d. *Assessments:* Assess intake of acrylamide-forming foods.
   e. *Tips on use:* Adding rosemary to dough prior to baking a portion of wheat buns at 225° C reduced the acrylamide content by up to 60%. Even rosemary

in small quantities in 1% of the dough was enough to reduce the acryl-amide content significantly.

  f. *Other considerations:* Flavonoids in vegetables, unsweetened chocolate, and tea (especially green tea) considerably reduce the acrylamide content. These antioxidants inhibit the formation of the free radicals formed when cooking that increase the acrylamide in certain foods. Other tests show that blanching and salting may reduce the acrylamide content in potato products.

  g. *References/other sources:*

  Technical University of Denmark. (2008, March 4). A little rosemary can go a long way to reducing acrylamide in food. *ScienceDaily.* Retrieved March 9, 2008, from http://www.sciencedaily.com/releases/2008/02/080229142817.htm

 2. Alcohol

  a. *Actions/expected responses:* Two drinks a day can increase risk of breast cancer by 10%; three of more drinks increases risk by 30% and is equal to smoking a pack of cigarettes a day.

  b. *Routes/dosages/frequencies:* Daily by mouth and includes beer, wine, or liquor.

  c. *Cautions:* Binge drinking can increase risk of breast cancer by 55%.

  d. *Assessments:* Assess use of alcohol.

  e. *Tips on use:* Although not drinking is preferable, sufficient folate intake can mitigate this excess risk. (See chapter 1, Nutrition section, #13 for more information.)

  f. *Other considerations:* Risk of breast cancer is strongest among women who drink and take postmenopausal hormones.

  g. *References/other sources:*

  Klatsky, A., & Li, Y. (2007). *Alcohol consumption—no matter the beverage type—is linked to breast cancer.* Presented to the European Cancer Conference, September 27, Barcelona, Spain.

  Linos, E., & Willett, W. C. (2007). Diet and breast cancer risk reduction. *Journal of National Comprehensive Cancer Network, 5*(8), 711–718.

  Zhang, S. M., Lee, I. M., Manson, J. E., Cook, N. R., Willett, W. C., & Buring, J. E. (2007). Alcohol consumption and breast cancer risk in the Women's Health Study. *American Journal of Epidemiology, 165*(6), 667–676.

 3. Aluminum in breast tissue

  a. *Actions/expected responses:* Recent research has linked breast cancer with the use of aluminum-based, underarm antiperspirants. The known, but unaccounted for, higher incidence of tumors in the upper outer quadrant of the breast seem to support this theory.

  b. *Routes/dosages/frequencies:* Daily, underarms.

  c. *Cautions:* Continuing to use underarm antiperspirants may increase risk for breast cancer.

  d. *Assessments:* Assess use of underarm antiperspirants.

  e. *Tips on use:* Recommend using deodorants, which don't contain aluminum salts.

  f. *Other considerations:* Aluminum is a metalloestrogen, is genotoxic, is bound by DNA, and has been shown to be carcinogenic.

g. *References/other sources:*

Keele University. (2007, September 2). Aluminum in breast tissue: A possible factor in the cause of breast cancer. *ScienceDaily*. Retrieved 12/7/07 from http://www.sciencedaily.com/release/2007/08/070831210302.htm

4. Catfish caught in polluted waters

a. *Actions/expected responses:* Exposing estrogen-sensitive breast cancer cells to extracts of channel catfish caught in areas with heavy sewer and industrial waste causes the cells to multiply.

b. *Routes/dosages/frequencies:* Eating any fish caught from polluted waters may expose women to risk of breast cancer.

c. *Cautions:* Researchers at the University of Pittsburgh found vast quantities of pharmaceutical and xeno-estrogenic waste in outflows from sewage treatment plants and from sewer overflows that end up concentrated and magnified in channel catfish.

d. *Assessments:* Assess amount of catfish eaten.

e. *Tips on use:* Eat only fish not caught in areas heavily polluted by industrial and municipal wastes.

f. *Other considerations:* The consumption of river-caught fish, especially by semi-subsistence anglers, may increase their risks for endocrine-related health issues.

g. *References/other sources:*

University of Pittsburgh School of the Health Sciences. (2007, November 9). Extracts of catfish caught in polluted waters cause breast cancer cells to multiply. *ScienceDaily*. Retrieved November 22, 2007, from http://www.sciencedaily.com/releases/2007/11/071107083910.htm

5. Circadian disruption

a. *Actions/expected responses:* Accumulating evidence that circadian disruption (shift work) increases the risk of breast cancer in women, possibly due to altered light exposure and reduced melatonin secretion.

b. *Routes/dosages/frequencies:* Working nights, changes in sleep and light exposure.

c. *Cautions:* Sleep at night and use measures to reduce breast cancer risk. See chapters 8, 25, and 27.

d. *Assessments:* Assess shift work, sleep patterns and breast cancer risk.

e. *Tips on use:* Discuss options, other than shift work, with employer.

f. *Other considerations:* None.

g. *References/other sources:*

Baker, F. C., & Driver, H. S. (2007). Circadian rhythms, sleep and the menstrual cycle. *Sleep Medicine, 8*(6), 613–622.

6. Cooked meat carcinogens

a. *Actions/expected responses:* During the cooking of meat, mutagenic and carcinogenic heterocyclic amines are formed, the most abundant of which, 2-amino-1-methyl-6-phenylimidazo[4–5-b]pyridine (PhIP), induces mammary gland tumors. PhIP acts as a tumor initiator and promoter, and dietary exposure could contribute to carcinogenesis in breast tissue.

b. *Routes/dosages/frequencies:* Humans are exposed to PhIP on a daily basis.

c. *Cautions:* PhIP can activate estrogen receptor–mediated signaling pathways following consumption of a cooked meat meal.

d. *Assessments:* Assess amount of meat eaten weekly.

e. *Tips on use:* Slowly replace cooked meat with other safer sources of protein.

f. *Other considerations:* Alternate sources of protein include fish, soy, beans and rice, and chicken.

g. *References/other sources:*

Creton, S. K., Zhu, H., & Gooderham, N. J. (2007). The cooked meat carcinogen 2-amino-1-methyl-t-phenylimidazo[4–5-b]pyridine activates the extracellular signal regulated kinase mitogen-activated protein kinase pathway. *Cancer Research, 67*(23), 11455–11462.

7. Dioxin

a. *Actions/expected response:* Dioxins are known human carcinogens and hormone mimickers.

b. *Routes/dosages/frequencies:* Dioxin is ubiquitous and is found in the body fat of every human being, including every newborn. It is formed by the incineration of products containing polyvinylchloride (PVC), PCBs, and other chlorinate compounds. Dioxin also comes from industrial processes that use chlorine and combustion of diesel and gasoline containing chlorinated additives.

c. *Cautions:* Women are exposed to dioxin primarily through consumption of animal products. Sources of dioxin include meat, poultry, dairy products, and human breast milk. Dioxin enters the food chain when vehicle exhaust or soot from incinerated chlorinated compounds falls on field crops later eaten by farm animals.

d. *Assessments:* Assess exposure to dioxin.

e. *Tips on use:* Exposure to dioxin can be reduced by reducing intake of meat, poultry, and dairy products and living far from incineration plants and highways.

f. *Other considerations:* Intrauterine exposure to dioxin can disrupt the development of mammary glands, which can predispose offspring to breast cancer.

g. *References/other sources:*

International Agency for Research on Cancer. (1997). *IARC monographs on the evaluation of carcinogenic risks to humans. Volume 69. Polychlorinated dibenzodioxins and polychlorinated dibenzofurans.* Lyon: IARC.

Warner, M. B., Eskenazi, B., Mocarelli, P., Gerthoux, P. M., Samuels, S., & Needham, L. (2002). Serum dioxin concentrations and breast cancer risk in the Seveso Women's Health Study. *Environmental Health Perspectives, 110,* 625–628.

World Health Organization. (2007). Dioxins and their effects on human health. Retrieved December 15, 2007 from http://www.who.int/mediacentre/factsheets/fs225/en/print.html

8. Electromagnetic fields

a. *Actions/expected responses:* Extremely low intensity electromagnetic field exposure is correlated with breast cancer.

b. *Routes/dosages/frequencies:* New guidelines for exposure to power lines, extremely low frequency electromagnetic fields, and to radiofrequency/microwave radiation emissions may be necessary.

c. *Cautions:* Use a headset and carry wireless phones away from their body, limit the duration and number of cells phone calls, and unplug or disconnect the microwave from electrical power before reaching inside.

d. *Assessments:* Assess use of cell phones and microwave ovens.

e. *Tips on use:* Follow safe use for cell phones and microwave ovens.

f. *Other considerations:* If purchasing or renting a house, opt for housing far away from cell phone antennas and new, high tension, or upgraded power lines.

g. *References/other sources:*

Hardell, L., & Sage, C. (2007). Biological effects from electromagnetic field exposure and public exposure standards. *Biomedicine and Pharmacotherapy, 62*(2), 104–109.

9. Mastectomy (preventive)

a. *Actions/expected responses:* The rate of voluntary preventive mastectomy doubled between 1998 and 2003.

b. *Routes/dosages/frequencies:* Women diagnosed with breast cancer who have a mastectomy are increasingly choosing to have their other, healthy breast removed as a preventive measure.

c. *Cautions:* Research has failed to show a survival benefit with the second mastectomy. The risk of cancer spread from the original breast to the other body sites often exceeds the risk of getting cancer in the second breast. A study of 296 women who opted for preventive mastectomy revealed the following regrets: poor cosmetic result (39%), diminished sexuality (22%), lack of education regarding alternative measures (22%), other reasons (17%).

d. *Assessments:* Assess wish to have a contralateral prophylactic mastectomy.

e. *Tips on use:* Avoid overestimating the risk for cancer in the healthy breast and convey information about the study of regrets after preventive mastectomy.

f. *Other considerations:* Increase vitamin D intake to keep the healthy breast healthy. See section 14.

g. *References/other sources:*

Montgomery, L. L., Tran, K. N., Heelan, M. C., Van Zee, K. J., Massie, M. J., Payne, D. K., et al. (1999). Issues of regret in women with contralateral prophylactic mastectomies. *Journal of Surgical Oncology, 6*(6), 546–552.

More women choosing "preventive" double mastectomy. (2008). Retrieved January 18, 2008, at www.healthday.com/Article.asp?AID= 609318.

10. Neighborhood conditions

a. *Actions/expected responses:* Women's vulnerability to stress and social isolation could lead to early-onset breast cancer.

b. *Routes/dosages/frequencies:* Living in a disadvantaged neighborhood that includes situations women can't control, seeing crime in their neighborhood, being afraid to go out, and not being able to form casual relationships with their neighbors that might make them feel safe.

c. *Cautions:* Environmental factors, such as social isolation, can have important effects on women's health.

d. *Assessments:* Assess social isolation and helplessness.

e. *Tips on use:* Find a way to establish networks that would give a greater feeling of control over environments.

f. *References/other sources:*

University of Chicago. (2008, March 20). Breast cancer in Black women may be connected to neighborhood conditions, study suggests.

ScienceDaily. Retrieved April 17, 2008, from http://www.sciencedaily. com/releases/2008/03/080317164342.htm

11. Pesticides
    a. *Actions/expected response:* Lawn and garden pesticide use is associated with breast cancer risk.
    b. *Routes/dosages/frequencies:* No known safe level.
    c. *Cautions:* Stay away from lawns and gardens where pesticides are used.
    d. *Assessments:* Assess exposure to lawns and gardens where pesticides are used.
    e. *Tips on use:* Xeriscape and use natural pesticides. Go to http://www. beyondpesticides.org/lawn/factsheets/
    f. *Other considerations:* Little or no association was found for nuisance-pest pesticides, insect repellants, or products used to control lice, fleas, and ticks on pets.
    g. *References/other sources:*
       Teitelbaum, S. L., Gammon, M. D., Britton, J. A., Neugut, A. I., Levin, B., & Stellman, S. D. (2007). Reported residential pesticide use and breast cancer risk on Long Island, New York. *American Journal of Epidemiology, 165*(6), 643–651.

12. Power-frequency fields and wireless communications
    a. *Actions/expected responses:* Breast cancer is associated with exposure to electromagnetic fields (EMFs).
    b. *Routes/dosages/frequencies:* Current levels of long-term exposure to some kinds of electromagnetic fields are not protective of public health.
    c. *Cautions:* Scientific evidence raises concerns about the health impacts of mobile or cell phone radiation, power lines, interior wiring and grounding of buildings, appliances such as microwaves, wireless technologies, and electric blankets.
    d. *Assessments:* Assess exposure to EMFs listed in item c.
    e. *Tips on use:* Until new public safety limits and limits on further deployment of risky technologies are warranted, avoid exposure to EMFs.
    f. *Other considerations:* An international working group of renowned scientists, researchers, and public health policy professionals (The Bioinitiative Working Group) has released its report on electromagnetic fields and health. It raises serious concerns about the safety of existing public limits that regulate how much EMF is allowable from power lines, cell phones, and many other EMF sources of exposure in daily life.
    g. *References/other sources:*
       Hardell, L., & Sage, C. (2008). Biological effects from electromagnetic field exposure and public exposure standards. *Biomedical Pharmacotherapy. 62*(2), 104–109.

13. Sexual assault
    a. *Actions/expected responses:* Sexual assault has been associated with an increased risk of breast cancer.
    b. *Routes/dosages/frequencies:* Multiple episodes of sexual assault carried a two- to three-fold increased risk of breast cancer compared with a single episode.
    c. *Cautions:* Individuals who have been sexually assaulted are at high risk for breast cancer.

d. *Assessments:* Every woman should be asked about being sexually assaulted as part of the history and intake process.

e. *Tips on use:* For more information on sexual assault and how to introduce the topic go to http://www.musc.edu/awprevention/research/screening.shtml

f. *Other considerations:* Although causality cannot be inferred, there is a definite link, and women who have been assaulted should be referred for or seek out counseling and/or to a shelter as appropriate to help prevent the development of breast cancer in the future.

g. *References/other sources:*

Stein, M. B., & Barrett-Connor, E. (2000). Sexual assault and physical health: Findings from a population-based study of older adults. *Psychosomatic Medicine, 62*(6), 838–843.

14. Vitamin D deficiency

a. *Actions/expected responses:* Vitamin D deficiency may precipitate or exacerbate breast cancer or may be a sign of the disease process.

b. *Routes/dosages/frequencies:* Daily sensible sun exposure (4–10 minutes with face and arms exposed for light-skinned women and 60–80 minutes for dark skin).

c. *Cautions:* Longer exposure can increase the risk of skin cancer. Vitamin D supplements are not recommended as they can promote a disease process already in effect.

d. *Assessments:* Assess daily sun exposure.

e. *Tips on use:* Sun exposure should be at solar noon when UVB rays are most directly penetrating.

f. *Other considerations:* Women residing at latitudes north of 35 degrees have a higher incidence of breast cancer. They may need to take a tablespoon of cod liver oil daily, eat fatty fish several times a week, eat eggs several times a week (the yolks are the portion that contain vitamin D), and/or take fish oil supplements.

g. *References/other sources:*

Autoimmunity Research Foundation. (2008, January 27). Vitamin D deficiency study raises new questions about disease and supplements. *ScienceDaily.* Retrieved February 13, 2008, from http://www.science daily.com/releases/2008/01/080125223302.htm

Jocker, B. S. (2007). Vitamin D sufficiency: An approach to disease prevention. *The American Journal for Nurse Practitioners, 11*(10), 43–60.

15. Workplace chemical exposures

a. *Actions/expected responses:* Current research provides evidence that workplace chemicals increase breast cancer risk among women.

b. *Routes/dosages/frequencies:* Dependent on source.

c. *Cautions:* Reduce the risk of environmental toxins from exposure to organic solvents, metals, acid mists, sterilizing agents, some pesticides, light during night shifts, and tobacco smoke.

d. *Assessments:* Evaluate which risks are being faced.

e. *Tips on use:* Consider ways to reduce risks.

f. *Other considerations:* Animal cancer bioassays conducted by the National Toxicology Program indicate more than 40 chemicals can induce mammary tumors, and most of these are still in production. A variety of occupations worldwide, including health care providers and metal, textile, dye, rubber, and plastic manufacturing workers, have been identified as having some evidence of higher breast cancer risk.

   g. *References/other sources:*
      Snedeker, S. M. (2006). Chemical exposures in the workplace: Effect on breast cancer risk among women. *American Association of Occupational Health Nursing Journal, 54*(6), 270–279.

16. X-rays, including mammograms
   a. *Actions/expected responses:* Low-dose medical radiation exposure and particularly exposures during childhood, increase breast cancer risk.
   b. *Routes/dosages/frequencies:* Elevated risk for breast cancer include multiple chest X-rays, seven or more mammograms, CT scans, and receiving dental X-rays without lead apron protection prior to age 20.
   c. *Cautions:* Evaluate the dangers of X-rays (including CAT scans).
   d. *Assessments:* Assess number of X-rays undergone.
   e. *Tips on use:* Weigh the dangers of X-rays against the need for diagnostic information, including whether other, safer methods of diagnosis are available.
   f. *Other considerations:* X-rays and y-rays have been added to the national list of carcinogens. Good alternatives are the AMAS Test and using a plastic syringe to extract a small amount of breast fluids (a test developed by Dr. Chandice Covington, RN).
   g. *References/other sources:*
      AMAS Test measures lethal replikin gene activity in lung and other cancers. (2008). Retrieved January 18, 2008, from http://www.reuters.com/article/pressRelease/idUS248597+06-Dec-2007+PRN20071206
      Brenner, D., & Hall, E. J. (2007). Computed tomography, an increasing source of radiation exposure. *New England Journal of Medicine, 357*(22), 2277–2284.
      Group Health Cooperative Center for Health Studies. (2007, December 12). Accuracy of diagnostic mammograms varies by radiologist, study finds. *ScienceDaily.* Retrieved December 23, 2007, from http://www.sciencedaily.com/releases/2007/12/071211234019.htm
      Ma, H., Hill, C. K., Bernstein, L., & Ursin, G. (2007). Low-dose medical radiation exposure and breast cancer risk in women under age 50 years overall and by estrogen and progesterone receptor status: Results from a case-control and case-case comparison. *Breast Cancer Research and Treatment, 109*(1), 77–90.
      Maloof, S. (2003). *Breast fluid a better option for detecting cancer.* (2003). Retrieved January 18, 2007, from http://www.medicalnewstoday.com/articles/3920.php

Exercise/Movement

1. Prevent breast cancer
   a. *Actions/expected responses:* A study of nearly 65,000 women found that those who were physically active had a 23% lower risk of breast cancer before menopause. In particular, high levels of physical activity from ages 12 to 22 contributed most strongly to the lower breast cancer risk.

b. *Routes/dosages/frequencies:* Running 3.25 hours a week or walking 13 hours a week.

c. *Cautions:* Discuss any new exercise program with primary health care provider.

d. *Assessments:* Assess readiness for high levels of physical activity.

e. *Tips for use:* Use appropriate clothes and shoes and stop exercising if any untoward signs occur. Use warm-ups and cooldowns to protect your body and prepare for exercise. For more information go to http://www.pponline.co.uk/encyc/warm-up-exercises.html

f. *Tips on use:* For more information go to walking.about.com/od/fitness/a/startrunning.htm

g. *Other considerations:* You should be able to exercise and carry on a conversation without becoming short of breath.

h. *References/other sources:*

Washington University School of Medicine. (2008, May 14). Girls, young women can cut risk of early breast cancer through regular exercise. *ScienceDaily.* Retrieved May 15, 2008, from http://www.sciencedaily.com/releases/2008/05/080513171443.htm

2. Survivor strategies

a. *Actions/expected responses:* Giving a breast cancer survivor an exercise workbook or step pedometer can improve their quality of life and fatigue levels. Women who exercised more than 7 hours per week lowered their risk for breast cancer by 20% more than those women who exercised less than 1 hour per week. In lean, regularly exercising premenopausal women, the risk for breast cancer was reduced by 72%. Exercise can also lower estrogen levels; high levels of estrogen contribute to an increased risk of breast cancer.

b. *Routes/dosages/frequencies:* 30 minutes of moderate to vigorous activity at least 5 days a week for premenopausal women (reduced risk of dying within a 10-year period) and occupational and household physical activity in postmenopausal women (reduced breast cancer risk by 30%). Best exercise formats are walking, jogging, running, playing tennis, bicycling, swimming, and aerobic dance.

c. *Cautions:* Start slowly with exercise and inform health care practitioners of exercise plans if over 35 years old and have chest pain or shortness of breath, have leg pain when walking, ankles that swell regularly, or have been diagnosed with heart disease.

d. *Assessments:* Assess for any of the symptoms mentioned in Cautions and contact health care practitioner if any of the signs are in evidence.

e. *Tips on use:* Use appropriate clothes and shoes and stop exercising if any untoward signs occur. You should be able to exercise and carry on a conversation without becoming short of breath.

f. *Other considerations:* Previous research has found that maintaining a healthy body weight is associated with reducing the risks of dying from breast cancer or having it recur. Exercise is a key component in maintaining healthy weight. See chapter 25 "Overweight/Obesity."

g. *References/other sources:*

American Association for Cancer Research. (2008, March 6). High levels of estrogen associated with breast cancer recurrence. *ScienceDaily.* Retrieved

March 9, 2008, http://www.sciencedaily.com/releases/2008/03/080306075218.htm

Friedenreich, C. M., Bryant, H. E., & Coumeya, K. S. (2001). Case-control study of life-time physical activity and breast cancer risk. *American Journal of Epidemiology, 154,* 336–347.

Rockhill, B., Willett, W. C., Hunter, D. J., Manson, J. E., Hankinson, S. E., & Colditz, G. A. (1999). A prospective study of recreational physical activity and breast cancer risk. *Archives of Internal Medicine, 159,* 2290–2296.

Thune, I., Brenn, T., Lund, E., & Gaard, M. (1997). Physical activity and the risk of breast cancer. *The New England Journal of Medicine, 336*(18), 1269–1274.

University of Alberta. (2007, June 19). Simple steps make breast cancer survivors eager to exercise, study shows. *ScienceDaily.* Retrieved December 9, 2007, from http://www.sciencedaily.com/releases/2007/06/070613120937.htm

Herbs/Essential Oils

1. Astragalus
   a. *Actions/expected responses:* A weak immune system is one of the major factors that promotes cancer metastases after an operation, chemotherapy, or radiation therapy. Fear and stress weaken the immune system. Adequate stress management prior to and after medical treatment may help to prevent metastases. Astragalus enhances immune response, stimulates the production of interferon, and protects against mammary tumors.
   b. *Routes/dosages/frequencies:* By mouth as a tincture, decoction, fluid extract, or in capsule form.
   c. *Cautions:* Avoid using astragalus during a fever, infection, or inflammation, pregnancy or lactation, or concurrently with antihypertensives, Cyclophosphamide, immunosuppressants, Interleukin-2, or interferon.
   d. *Assessments:* Assess use of any of the items listed in "Cautions" and for allergic reactions to astragalus.
   e. *Tips on use:* This herb is generally safe.
   f. *Other considerations:* Allergic reactions are rare.
   g. *References/other sources:*

   Nagasawa, H., Watanabe, K., Yoshida, M., & Inatomi, H. (2001). Effects of gold banded lily (Lillium auratum Lindl) or Chinese milk vetch (Astragalus sinicus L) on spontaneous mammary tumourigenesis in SHN mice. *Anticancer Research, 21*(4A), 2323–2328.

   Tel Aviv University. (2008, February 29). Stress and fear can affect cancer's recurrence. *ScienceDaily.* Retrieved March 9, 2008, from http://www.sciencedaily.com/releases/2008/02/080227142656.htm

2. Black cohosh
   a. *Actions/expected responses:* An in vitro study has shown that extracts from black cohosh can kill breast cancer cells. A growing body of research suggests that black cohosh may provide breast cancer prevention. The studies indicate the growth-inhibitory effect of actein or an extract of black cohosh is associated with activation of a specific stress response pathway

and cell death. An epidemiology study found that black cohosh may cut risk of breast cancer by 61%.

b. *Routes/dosages/frequencies*: 40–80 mg a day standardized triterpines per caplet/capsule or Remifemin, a herbal preparation derived from black cohosh reduced the risk of breast cancer by 53%.

c. *Cautions*: Should not be used during pregnancy as it is a uterine stimulant that can lead to miscarriage. Avoid if hypotensive or have a slow heart rate. Do not give to children or leave in a place where children might take it.

d. *Assessments:* Assess for concurrent use of other hormonal products: estrogen, rogesterone, oral contraceptives, thyroid products, steroids, and/or androgens.

e. *Tips on use:* Discuss with prescribing health care practitioner prior to using. Keep black cohosh in a cool dry place.

f. *Other considerations:* Take under supervision of a qualified herbalist.

g. *References/other sources:*

Einbond, L. S., Shimizu, M., Xiao, D., Nuntanakorn, P., Lim, J. T., Suzui, M., et al. (2004). Growth inhibitory activity of extracts and purified components of black cohosh on human breast cancer cells. *Breast Cancer Research and Treatment, 83*(3), 221–231.

Einbond, L. S., Wen-Cai, Y., He, K., Wu, H. A., Cruz, E., Roller, M., et al. (2008). Growth inhibitory activity of extracts and compounds from Cimicifuga species on human breast cancer cells. *Phytomedicine, 15* (6-7), 504–511.

Rebbeck, T. R., Troxel, A. B., Norman, G. R., Bunin, A., DeMichele, M., Bauymgarten, M., et al. (2007). A retrospective case-control study of the use of hormone-related supplements and association with breast cancer. *International Journal of Cancer, 120*(7), 1523–1528.

3. Curcumin (turmeric)

a. *Actions/expected responses:* Curcumin has antiproliferative and antiangiogenic activities that make it therapeutically efficacious for treating cancer.

b. *Routes/dosages/frequencies:* 400–600 mg three times a day standardized to curcumin content or tincture, 10 ml (1:5 dilution).

c. *Cautions:* Pregnant and lactating women or women with bile duct obstruction, peptic ulcer, hyperacidity, gallstones, bleeding disorders, or hypersensitivity to the herb should not use curcumin. Women who take the following drugs should also not use curcumin: anticoagulants, immunosuppressants, or NSAIDs. May potentiate warfarin and antiplatelet medications as well as nonsteroidal anti-inflammatory drugs.

d. *Assessments:* Assess for hypersensitivity reactions including dermatitis and monitor coagulant studies for long-term use of the herb.

e. *Tips on use:* Store curcumin in a cool, dry place. Do not take on an empty stomach. Turmeric/curcumin can be sprinkled on food as a spice.

f. *Other considerations:* Report bleeding gums, blood in the urine or stool, or bruising to health care practitioner. Curcumin can potentiate Taxol, preventing the metastasis of breast cancer.

g. *References/other sources:*

Anand, P., Kunnumakkara, A. B., Newman, R. A., & Aggarwal, B. B. (2007). Bioavailability of curcumin: Problems and promises. *Molecular Pharmacology, 4*(6), 807–818.

Corona-Rivera, A., Urbina-Cano, P., Bobadilla-Moralies, L., Vargas-Lares J., Ramirez-Herrera, M.A., Mendoza-Magaua, M. L., et al. (2007). Protective in vivo effect of curcumin on copper genotoxicity evaluated by comet and micronucleus assays. *Journal of Applied Genetics, 48*(4), 389–396.

Sego, S. (2008, July). Turmeric. *The Clinical Advisor,* 109–110.

Skidmore-Roth, L. (2006). Turmeric. In *Mosby's handbook of herbs & natural supplements* (pp. 974–977). St. Louis, MO: ElsevierMosby.

4. Licorice (Glycyrrhiza uralensis)
   a. *Actions/expected responses:* Chinese licorice has anticancer effects against human breast cancer cells.
   b. *Routes/dosages/frequencies:* 1 tsp of the cut and sifted root in a cup of boiling water. Allow to simmer for 5 minutes. Cool and drink 1 cup a day.
   c. *Cautions:* Avoid licorice when pregnant or lactating, during hepatic or liver disease, during a state of hypokalemia, hypertension, arrhythmia, congestive heart failure, if there is a hypersensitivity to the herb, or when taking aloe, buckthorn, cascara, Chinese rhubarb, grapefruit, or diuretics.
   d. *Assessments:* Assess for all the conditions listed under "Cautions," as well as for taking cardiac glycosides, antihypertensives, antiarrhythmics, azole antifungals, cytochrome P450 or coricosteroids, which may interact with this herb.
   e. *Tips on use:* Keep licorice in a cool, dry place and avoid using this herb for longer than 6 weeks at a time.
   f. *Other considerations:* Increase potassium intake if it becomes necessary to take this herb for longer than 6 weeks.
   g. *References/other sources:*

   Dong, S., Inoue, A., Zhu, Y., Tanji, M., & Kiyama, R. (2007). Activation of rapid signaling pathways and the subsequent transcriptional regulation for the proliferation of breast cancer. *Food and Chemical Toxicology, 45*(12), 2470–2478.

   Jo, E. H., Kim, S. H., Ra, J. C., Kim, S. R., Cho, S. D., Jung, J. W., et al. (2005). Chemopreventive properties of the ethanol extract of Chinese licorice (Glycyrrhiza uralensis) root: Induction of apoptosis and GI cell cycle arrest in MCF-7 human breast cancer cells. *Cancer Letters 230*(2), 239–247.

5. Milk thistle
   a. *Actions/expected responses:* Silymarin, the active substance in milk thistle, stimulates detoxification pathways, inhibits the growth of certain cancer cell lines, exerts direct cytotoxic activity toward certain cancer cell lines, and may increase the efficacy of certain chemotherapy agents. Milk thistle also protects the liver from drug or alcohol-related injury. Silibinin, a compound of milk thistle, may even prevent the development of liver cancer.
   b. *Routes/dosages/frequencies:* 200–400 mg silymarin per day.
   c. *Cautions:* Milk thistle is considered safe and well-tolerated, with GI upset, a mild laxative effect, and rare allergic reaction being the only adverse events reported when taken within the recommended dose range. Pregnant and lactating women or those who are hypersensitive (have a known sensitivity to ragweed, marigolds, or chrysanthemums) should not use milk thistle.
   d. *Assessments:* Assess hypersensitivity to milk thistle.
   e. *Tips on use:* Milk thistle may protect against liver damage from antipsychotics, acetaminophen, phenytoin, and halothane.

f. *Other considerations:* Preliminary research suggests that silibinin may enhance the tumor-fighting effects of cisplatin and doxorubicin.

g. *References/other sources:*

Bokemeyer, C., Fells, L. M., & Dunn, T. (1996). Silibinin protects against cisplatin-induced nephrotoxicity without compromising cisplatin on isosfamide anti-tumor activity. *British Journal of Cancer, 74,* 2036–2041.

Post-White, J., Ladas, E. J., & Kelly, K. M. (2007). Advances in the use of milk thistle (Silybum marianum). *Integrative Cancer Therapy, 6*(2), 104–109.

Zi, X., Feyes, D. K., & Agarwal, R. (1998). Anticarcinogenic effect of a flavonoid antioxidant, silymarin, in human breast cancer cells MDA-MB 468: Induction of G1 arrest through an increase in Cip1/p21 concomitant with a decrease in kinase activity of cyclin-dependent kinases and associated cyclins. *Clinical Cancer Research, 239*(1), 334–339.

Zi, X., Mukhtar, H., & Agarwal, R. (1997). Novel cancer chemopreventive effects of a flavonoid antioxidant silymarin: Inhibition of RNA expression of an endogenous tumor promoter TNF-alpha. *Biochemical Biophysical Research Communication, 239,* 334–339.

6. Rosemary

a. *Actions/expected responses:* Constituents in rosemary have shown a variety of pharmacological activities for breast cancer prevention.

b. *Routes/dosages/frequencies:* Use as a spice in cooking or drink as a tea.

c. *Cautions:* In culinary amounts, rosemary poses no dangers. Use herbs that have not been treated with pesticides or irradiated. Nonirradiated spices can be found in health food stores or online.

d. *Assessments:* Assess for an allergic reaction to rosemary.

e. *Tips on use:* Use 1 tsp of crushed rosemary leaves in one cup of boiled water. Steep for 10 minutes and let cool to a safe drinking temperature. Drink up to three cups a day. Sprinkle on stews, poultry, soups or salads.

f. *Other considerations:* Rosemary contains chemicals that help fight infection caused by bacteria and fungi.

g. *References/other sources:*

Cheung, S., & Tai, J. (2007). Anti-proliferative and antioxidant properties of rosemary. *Oncology Reports, 17*(6), 1525–1531.

Vittum, B. (2002). *Rosemary.* Cornell University, Cornell Cooperative Extension. Retrieved December 9, 2007, http://counties.cce.cornell.edu/yates/MG2.20.02.htm

Mindset

1. Affirmations

a. *Actions/expected responses:* Self-affirmation of personal values and beliefs buffers neuroendocrine and psychological stress.

b. *Routes/dosages/frequencies:* Repeat aloud or write positive affirmations up to 20 times a day such as "I lovingly forgive and release all of the past," "I choose to fill my world with joy," and "I love and approve of myself."

c. *Cautions:* Ensure affirmations are positive and acceptable to the woman.

d. *Assessments:* Assess anxiety prior to and after completing affirmations for a week.

e. *Tips on use:* Ask women to write their favorite affirmations on 3 by 5 cards and place them in places where they will be read frequently.

f. *Other considerations:* Find more affirmations information at www.success consciousness.com/index_00000a.htm

g. *References/other sources:*

Hay, L. (2000). *Heal your body.* Carlsbad, CA: Hay House.

Schwarzer, R., Babler, J., Kwiatek, P., Schroder, K., & Zang, J. W. (1997). The assessment of optimistic self-beliefs: Assessment of general perceived self-efficacy in thirteen cultures. *World Psychology, 3*(1–2), 177–190.

2. Cognitive-behavioral therapy (CBT)

a. *Actions/expected responses:* Survivors of breast cancer often suffer from insomnia. CBT has significantly improved insomnia.

b. *Routes/dosages/frequencies:* 6 weeks of group CBT.

c. *Cautions:* None.

d. *Assessments:* Assess insomnia prior to and after taking part in CBT.

e. *Tips on use:* For more information, go to http://www.mind.org.uk/Infor mation/Booklets/Making+sense/MakingSenseCBT.htm

f. *Other considerations:* CBT can reduce depression and anxiety and can enhance quality of life in breast cancer survivors.

g. *References/other sources:*

Epstein, D., & Dirksen, S. (2008). Efficacy of an insomnia intervention on fatigue, mood and quality of life in breast cancer survivors. *Journal of Advanced Nursing, 51*(6), 664–675.

Fiorentino, L. (2005). Treating insomnia with CBT in women with breast cancer. *Journal of Cancer Education, 21*(2), 12–56.

Nutrition

1. Berries

a. *Actions/expected responses:* Black raspberry and strawberry extracts showed the most significant ability to inhibit the growth of breast cancer cells.

b. *Routes/dosages/frequencies:* Eat raspberries or strawberries daily if risk of breast cancer is high.

c. *Cautions:* Avoid raspberries or strawberries if hypersensitive to them.

d. *Assessments:* Assess hypersensitivity to raspberries and strawberries.

e. *Tips on use.* Use local berries in the summer and rely on frozen berries the rest of the year.

f. *References/other sources:*

Seeram, N. P., Adams, L. S., Zhang, Y., Lee, R., Sand, D., Scheuller, H. S., et al. (2006). Blackberry, black raspberry, blueberry, cranberry, red raspberry, and strawberry extract inhibit growth and stimulate apoptosis of human cancer cells in vitro. *Journal of Agriculture and Food Chemistry, 54*(25), 9329–9339.

2. Flaxseed

a. *Actions/expected responses:* Flaxseed reduced the growth and metastasis of established estrogen receptor human breast cancer in part due to its lignan and oil components.

b. *Routes/dosages/frequencies:* 2 1/2 tsp of ground seeds twice or three times a day in salad, soup, other foods, or water.

c. *Cautions:* Until more research is available, pregnant and lactating women should not use flaxseeds nor give them to children. Women with bowel obstruction, dehydration, or sensitivity to flaxseed should avoid using it. Flax can decrease the absorption of other medications, so separate by several hours.

d. *Assessments:* Assess for hypersensitivity (integumentary/skin) reactions and gastrointestinal reactions (nausea, vomiting, anorexia, diarrhea, and flatulence).

e. *Tips on use:* Use only mature seeds; immature seeds are toxic. Keep flaxseeds in the refrigerator to prevent fatty acid breakdown. Adequate levels of zinc and acidophilus are needed to metabolize flax.

f. *Other considerations:* Flax may increase risk of bleeding if taken with anticoagulants/antiplatelets or antidiabetes agents.

g. *References/other sources:*

Haggans, C. J., Travelli, E. J., Thomas, W., Martini, M. C., & Slavin, H. (2000). The effect of flaxseed and wheat bran consumption on urinary estrogen metabolites in premenopausal women. *Cancer Epidemiology Biomarkers and Prevention 9*(7), 719–725.

Skidmore-Roth, L. (2006). Flax. In *Mosby's handbook of herbs and natural supplements* (pp. 450–454). St. Louis, MO: ElsevierMosby.

Wang, L., Chen, J., & Thompson, L. U. (2005). The inhibitory effect of flaxseed on the growth and metastasis of estrogen receptor negative human breast cancer xenografts is attributed to both its lignan and oil components. *International Journal of Cancer, 116*(5), 793–798.

3. Green tea

a. *Actions/expected responses:* Green tea is protective against breast cancer before disease occurs and after onset, possibly by creating a detoxifying effect.

b. *Routes/dosages/frequencies:* Two to five cups of decaffeinated tea daily (1 tsp tea leaves in 8 ounces of hot water).

c. *Cautions:* May decrease iron absorption, so separate iron-rich foods or iron pills by at least 2 hours from green tea ingestion.

d. *Assessments:* Assess for hypersensitivity reactions. Also assess for cardiovascular (increased blood pressure, palpitations, and irregular heartbeat), central nervous system (anxiety, nervousness, insomnia), and gastrointestinal (nausea, heartburn, increased stomach acid) reactions.

e. *Tips on use:* Caffeinated green tea can interact with MAOIs and lead to a hypertensive crisis. Counsel women not to take green tea with anticoagulants/antiplatelets (may increase risk of bleeding), beta-adrenergic blockers (can lead to increased inotropic effects), or benzodiazepines (may increase sedation). Teach women to store green tea in a cool, dry place.

f. *Other considerations:* Dairy products may decrease the therapeutic effects of green tea, so separate their intake by several hours. Digestive process affects anticancer activity of tea in gastrointestinal cells; add citrus (such as lemon juice) or take ascorbic acid (vitamin C) to protect the catechins in green tea from digestive degradation.

g. *References/other sources:*

American Association for Cancer Research. (2007, August 12). Green tea boosts production of detox enzymes, rendering cancerous chemicals harmless. *ScienceDaily.* Retrieved December 20, 2007, from http://www.sciencedaily.com/releases/2007/08/070810194923.htm

Federation of American Societies for Experimental Biology. (2008, April 10). Digestive process affects anti-cancer activity of tea in gastrointestinal cells. *ScienceDaily.* Retrieved April 20, 2008, from http://www.sciencedaily.com/releases/2008/04/080407172713.htm

Skidmore-Roth, L. (2006). Green tea. In *Mosby's handbook of herbs and natural supplements* (pp. 535–539). St. Louis, MO: ElsevierMosby.

4. Mediterranean diet

a. *Actions/expected responses:* Mediterranean diet is linked with prevention of breast cancer.

b. *Routes/dosages/frequencies:* High daily intake of vegetables, legumes, fruits (high in protective fiber associated with a 40% reduced risk in developing breast cancer; black raspberry and strawberry showed the most significant ability to inhibit growth of cancer cells), antioxidants and antiproliferatives, whole grain foods (high fiber), fish, and unsaturated fatty acids such as olive oil; low intake of saturated fatty acids, dairy products, meat (diets high in red and processed meat increase risk), and poultry; and low to moderate intake of alcohol. For more information, go to http://www.mayoclinic.com/health/mediteraneandiet/CL00011

c. *Cautions:* Drink no more than one 5-ounce glass of red wine a day; drinking more has been linked with health problems including cancers. Excessive dietary intake of sugar, refined carbohydrates, and animal products (meat and dairy products with high content of saturated fat), also known as a traditional Western diet, is linked with breast cancer. Make sure to eat only whole grains and to check labels carefully; to ensure whole grains are being ingested, eat brown rice, barley, and oats.

d. *Assessments:* Assess intake of foods listed in "Other considerations." Sixty-eight percent of women do not eat five portions of fruits and vegetables a day.

e. *Tips on use:* If you must have sweet foods, use stevia as a sweetener. It's been shown to repair DNA, has no calories, and no side effects.

f. *Other considerations:* Eat foods that are especially protective for breast cancer, including: apples with their peelings (number of breast tumors was reduced by 25% after eating one apple a day, and 61% after eating six apples a day); pineapple (bromelain), cranberries, red grapes, strawberries, peaches, citrus fruits (contain limonene, which increases the production of enzymes that help the body dispose of carcinogens), pears, bananas (contain caffeic acid, which aids the production of an enzyme that makes it easier for the body to get rid of carcinogens, and ferulic acid, which binds to nitrates, possibly preventing them from converting to cancer-causing nitrosamines), carrots (vitamin A, a retinoid), tomatoes, squash, corn, peanuts, oats, and barley. Also counsel women to eat daily servings of leafy green vegetables (like spinach and turnip greens), and soybeans and other dried beans and peas (high in protective fiber, provide protease inhibitors that suppress enzyme production in cancer cells to slow tumor growth), which are all natural sources of folate, which prevents changes to DNA that can lead to cancer. Encourage women to eat daily portions of brassica vegetables, including broccoli, cauliflower, cabbage, Brussels sprouts and kohlrabi, which contain sulforaphane and other isothiocyantestes that stimulate the production of anticancer enzymes to bolster the body's natural ability to ward off cancer, and indoles that stimulate enzymes that make the hormone estrogen less effective. Eat allium vegetables daily, including garlic, onions, leeks, and chives, which can help block the action of cancer-causing chemicals, as can watercress. Buy organic foods. They are grown in selenium-rich soils, giving them greater anticarcinogenic potential. Avoid microwaving vegetables and fruits; microwaving broccoli resulted in a loss of 97%, 74%, and 87% of its three major antioxidant compounds, respectively; steaming for 5 minutes resulted in a loss of only 11%, 0%, and 8%, respectively, of the same antioxidants.

g. *References/other sources:*

Aggarwal, B. B., & Ichikawa, H. (2005). Molecular targets and anticancer potential of indole-3-carbinol and its derivatives. *Cell Cycle, 4*(9), 1201–1215.

Cornblatt, B. S., Ye, L., Dinkova-Kostova, A. T., Erb, M., Fahey, J. W., & Singh, N. K. (2007). Preclinical and clinical evaluation of sulforaphane for chemoprevention in the breast. *Carcinogenesis, 28*(7), 1485–1490.

Do, M. H., Lee, S. S., Kim, J. Y., Jung, P. H., & Lee, M. H. (2007). Fruits, vegetables, soy foods and breast cancer in pre- and postmenopausal Korean women: A case-control study. *International Journal of Vitamin and Nutrition Research, 77*(2), 130–141.

Fields, A. L., Soprano, D. R., & Soprano, K. J. (2007). Retinoids in biological control and cancer. *Journal of Cell Biochemistry, 102*(4), 886–898.

Ghanta, S., Banerjee, A., Poddar, A., & Chattopadhyay, S. (2007). Oxidative DNA damage preventive activity and antioxidant potential of Stevia rebaudiana (Bertoni) Bertoni, a natural sweetener. *55*(26), 10962–10967.

Gill, C. I., Haldar, S., Boyd, L. A., Bennett, R., Whiteford, J., Butler, M., et al. (2007). Watercress supplementation in diet reduces lymphocyte DNA damage and alters blood antioxidant status in healthy adults. *American Journal of Clinical Nutrition, 85*(2), 504–510.

Irion, C. W. (1999). Growing alliums and brassicas in selenium-enriched soils increases their anticarcinogenic potentials. *Medical Hypotheses, 53*(3), 232–235.

Liu, R. H., Liu, J., & Chen, B. (2005). Apples prevent mammary tumors in rats. *Journal of Agricultural and Food Chemistry, 53*(6), 2341–2343.

Maurer, H. R. (2001). Bromelain: Biochemistry, pharmacology and medical use. *Cell and Molecular Life Science, 58*(9), 1234–1245.

Mitrou, P. N., Kipnis, V., Thiebaut, A. C., Reedy, J., Subar, A. F., Wirfalt, E., et al. (2007). Mediterranean dietary pattern and prediction of all-cause mortality in a US population: Results from the NIH-AARP Diet and Health Study. *Archives of Internal Medicine, 167*(22), 2461–2468.

Seeram, N. P., Adams, L. S., Zhang, Y., Lee, R., Sand, D., Scheuller, H. S., et al. (2006). Blackberry, black raspberry, blueberry, cranberry, red raspberry, and strawberry extracts inhibit growth and stimulate apoptosis of human cancer cells in vitro. *Journal of Agriculture and Food Chemistry, 54*(25), 9329–9339.

Sun, J., Chu, Y. F., Wu, X., & Liu, R. H. (2002). Antioxidant and antiproliferative activities of common fruits. *Journal of Agricultural and Food Chemistry, 50*(23), 6910–6916.

Taylor, E. F., Burley, V. J., & Cade, J. E. (2007). Meat consumption and risk of breast cancer in the UK Women's Cohort Study. *British Journal of Cancer, 96*(7), 1139–1146.

Vallejo, F., Tomas-Barberan, F. A., & Garcia-Viguera, C. (2003). Phenolic compounds content in edible parts of broccoli inflorescences after domestic cooking. *Journal of Science and Food Agriculture, 83*(14), 1151–1156.

Zhang, S., Hunger, D. J., Hankinson, S. E., Giovannucci, E. L., Rosner, B. A., Colditz, G. A., et al. (1999). A prospective study of folate intake and the risk of breast cancer. *Journal of the American Medical Association, 281*(17), 1632–1637.

5. Probiotics

   a. *Actions/expected responses:* Probiotics (lactic acid bacteria or LAB) are present in many foods such as yogurt. Probiotics increase immune cell activity and may suppress the growth of bacteria that convert procarcinogens into carcinogens.

   b. *Routes/dosages/frequencies:* Eat plain yogurt with active organisms daily to reduce the proliferation of cancer cells.

   c. *Cautions:* None unless women are sensitive to yogurt.

   d. *Assessments:* Assess intake of yogurt.

   e. *Tips on use:* Obtain plain, nonsweetened yogurt and sweeten it with banana, raisins, or molasses. Stevia is also a healthy sweetener that can help repair your DNA.

   f. *Other considerations:* Milk products may contain growth hormones. Use organic yogurt.

   g. *References/other sources:*

   Matar, C., & Perdigon, G. (2007). The application of probiotics in cancer. *British Journal of Nutrition* (1 Suppl.), *98*, S105–S110.

6. Soy

   a. *Actions/expected responses:* Soyasaponins have been shown to inhibit the proliferation of cancer cells. A meta-analysis of the eight studies conducted in high-soy-consuming Asians show a significant trend of decreasing risk with increasing soy food intake. Eating soy foods in puberty protects against breast cancer.

   b. *Routes/dosages/frequencies:* Eat soy foods daily to reduce the proliferation of cancer cells.

   c. *Cautions:* Nonfermented forms of soy foods may reduce assimilation of calcium, magnesium, copper, iron, and zinc because of their high levels of phytic acid.

   d. *Assessments:* Assess intake of soy foods.

   e. *Tips on use:* The best sources are organic fermented products like tempeh or miso. Counsel women to give their teenagers soy foods to prevent breast cancer.

f. *Other considerations:* Many nonorganic soy beans have been genetically modified (never researched for their long-term effects) and treated with dangerous chemicals, so they should be avoided.

g. *References/other sources:*

Georgetown University Medical Center. (2008, April 9). Eating soy foods in puberty protects against breast cancer, evidence now suggests. *ScienceDaily*. Retrieved April 20, 2008, from http://www.sciencedaily.com/releases/2008/04/080409091727.htm

Ghanta, S., Banerjee, A., Poddar, A., & Chattopadhyay, S. (2007). Oxidative DNA damage preventive activity and antioxidant potential of Stevia rebaudiana (Bertoni) Bertoni, a natural sweetener. *55*(26), 10962–10967.

Wu, A. H., Yu, M. C., Tseng, C. C., & Pike, M. C. (2008). Epidemiology of soy exposures and breast cancer risk. *British Journal of Cancer, 98*(1), 9–14.

Xiao, J. X., Huang, G. Q., & Zhang, S. H. (2007). Soyasaponins inhibit the proliferation of Hela cells by inducing apoptosis. *Experimental Toxicology and Pathology, 59*(1), 35–42.

Stress Management

1. Affirmations

a. *Actions/expected responses:* A weak immune system is one of the major factors that promotes cancer metastases after an operation, chemotherapy, or radiation therapy. Fear and stress weaken the immune system. Psychological stress has been linked to breast cancer. Adequate stress management prior to and after medical treatment may help to prevent metastases. Self-affirmation of personal values and beliefs buffers neuroendocrine and psychological stress surrounding cancer risk, diagnosis and treatment.

b. *Routes/dosages/frequencies:* Affirmations are repeated aloud or written in positive language up to 20 times a day. Some suggested affirmations are: "I let go, forgive myself and others," "I fill my world with joy and peace," and "I love and approve of my life and myself."

c. *Cautions:* Ensure affirmations are positive and acceptable to the women by asking them to participate in composing their own affirmations.

d. *Assessments:* Assess reactions prior to and after completing affirmations for a week.

e. *Tips on use:* Ask women to write their favorite affirmations on 3 by 5 cards and place them in spots where they will be read frequently.

f. *Other considerations:* See affirmations information at www.successconsciousness.com/index_00000a.htm

g. *References/other sources:*

Hay, L. (2000). *Heal your body*. Carlsbad, CA: Hay House.

Queen's University. (2008, March 9). Severe psychological stress may be linked to breast cancer. *ScienceDaily*. Retrieved March 23, 2008, from http://www.sciencedaily.com/releases/2008/03/080308103341.htm

Schwarzer, R., Babler, J., Kwiatek, P., Schroder, K., & Zang, J. W. (1997). The assessment of optimistic self-beliefs: Assessment of general perceived self-efficacy in thirteen cultures. *World Psychology, 3*(1–2), 177–190.

Tel Aviv University. (2008, February 29). Stress and fear can affect cancer's recurrence. *ScienceDaily*. Retrieved March 9, 2008, from http://www.sciencedaily.com/releases/2008/02/080227142656.htm

2. Aromatherapy
   a. *Actions/expected responses:* Laboratory and clinical research with women has shown that the use of essential oils from plants (typically chamomile, geranium, and lavender) support and balance the mind, body, and spirit and can enhance quality of life.
   b. *Routes/dosages/frequencies:* Inhalation or skin application as requested after initial treatment.
   c. *Cautions:* None known. Safety testing on essential oils has found very few if any bad effects.
   d. *Assessments:* Assess stress level prior to and after using aromatherapy.
   e. *Tips on use:* Allow women to choose the oils or combinations that work best for them.
   f. *Other considerations:* Suggest women either inhale a specific essential oil(s) or add a few drops to bath oil or pillow.
   g. *References/other sources:*
      National Cancer Institute. (2008). *Aromatherapy and essential oils*. Accessed July 29, 2008 at http://www.cancer.gov/cancertopics/pdq/cam/aromatherapy/patient

3. Journaling
   a. *Actions/expected responses:* A weak immune system is one of the major factors that promotes cancer metastases after an operation, chemotherapy, or radiation therapy. Fear and stress weaken the immune system. Adequate stress management prior to and after medical treatment may help to prevent metastases. Expressing emotions (for example, by journaling) and finding benefit in stressful experiences have been associated with positive adjustment.
   b. *Routes/dosages/frequencies:* Women write for at least four sessions about their deepest thoughts and feelings, or positive thoughts and feelings, or about their treatment.
   c. *Cautions:* Women high in avoidance may not respond well to being asked to write about their deepest thoughts and feelings about breast cancer.
   d. *Assessments:* Assess avoidance of and wish not to talk about their breast cancer experience.
   e. *Tips on use:* Ask women high in avoidance to journal about their positive thoughts and feelings regarding their experience with breast cancer. Ask women low in avoidance to write about their deepest thoughts and feelings regarding breast cancer.
   f. *Other considerations:* Expect women who write about their deepest thoughts and feelings regarding breast cancer to report significantly decreased physical symptoms, and women who write about their deepest thoughts and feelings and positive thoughts and feelings to have significantly fewer appointments for cancer-related morbidities.
   g. *References/other sources:*
      Stanton, A. L., Danoff-Burg, S., Sworowski, L. A., Collins, C. A., Branstetter, A. D., Rodriguez-Hanley, A., et al. (2002). Randomized, controlled trial

of written emotional expression and benefit finding in breast cancer patients. *Journal of Clinical Oncology, 20*(20), 4160–4168.

Tel Aviv University. (2008, February 29). Stress and fear can affect cancer's recurrence. *ScienceDaily*. Retrieved March 9, 2008, from http://www.sciencedaily.com/releases/2008/02/080227142656.htm

4. Mindfulness-based stress reduction program (MBSR)

a. *Actions/expected responses:* A weak immune system is one of the major factors that promotes cancer metastases after an operation, chemotherapy, or radiation therapy. Fear and stress weaken the immune system. Adequate stress management prior to and after medical treatment may help to prevent metastases. MBSR is a program that incorporates relaxation, meditation, gentle yoga, and daily home practice. MBSR is associated with enhanced quality of life and decreased stress symptoms in women with breast cancer.

b. *Routes/dosages/frequencies:* MBSR is an 8-week program.

c. *Cautions:* May not be congruent with the following diagnoses: antisocial personality disorder, borderline personality disorder, current major depressive disorder, physical impairment that precludes attending class, posttraumatic stress disorder, psychosis, social anxiety (if it interferes with participation in class), substance abuse or addiction (current or recovery within the past year), suicidal intent or plan, or unstable medical diagnosis.

d. *Assessments*: Rate quality of life and stress symptoms from 0 (none) to 10 (high amount) prior to and after participating in mindfulness sessions.

e. *Tips on use:* For more information go to http://www.stjohn.org/innerpage.aspx?PageID=1779

f. *Other considerations:* Other Web sites that may be useful are http://www.mindfulnessmeditationcentre.org/breathingGathas.htm or http://www.meditationcenter.com

g. *References/other sources:*

Carlson, L. E., Speca, M., Patel, K. D., & Goodey, E. (2004). Mindfulness-based stress reduction in relation to quality of life, mood, symptoms of stress and levels of cortisol, dehydroepiandrosterone sulfate (DHEAS) and melatonin in breast and prostate cancer outpatients. *Psychoneuroendocrinology, 29*(4), 448–474.

Tel Aviv University. (2008, February 29). Stress and fear can affect cancer's recurrence. *ScienceDaily*. Retrieved March 9, 2008, from http://www.sciencedaily.com/releases/2008/02/080227142656.htm

5. Yoga

a. *Actions/expected responses:* A weak immune system is one of the major factors that promotes cancer metastases after an operation, chemotherapy, or radiation therapy. Fear and stress weaken the immune system. Adequate stress management prior to and after medical treatment may help to prevent metastases. Yoga reduces perceived stress in women diagnosed with breast cancer as measured by the Hospital Anxiety and Depression Scale (HADS) and Perceived Stress Scale (PSS). Compared to a control group, among women not receiving chemotherapy, yoga appears to enhance emotional well-being and mood and may serve to buffer deterioration in both overall and specific domains of quality of life.

b. *Routes/dosages/frequencies:* 1 hour weekly.

   c. *Cautions:* Go to http://yoga.lifetips.com/cat/56770/yoga-cautions/

   d. *Assessments:* Assess interest in and ability to participate in yoga. Assess for extreme menstrual flow, pregnancy, knee problems, and conditions that may affect yoga practice. Self-assess stress following each yoga session.

   e. *Tips on use:* Because yoga exerts pressure on internal organs, wait at least 2 hours after a meal and 30 minutes to 1 hour after a snack to practice.

   f. *Other considerations:* To avoid knee injury when doing yoga, keep the knees straight (especially in standing poses). The knees should be forward in line with the ankle and foot and should not be allowed to twist inward or outward. For more information about yoga, go to http://www.mother nature.com/Library/Bookshelf/Books/21/54.cfm. For poses that free up the shoulder, go to http://www.yogajournal.com/practice/955

   g. *References/other sources:*

      Banerjee, B., Vadiraj, H. S., Ram, A., Rao, R., Jayapal, M., Gopinath, K. S., et al. (2007). Effects of an integrated yoga program in modulating psychological stress and radiation-induced genotoxic stress in breast cancer patients undergoing radiotherapy. *Integrative Cancer Therapies, 6*(3), 242–250.

      Moadel, A. B., Shah, C., Wylie-Rosett, J., Harris, M. S., Patel, S. R., Hall, C. B., et al. (2007). Randomized controlled trial of yoga among a multiethnic sample of breast cancer patients: Effects on quality of life. *Journal of Clinical Oncology, 25*(28), 4387–4395.

      Tel Aviv University. (2008, February 29). Stress and fear can affect cancer's recurrence. *ScienceDaily.* Retrieved March 9, 2008, from http://www.sciencedaily.com/releases/2008/02/080227142656.htm

Supplements

1. Coenzyme Q10/riboflavin/niacin

   a. *Actions/expected responses:* A combination of coenzyme Q10 (CoQ10) and two vitamins (riboflavin and niacin) suggest a good prognosis and a significant reduction in cytokine levels, and might even offer protection from metastases and recurrence of cancer.

   b. *Routes/dosages/frequencies:* 100 mg CoQ10, 10 mg riboflavin, and 50 mg niacin by mouth per day.

   c. *Cautions:* Until more research is available, these supplements should not be used by pregnant or lactating women or by those with hypersensitivity to the combination.

   d. *Assessments:* Assess for concurrent use with anticoagulants, antidiabetes agents, beta-blockers, HMG-CoA reductase inhibitors, phenothiazines, tricylic antidepressants or l-carnitine, any of which can interact with CoQ10.

   e. *Tips on use:* Keep supplements in a cool, dark place.

   f. *Other considerations:* Have lab parameters monitored carefully when taking any of the medications that interact with CoQ10. Avoid using CoQ10 with phenothiazines, tricyclics, beta-blockers, and cholesterol-lowering agents.

g. *References/other sources:*

Premkumar, V. G., Yuvaraj, S., Vijayasarathy, K., Gangadaran, S. G., & Sachdanandam, P. (2007). Serum cytokine levels of interleukin-1beta, -6,-8, a tumour necrosis factor-alpha and vascular endothelial growth factor in breast cancer patients treated with tamoxifen and supplemented with co-enzyme Q(10), riboflavin, and niacin. *Basic Clinical Pharmacology Toxicology, 100*(6), 387–391.

Skidmore-Roth, L. (2006). Coenzyme Q10. In *Mosby's handbook of herbs and natural supplements* (pp. 315–319). St. Louis, MO: Elsevier-Mosby.

2. Grapeseed extract (GSPE)

   a. *Actions/expected responses:* Inhibits the growth of breast cancer cells.

   b. *Routes/dosages/frequencies:* Capsules/tablets; 150–300 mg per day for 21 days, then 50–80 mg per day, maintenance.

   c. *Cautions:* Should not be used during pregnancy or lactation or given to children.

   d. *Assessments:* Assess for hepatoxicity; assess women's use of anticoagulants and antiplatelets, which could increase the risk of bleeding if taken concurrently.

   e. *Tips on use:* Take grapeseed only once a day.

   f. *Other considerations:* Keep grapeseed capsules/tablets in a cool, dry place.

   g. *References/other sources:*

   Agarwal, C., Sharma, Y., Zhao, J., & Agarwall, R. (2000). A polyphenolic fraction from grape seeds causes irreversible growth inhibition of breast carcinoma MDA-MB468 cells by inhibiting mitogen-activated protein kinases activation and inducing G1 arrest and differentiation. *Clinical Cancer Research, 6*, 2921–2930.

3. Maitake extract

   a. *Actions/expected responses:* A weak immune system is one of the major factors that promotes cancer metastases after an operation, chemotherapy, or radiation therapy. Fear and stress weaken the immune system. Adequate stress management prior to and after medical treatment may help to prevent metastases. This mushroom exerts an antitumor effect by enhancing the immune system through activation of macrophages.

   b. *Routes/dosages/frequencies:* 250–500 mg by mouth per day.

   c. *Cautions:* Until more information is available, maitake should not be used by pregnant or lactating women or be given to children.

   d. *Assessments:* Assess for sensitivity to maitake. Assess for concurrent use with antidiabetes agents or immunosuppressants.

   e. *Tips on use:* Keep maitake in a cool, dry place.

   f. *Other considerations:* May have the potential to decrease the size of breast tumors.

   g. *References/other sources:*

   Kodama, N., Komuta, K., & Nanba, H. (2003). Effect of maitake (Grifola frondosa) D-fraction on the activation of NK cells in patients. *Journal of Medicinal Food, 6*(4), 371–377.

   Skidmore-Roth, L. (2006). Maitake. In *Mosby's handbook of herbs and natural supplements* (pp. 683–686). St. Louis, MO: ElsevierMosby.

Tel Aviv University. (2008, February 29). Stress and fear can affect cancer's recurrence. *ScienceDaily*. Retrieved March 9, 2008, from http://www.sciencedaily.com/releases/2008/02/080227142656.htm

4. Milk thistle (silymarin)
   a. *Actions/expected responses:* Milk thistle exerts anticarcinogenic effects, including inhibition of cancer cell growth in human breast cells. The herb protects liver and kidney from toxic effects of drugs, including chemotherapy.
   b. *Routes/dosages/frequencies:* 200–400 mg tincture by mouth three times daily (dosage standardized to silymarin content).
   c. *Cautions:* Considered safe and well-tolerated, with gastrointestinal upset, a mild laxative effect, and rare allergic reactions being the only adverse events reported when taken in the recommended dose range.
   d. *Assessments:* Assess reactions to milk thistle.
   e. *Tips on use:* Keep milk thistle in a cool, dry place.
   f. *Other considerations:* Until more research is available, pregnant and lactating women should not use milk thistle or give it to children.
   g. *References/other sources:*
      Post-White, J., Ladas, E. J., & Kelly, K. M. (2007). Advances in the use of milk thistle. *Integrative Cancer Therapies, 6*(2), 104–109.
5. Pycnogenol and ginkgo biloba extract
   a. *Actions/expected responses:* Either pycnogenol or ginkgo biloba extract can protect against antimutagenic activity in animal studies. They have potential as antimutagenic agents for lung cancer.
   b. *Routes/dosages/frequencies:* 5–100 microgram/mL.
   c. *Cautions:* Until more research is completed, pregnant and lactating women should not use these supplements, nor should they be given to children. Ginkgo should not be taken concurrently with anticoagulants.
   d. *Assessments:* Assess reaction to pycnogenol and ginkgo.
   e. *Tips on use:* Store supplements in a cool, dry place.
   f. *Other considerations:* Pycnogenol has also been found useful in preventing venous thrombosis, thrombophlebitis, gingival bleeding and plaque, inflammatory bowel disease, venous insufficiency, digestive conditions, and menopause symptoms.
   g. *References/other sources:*
      Krizkova, L., Chovanova, Z., Durackova, Z., & Krajcovic, J. (2008). Antimutagenic in vitro activity of plan polyphenols: Pycnogenol and Ginkgo biloba extract. *Phytotherapy Research, 22*(3), 384–388.
6. Selenium
   a. *Actions/expected responses:* Selenium has been associated with decreased risk of cancer.
   b. *Routes/dosages/frequencies*: 300 micrograms (mcg) per day.
   c. *Cautions:* Avoid taking more than 300 mcg per day.
   d. *Assessments:* Assess use of selenium and remind them not to take more than the suggested amount.
   e. *Tips on use:* Keep the supplement in a cool, dry place.
   f. *Other considerations:* Selenium-enriched yeast and selenium-enriched milk are also available. For food sources, go to http://ods.od.nih.gov/factsheets/selenium.asp

g. *References/other sources:*

Rayn-Haren, G., Bugel, S., Krath, B. N., Hoac, R., Stagsted, J., Jorgensen, K., et al. (2007). A short-term intervention trial with selenate, selenium-enriched yeast and selenium-enriched milk: Effects on oxidative defence regulation. *British Journal of Nutrition, 21,* 1–10.

7. Vitamins A, B, C, D, and E

a. *Actions/expected responses:* Intake of additional vitamins A, B, C, D, and E can confer protection against breast cancer among women who have low intake of these vitamins.

b. *Routes/dosages/frequencies:* Daily intake of 10,000 by mouth IU vitamin A, 1 B-50 capsule, up to 10 grams of vitamin C, between 400 and 600 IU of vitamins D and E.

c. *Cautions:* Avoid vitamin C after eating anything containing fat and to wait at least 2 hours after eating before taking the supplement. Vitamin C can cause loose bowels when taken at high levels.

d. *Assessments:* Complete a food diary to assess intake of these vitamins (see f).

e. *Tips on use:* Follow directions on the bottles and to keep supplements in a cool, dry place.

f. *Other considerations:* Eating a combined amount of 8–10 servings (1/2 cup) a day of fresh fruits (especially citrus and berries), vegetables (especially leafy greens), legumes (dried beans and peas), and whole grain cereals may provide sufficient levels of vitamins necessary to provide protection.

g. *References/other sources:*

Dembrow, M. (2007, June). High vitamin D: Treatment for cancer prevention? *The Clinical Advisor, 54,* 57.

Dorjgochoo, T., Shrubsole, M. J., Shu, X. O., Lu, W., Ruan, Z., Zheng, Y., et al. (2007). Vitamin supplement use and risk for breast cancer: The Shanghai Breast Cancer Study. *Breast Cancer Research and Treatment.* Retrieved December 26, 2007, from http://www.springerlink.com/content/9147635438972118

Head, K. A. (1998). Ascorbic acid in the prevention and treatment of cancer. *Alternative Medicine Review, 3*(3), 174–186.

Sylvester, P. W. (2007). Vitamin E and apoptosis. *Vitamins and Hormones, 76,* 329–356.

Touch

1. Acupressure

a. *Actions/expected responses:* Acupressure can relieve nausea, vomiting, and retching associated with chemotherapy.

b. *Routes/dosages/frequencies:* Finger acupressure treatment is given bilaterally at the acupressure points P6 and ST36, located on the forearm and by the knee.

c. *Cautions:* Use gentle acupressure if knee or forearm conditions are apparent.

    d. *Assessments:* Collect baseline and posttreatment questions about amount of nausea, vomiting, and retching, and ask women to keep a daily log of the intensity of these symptoms.

    e. *Tips on use:* Gentle acupressure means holding the spot with the middle three fingers until a strong pulsation is felt (signaling a blockage has opened), and then moving to the next spot. For more information on using acupressure, go to http://www.eclecticenergies.com/acupressure/howto.php

    f. *Other considerations:* Changes will begin to occur immediately and will continue for several days. Gentle acupressure points that can strengthen the breast include the inside of the knees, on either side of the spine about 4 inches down, back of the head on bony crest on either side of the spine, back of big toes, back of knees, and mid-chest (above breasts) on both sides.

    g. *References/other sources:*

        Dayton, B. R. (1987). *Caregiver's introduction to High Touch acupressure.* Friday Harbor, WA: High Touch Network.

        Dribble, S. L., Luce, J., Cooper, B. A., Israel, J., Cohen, M., Nussey, B., et al. (2007). Acupressure for chemotherapy-induced nausea and vomiting: A randomized clinical trial. *Oncology Nursing Forum, 34*(4), 813–820.

2. Foot reflexology

    a. *Actions/expected responses:* Foot reflexology significantly reduced nausea, vomiting, and fatigue in women with breast cancer undergoing chemotherapy. Self-administered foot reflexology also enhances natural killer cells and IgG, strengthening the immune system against cancer and possibly preventing tumor development.

    b. *Routes/dosages/frequencies:* Four 40-minute treatments.

    c. *Cautions:* None unless the feet have been injured.

    d. *Assessments:* Obtain a baseline for nausea, vomiting, and fatigue.

    e. *Tips on use:* See http://groups.msn.com/AlternativesToPainandDisease/reflexologyinstructionspg1.msnw and http://groups.msn.com/AlternativesToPainandDisease/reflexologyinstructionspg2.msnw.

    f. *Other considerations:* Foot reflexology has been shown to significantly improve life satisfaction, the most important predictor of survival for women with advanced cancer.

    g. *References/other sources:*

        Fox Chase Cancer Center. (2007, November 1). Quality of life is the most important predictor of survival for advanced cancer patients. *ScienceDaily.* Retrieved November 12, 2007, from http://www.sciencedaily.com/releases/2007/10/07/071030170208.htm

        National Cancer Center. (2006). *Immunity and cancer.* Retrieved February 6, 2008, from http://www.nci.nih.go/cancertopics/understandingcancer/immunesystem/Slide32

        Park, H. S., & Cho, G. Y. (2004). Effects of foot reflexology on essential hypertension patients. *Tachan Kanho Hakhoe Chi, 34*(5), 739–750.

        Yang, J. H. (2005). The effects of foot reflexology on nausea, vomiting, and fatigue of breast cancer patients undergoing chemotherapy. *Taehan Kanho Hakkoe Chi, 35*(1), 177–185.

3. Massage therapy
   a. *Actions/expected responses:* Women diagnosed with breast cancer reported being less depressed and less angry and having more vigor after receiving massage therapy.
   b. *Routes/dosages/frequencies:* 30-minute sessions three times a week for 5 weeks.
   c. *Cautions:* No adverse effects were reported.
   d. *Assessments:* Urine tests showed increased dopamine levels, natural killer cells, and lymphocytes as well.
   e. *Tips on use:* Stroking, squeezing, and stretching techniques are used on the head, arms, legs, feet, and back. For techniques to use, go to http://www.videojug.com/film/how-to-do-a-relaxing-hand-and-arm-massage, http://www.ifilm.com/video/28622378, http://www.ifilm.com/video/2797488 and http://www.drfoot.co.uk/foot_massage.htm
   f. *Other considerations:* Women receiving massage therapy or progressive muscle relaxation reported less depressed mood, anxiety, and pain immediately after their first and last sessions. By the end of one study, only the massage therapy group reported being less depressed and less angry and having more vigor.
   g. *References/other sources:*

   Hernandez-Reif, M., Field, T., Ironson, G., Beutler, J., Vera, Y., Hurley, J., et al. (2005). Natural killer cells and lymphocytes increase in women with breast cancer following massage therapy. *International Journal of Neuroscience, 115,* 495–510.

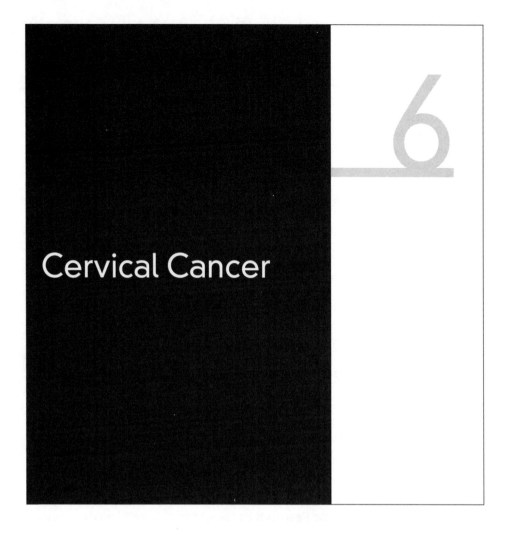

Cervical Cancer

Environment

1. Computed Tomography (CT) scans
   a. *Actions/expected responses:* CT scans could be responsible for raising the risk of cancer.
   b. *Routes/dosages/frequencies:* A typical CT scan delivers 50 to 100 times more radiation than a conventional X-ray.
   c. *Cautions:* Brenner and Hall (2007) estimate that one-third of all CT scans might not be necessary.
   d. *Assessments:* Assess number of CT scans.
   e. *Tips on use:* Use the safer options of ultrasound and magnetic resonance imaging, which do not expose women to radiation.
   f. *Other considerations:* An estimated 62 million CT scans were performed in 2006 compared to only 3 million in 1980.
   g. *References/other sources:*
      Brenner, D., & Hall, E. J. (2007). Computed tomography, an increasing source of radiation exposure. *New England Journal of Medicine, 357*(22), 2277–2284.

2. Music
   a. *Actions/expected responses:* Listening to music during colposcopy produced a significant reduction in anxiety levels as compared to pretest counseling, information leaflets, and video information.
   b. *Routes/dosages/frequencies:* Listening during colposcopy screening.
   c. *Cautions:* Select music that is calming to the woman.
   d. *Assessments:* Assess anxiety prior to, during, and after colposcopy.
   e. *Tips on use:* Although not all sources agree, classical music, ballroom dance music, and familiar songs from pleasant situations may be best.
   f. *Other considerations:* Many women find the procedure highly stressful and have particularly high levels of anxiety before and during colposcopy.
   g. *References/other sources:*
      Campbell, D. (1997). *The Mozart effect: Tapping the power of music to heal the body, strengthen the mind and unlock the creative spirit.* New York: Avon.
      John Wiley & Sons, Inc. (2007, July 18). Colposcopy: Playing music helps women relax. *ScienceDaily.* Retrieved November 10, 2007, from http://www.sciencedaily.com/releases/2007/07/070718002440.htm
3. Oral contraceptive use
   a. *Actions/expected responses:* The use of oral contraceptive use is linked to an increase in cervical cancer.
   b. *Routes/dosages/frequencies:* The relative risk for cancer rises with increasing duration of oral contraceptive use.
   c. *Cautions:* Counsel women to use other forms of birth control that are less risky.
   d. *Assessments:* Assess women's use of oral contraceptives.
   e. *Tips on use:* None.
   f. *Other considerations:* Combined oral contraceptives are classified by the International Agency for Research on Cancer as a cause of cervical cancer. The risk declines after use ceases.
   g. *References/other sources:*
      Appleby, P., Beral, V., Berrington de Gonzalez, A., Colin, D., Franceschi, S., Goodhill, A., et al. (2007). Cervical cancer and hormonal contraceptives: Collaborative reanalysis of individual data for 16,573 women with cervical cancer and 35,509 women without cervical cancer from 24 epidemiological studies. *Lancet, 370*(9599), 1591–1592.

Exercise/Movement

1. Yoga
   a. *Actions/expected responses:* Yoga improves the quality of life and provides the energy lacking in most cancers.
   b. *Routes/dosages/frequencies:* Daily abdominal breathing can increase calm
   c. *Cautions:* None.
   d. *Assessments:* Assess quality of life and energy levels prior to and after completing abdominal breathing.
   e. *Tips on use:* See http://www.yogajournal.com/basics/614.
   f. *Other considerations:* See http://www.santosha.com/asanas/asana.html.

g. *References/other sources:*

Rosenbaum, E., Gautier, H., Fobair, P., Neri, E., Festa, B., Hawn, M., et al. (2004). Cancer supportive care, improving the quality of life for cancer patients. A program evaluation report. *Support Care Cancer, 12*(5), 293–301.

Herbs/Essential Oils

1. Aromatherapy
   a. *Actions/expected responses:* Laboratory and clinical research with women has shown that the use of essential oils from plants (typically chamomile, geranium, and lavender) support and balance the mind, body, and spirit and can enhance quality of life and reduce pain.
   b. *Routes/dosages/frequencies:* Inhalation or skin application (in a carrier oil) as requested after initial treatment.
   c. *Cautions:* None known. Safety testing on essential oils has found very few if any adverse effects.
   d. *Assessments:* Assess quality of life and pain prior to and after using aromatherapy.
   e. *Tips on use:* Allow women to choose the oils or combinations that work best for them.
   f. *Other considerations:* Inhale a specific essential oil(s) or add a few drops to bath or pillow. Aromatherapy has been shown to significantly improve life satisfaction, the most important predictor of survival for women with advanced cancer.
   g. *References/other sources:*
      Fox Chase Cancer Center. (2007, November 1). Quality of life is the most important predictor of survival for advanced cancer patients. *Science-Daily.* Retrieved November 12, 2007, from http://www.sciencedaily. com/releases/2007/10/07/071030170208.htm

      Gatlin, C. G., & Schulmeister, L. (2007). When medication is not enough: Nonpharmalogic management of pain. *Clinical Journal of Oncology Nursing, 11*(5), 699–704.
2. Milk thistle (Silybum marianum)
   a. *Actions/expected responses:* Milk thistle inhibits cancer cell growth in human cervical cells.
   b. *Routes/dosages/frequencies:* 200 to 400 mg silymarin per day.
   c. *Cautions:* Adverse effects are rare, but may include stomach pain, nausea, vomiting, diarrhea, headache, rash, joint pain, and anaphylaxis in allergic women. Avoid if pregnant or lactating or if hypersensitive (have a known sensitivity to ragweed, marigolds, or chrysanthemums).
   d. *Assessments:* Assess hypersensitivity to milk thistle.
   e. *Tips on use:* Milk thistle may protect against liver damage from antipsychotics, acetaminophen, phenytoin, and halothane.
   f. *Other considerations:* Preliminary research suggests that silybin may enhance the tumor-fighting effects of cisplatin and doxorubicin.
   g. *References/other sources:*
      Post-White, J., Ladas, E. J., & Kelly, K. M. (2007). Advances in the use of milk thistle (Silybum marianum). *Integrative Cancer Therapy, 6*(2), 104–109.

Mindset

1. Affirmations
   a. *Actions/expected responses:* Self-affirmation of personal values and beliefs buffers neuroendocrine and psychological stress such as not trusting the flow of life.
   b. *Routes/dosages/frequencies:* Repeat aloud or write positive affirmations up to 20 times a day such as "I now care for and nourish myself with love and joy," "I love and approve of myself," "I allow others to be who they are," and "I trust the process of life."
   c. *Cautions:* Give yourself permission to be positive and heal; think about being positive or think about feeling safe.
   d. *Assessments:* Assess resistance to using affirmations. This may be an important warning sign that you need containment and support, not exposure to feared situations. If unable to contemplate the actual change, the affirmations, "I can think about loving and approving of myself" or "I can allow others to be" or "I can think about trusting processes of life," may be useful as beginning affirmations. When ready, move to "I love and approve of myself," and/or "I trust the processes of life."
   e. *Tips on use:* Develop your own positive affirmations.
   f. *Other considerations:* For ideas, see affirmations information at www.success consciousness.com/index_00000a.htm
   g. *References/other sources:*
   Hay, L. (2000). *Heal your body.* Carlsbad, CA: Hay House.
   Schwarzer, R., Babler, J., Kwiatek, P., Schroder, K., & Zang, J. W. (1997). The assessment of optimistic self-beliefs: Assessment of general perceived self-efficacy in thirteen cultures. *World Psychology, 3*(1–2), 177–190.

Nutrition

1. Cruciferous vegetables
   a. *Actions/expected responses:* Cruciferous vegetables suppressed the proliferation of cervical tumor cells in initial clinical trials in women.
   b. *Routes/dosages/frequencies:* Eat 1/2 to 1 cup of one or more of the following vegetables: cabbage, radishes, cauliflower, broccoli, Brussels sprouts, and daikon.
   c. *Cautions:* None.
   d. *Assessments:* Assess intake of these vegetables.
   e. *Tips on use:* Except for daikon and radishes, which are eaten raw, cauliflower and broccoli florets and small heads of cabbage should be quartered and gently steamed for no more than 5 minutes to release the cancer-protective substances.
   f. *Other considerations:* To enhance taste, dribble vegetables with olive oil and lemon juice.
   g. *References/other sources:*
   Aggarwall, B. B., & Ichikawa, H. (2005). Molecular targets and anticancer potential of indole-4-carbinol and its derivatives. *Cell Cycle, 4*(9), 1201–1215.

Chen, D. Z., Qi, M., Auborn, K. J., & Carter, T. H. (2001). Indole-3-carbinol and diindolymethane induce apoptosis of human cervical cancer cells and in murine HPV16-transgenic preneoplastic cervical epithelium. *Journal of Nutrition, 131*(12), 3294–3230.

Jin, L., Qi, M., Chen, D. Z., Anderson, A., Yang, G. Y., Arbeit, J. M., et al. (1999). Indole-3-carbinol prevents cervical cancer in human papilloma virus type 16 (HPV16) transgenic mice. *Cancer Research, 59*(16), 3991–3997.

Vallejo, F., Tomas-Barberan, F. A., & Garcia-Viguera, C. (2003). Phenolic compounds content in edible parts of broccoli inflorescences after domestic cooking. *Journal of Science and Food Agriculture, 83*(14), 1151–1156.

2. Folate
   a. *Actions/expected responses:* Women with human papillomavirus may reduce their risk of cervical cancer by increasing their intake of folate. Because national surveys revealed most women did not consume adequate folate, a grain fortification program is in place.
   b. *Routes/dosages/frequencies:* Leafy green vegetables (like spinach and turnip greens), fruits (citrus fruits and juices), and dried beans and peas are all natural sources of folate that can help meet the suggested amount of 1,000 mcg a day. Women on diets who do not eat breads, cereals, or pasta, who abuse alcohol, or who take medications that interfere with folate absorption may not receive sufficient amounts of the nutrient and may need additional amounts.
   c. *Cautions:* Medications and medical conditions that increase the need for folate or result in an increased excretion of folate include: anticonvulsant medications, metformin, sulfasalazine, triamterene, methotrexate, barbiturates, pregnancy and lactation, alcohol abuse, malabsorption, kidney dialysis, liver disease, and certain anemias. Because folate is a water soluble B-vitamin, unneeded amounts will be eliminated in the urine.
   d. *Assessments:* Assess for signs of folate deficiency: anemia, diarrhea, loss of appetite, weight loss, weakness, sore tongue, headaches, heart palpitations, irritability, forgetfulness, behavioral disorders, and an elevated level of homocysteine.
   e. *Tips on use:* Avoid fortified foods as a source of folic acid; new research has shown the introduction of flour fortified with folic acid into common foods has been linked to colon cancer.
   f. *Other considerations:* Exceeding 1,000 mcg (micrograms) per day of folate may trigger vitamin B12 deficiency. To compensate, take a multivitamin that contains B12 or eat at least one food daily that contains B12: nutritional yeast (unless susceptible to candida), clams, eggs, herring, kidney, liver, mackerel, seafood, milk, or dairy products.
   g. *References/other sources:*

Blackwell Publishing Ltd. (2007, November 5). Folic acid linked to increased cancer rate, historical review suggests. *ScienceDaily.* Retrieved November 29, 2007, from http://www.sciencedaily.com-/releases/2007/11/07/071102111956.htm

Piyathilake, C. J., Macaluso, M., Brill, I., Heimburger, D. C., & Partridge, E. E. (2007). Lower red blood cell folate enhances the HPV-16-associated risk of cervical intraepithelial neoplasia. *Nutrition, 23*(3), 203–210.

3. Selenium
   a. *Actions/expected responses:* Increased selenium intake has been associated with decreased risk of cancer. Garlic and onions and members of the brassica family (broccoli, cauliflower, cabbage, Brussels sprouts, and kohlrabi) are able to extract selenium from the soil, providing selenium-containing phytochemicals that show anticarcinogenic potentials.
   b. *Routes/dosages/frequencies:* Most soils worldwide are deficient in this mineral. Eat as many of these foods as possible from selenium-rich soils, such as organic sources.
   c. *Cautions:* Selenium can be toxic when taken as a supplement instead of in food. Avoid selenium marked "sodium selenite." Selenium labeled "1-selenomethionine" is less likely to cause side effects and won't react with vitamin C to block selenium absorption. Consult a physician before taking doses over 100 micrograms (mcg).
   d. *Assessments:* Assess intake of selenium-rich foods.
   e. *Tips on use:* Other food sources of selenium include shellfish, Brazil nuts, vegetables, eggs, brewer's yeast, broccoli, brown rice, chicken, dairy products, liver, molasses, salmon, tuna, vegetables, wheat germ, and whole grains. No harm has been reported from obtaining selenium via food.
   f. *Other considerations:* Selenium deficiency can cause anemia, immune inactivity, infertility in men, hair loss, chest pains, heart muscle enlargement, irregular heartbeat, and is linked to cancer and heart disease.
   g. *References/other sources:*
      Irion, C. W. (1999). Growing alliums and brassicas in selenium-enriched soils increases their anti-carcinogenic potentials. *Medical Hypotheses, 53*(3), 232–235.
      Ravn-Haren, G., Bugel, S., Krath, B. N., Hoac, T., Stagsted, J., Jorgensen, K., et al. (2007). A short-term intervention trial with selenate, selenium-enriched yeast and selenium-enriched milk: Effects on oxidative defence regulation. *British Journal of Nutrition, 99*(4), 883–892.

4. Soy
   a. *Actions/expected responses:* Soyasaponins have been shown to inhibit the proliferation of cancer cells.
   b. *Routes/dosages/frequencies:* Eat soy foods daily to reduce the proliferation of cancer cells.
   c. *Cautions:* Nonfermented forms of soy foods may reduce assimilation of calcium, magnesium, copper, iron, and zinc because of their high levels of phytic acid.
   d. *Assessments:* Assess intake of soy foods.
   e. *Tips on use:* The best sources are organic fermented products like tempeh or miso.
   f. *Other considerations:* Many nonorganic soy beans have been genetically modified (never researched for their long-term effects) and treated with dangerous chemicals, so they should be avoided.
   g. *References/other sources:*
      Xiao, J. X., Huang, G. Q., & Zhang, S. H. (2007). Soyasaponins inhibit the proliferation of Hela cells by inducing apoptosis. *Experimental Toxicology and Pathology, 59*(1), 35–42.

5. Vegetables (other)
   a. *Actions/expected responses:* Oncogenic human papillomavirus (HPV) infection is the main factor in cervical cancer, although infection alone is insufficient to produce disease. Cofactors such as nutrition may be necessary for viral progression to neoplasia. Results from previous studies have suggested that higher dietary consumption and circulating levels of certain micronutrients, such as vitamin A and carotenoids, may be protective against cervical cancer, as may watercress.
   b. *Routes/dosages/frequencies:* Eat 5–10 vegetables daily, especially orange and dark green versions, including pumpkin, squash, cantaloupe, spinach, sweet potato, apricot, kale, broccoli, mango, cooked greens, sweet red peppers, turnip greens, and carrots. For more information on beta-carotene, go to http://www.ynhh.org/online/nutrition/advisor/beta_carotene.html. Watercress can reduce the risk of cancer via decreased damage to DNA and possible modulation of antioxidant status by increasing carotenoid concentrations.
   c. *Cautions:* None.
   d. *Assessments:* Assess intake of vegetables at baseline and 3 and 9 months postbaseline.
   e. *Tips on use:* Lightly steam (5 minutes) chopped vegetables. Eat cooked tomatoes (juice, ketchup, sauce, soup) or cook only the reddest to obtain sufficient lycopene.
   f. *Other considerations:* Higher levels of vegetable consumption were associated with a 54% decreased risk of HPV. A 56% reduction in HPV risk was observed in women with the highest plasma cis-lycopene concentrations compared with women with the lowest plasma cis-lycopene concentrations.
   g. *References/other sources:*
      Gill, C. I., Haldar, S., Boyd, L.A., Bennett, R., Whiteford, J., Butler, M., et al. (2007). Watercress supplementation in diet reduces lymphocyte DNA damage and alters blood antioxidant status in healthy adults. *American Journal of Clinical Nutrition 85*(2), 504–510.
      Peng, Y. M., Peng, Y. S., Childers, J. M., Hatch, K. D., Roe, D. J., Lin, Y., et al. (1998). Concentrations of carotenoids, tocopherols, and retinol in paired plasma and cervical tissue of patients with cervical cancer, precancer, and noncancerous diseases. *Cancer Epidemiological Biomarkers and and Prevention, 7*(4), 347–350.
      Sedjo, R. L., Roe, D. J., Abrahamsen, M., Harris, R. B., Craft, N., Baldwin, S., et al. (2002). Vitamin A, carotenoids and risk of persistent oncogenic human papillomavirus infection. *Cancer Epidemiology Biomarkers and Prevention, 11*, 876–884.

6. Vitamin-rich foods
   a. *Actions/expected responses:* Vitamin A, B12, D, and E foods have been shown to protect against cervical cancer.
   b. *Routes/dosages/frequencies:* Vitamin A is available in animal livers, fish liver oils, apricot, asparagus, beet greens, broccoli, cantaloupe, carrots, collards, dandelion greens, garlic, kale, mustard greens, papayas, peaches, pumpkin, red peppers, spinach, sweet potatoes, Swiss chard, turnip greens,

watercress, and yellow squash. Vitamin B12 is available in clams, eggs, herring, kidney, liver, mackerel, milk and dairy products, seafood, soybeans and soy products, and sea vegetables (dulse, kelp, kombu, and nori). Vitamin E is found in green leafy vegetables, legumes (peanuts, dried beans, and peas), seeds (e.g., sunflower and pumpkin), whole grains, brown rice, cornmeal, eggs, milk, soybeans, sweet potatoes, watercress, wheat, and wheat germ.

c. *Cautions:* Avoid genetically engineered products and produce as they have not been tested for long-term effects.

d. *Assessments:* Assess intake for vitamin A, vitamin B12, and vitamin E foods.

e. *Tips on use:* Most vegetables (except spinach) should be cut and lightly steamed to obtain the most nutrients.

f. *Other considerations:* A vitamin B-12 deficiency can be caused by malabsorption, which is most common in older women and those with digestive disorders.

g. *References/other sources:*

Friedrich, M., Villena-Heinsen, C., Axt-Fliedner, R., Meyberg, R., Tilgen, W., Schmidt, W., et al. (2002). Analysis of 25-hydroxyvitamin D3–1alpha-hydroxylase in cervical tissue. *Anticancer Research, 22*(1A), 183–186.

Lwanbunjan, K., Saengkar, P., Cheeramakara, C., Tangjitgamol, S., & Chitcharoenrung, K. (2006). Vitamin B12 status of Thai women with neoplasia of the cervix uteri. *Southeast Asian Journal of Tropical Medicine and Public Health, 37*(3 Suppl.), 178–183.

Shannon, J., Thomas, D. B., Ray, R. M., Kestin, M., Koetsawang, A., Koetsawang, S., et al. (2002). Dietary risk factors for invasive and in-situ cervical carcinomas in Bangkok, Thailand. *Cancer Causes Control, 13*(8), 691–699.

Siegel, E. M., Craft, N. E., Duarte-Franco, E., Villa L. L., Franco, E. L., & Giuliano, A. R. (2007). Associations between serum carotenoids and tocopherols and type-specific HPV persistence: The Ludwig-McGill cohort study. *International Journal of Cancer, 120*(3), 672–680.

Stress Management

1. Mindfulness-based stress reduction

a. *Actions/expected responses:* A weak immune system is one of the major factors that promotes cancer metastases after an operation, chemotherapy, or radiation therapy. Fear and stress weaken the immune system. Adequate stress management prior to and after medical treatment may help to prevent metastases. Women with abnormal pap smear participated in a mindfulness-based stress reduction (MBSR) program that was evaluated very positively by participants, and there was a significant reduction in anxiety.

b. *Routes/dosages/frequencies:* 2 hours each week over 6 consecutive weeks.

c. *Cautions:* May not be congruent with the following diagnoses: antisocial personality disorder, borderline personality disorder, current major depressive disorder, physical impairment that precludes attending class, posttraumatic stress disorder, psychosis, social anxiety (if it interferes with participation in class), substance abuse or addiction (current or recovery within the past year), suicidal intent or plan, or unstable medical diagnosis.

d. *Assessments:* Rate quality of life and stress symptoms from 0 (none) to 10 (high amount) prior to and after participating in mindfulness sessions.

e. *Tips on use:* Go to http://www.stjohn.org/innerpage.aspx?PageID=1779

f. *Other considerations:* Other Web sites that may be useful are http://www.mindfulnessmeditationcentre.org/breathingGathas.htm and http://www.meditationcenter.com

g. *References/other sources:*

Abercrombie, P. D., Zamora, A., & Korn, A. P. (2007). Lessons learned: Providing a mindfulness-based stress reduction program for low-income multiethnic women with abnormal pap smears. *Holistic Nursing Practitioner, 21*(1), 26–34.

Tel Aviv University. (2008, February 29). Stress and fear can affect cancer's recurrence. *ScienceDaily.* Retrieved March 9, 2008, from http://www.sciencedaily.com/releases/2008/02/080227142656.htm

Supplements

1. Cactus pear

a. *Actions/expected responses:* Cactus pear inhibits growth of cervical cancer cells in cultured cells and in an animal model, and modulates the expression of tumor-related genes.

b. *Routes/dosages/frequencies:* Two capsules with meals three times a day (or eat the fruit).

c. *Cautions:* None known. Cactus pear contains numerous antioxidants.

d. *Assessments:* Assess the effects of cactus pear on cancer cell growth.

e. *Tips on use:* Store supplements in a cool, dry place.

f. *Other considerations:* Cactus pear fruit can also be eaten; it is found in the produce section of grocery stores. Cactus pear effects are comparable with those caused by a synthetic retinoid currently used in chemoprevention trials.

g. *References/other sources:*

Tesoriere, L. (2004). Supplementation with cactus pear fruit decreases oxidative stress in healthy humans: A comparative study with vitamin C. *Journal of Clinical Nutrition, 80*(2), 391–395.

Zou, D. M., Brewer, M., Garcia, F., Feugang, J. M., Wang, R., Liu, H., et al. (2005). Cactus pear: A natural product in cancer chemoprevention. *Nutrition Journal, 8*(4), 25.

2. Mistletoe

a. *Actions/expected responses:* Mistletoe lengthens the survival time of women with cervical cancer and increases psychosomatic self-regulation more markedly than does conventional therapy alone.

b. *Routes/dosages/frequencies:* Dried leaves, 3–6 grams three times a day, fluid extract, 2–3 ml three times a day (1:1 dilution in 25% alcohol), or tincture, 0.5 ml twice to three times a day (1:5 dilution in 45% alcohol).

   c. *Cautions:* Because mistletoe is a uterine stimulant, it should not be used during pregnancy. Avoid mistletoe if hypersensitive, lactating, or during progressive infections. Mistletoe is a toxic plant and should be kept out of reach of children. Possible adverse reactions include change in blood pressure and cardiac arrest, nausea, vomiting, anorexia, diarrhea, gastritis, and hepatitis.

   d. *Assessments:* Assess for any adverse reaction to mistletoe.

   e. *Tips on use:* Store mistletoe away from heat, light, and moisture.

   f. *Other considerations:* Mistletoe may increase the hypotensive effect of antihypertensives and should not be taken with cardiac glycosides (digoxin, digitoxin, and calcium channel blockers), immunosuppressants, or iron salts. This supplement can also be used to reduce cancer-related fatigue.

   g. *References/other sources:*

       Grossarth-Maticek, R., & Ziegler, R. (2006). Prospective controlled cohort studies on long-term therapy of cervical cancer patients with a mistletoe preparation. *Forsch Komplement Med, 14*(3), 140–147.

       Sood, A., Barton, D. L., Bauer, B. A., & Loprinzi, C. I. (2007). A critical review of complementary therapies for cancer-related fatigue. *Integrative Cancer Therapies, 6*(1), 8–13.

3. Pycnogenol and ginkgo biloba extract

   a. *Actions/expected responses:* Either pycnogenol or ginkgo biloba extract can protect against antimutagenic activity in animal studies.

   b. *Routes/dosages/frequencies:* 5–100 microgram/mL.

   c. *Cautions:* Until more research is completed, pregnant and lactating women should not use these supplements, nor should they be given to children. Avoid taking ginkgo concurrently with anticoagultants.

   d. *Assessments:* Assess reaction to pycnogenol and ginkgo.

   e. *Tips on use:* Store supplements in a cool, dry place.

   f. *Other considerations:* Pycnogenol has also been found useful in preventing venous thrombosis, thrombophlebitis, gingival bleeding and plaque, inflammatory bowel disease, venous insufficiency, digestive conditions, and menopause symptoms.

   g. *References/other sources:*

       Krizkova, L., Chovanova, Z., Durackova, Z., & Krajcovic, J. (2008). Antimutagenic in vitro activity of plan polyphenols: Pycnogenol and Ginkgo biloba extract. *Phytotherapy Research, 22*(3), 384–388.

Touch

1. Foot reflexology

   a. *Actions/expected responses:* Life satisfaction was significantly improved in the experimental group after foot reflexology. Combined with aromatherapy and foot soak, reflexology also relieves fatigue in clients with cancer. Foot reflexology or self-administered foot reflexology also significantly enhances and strengthens the immune system so it can catch and eliminate cancer cells and prevent tumors from developing.

b. *Routes/dosages/frequencies:* Twice a week for 4 weeks. Three-minute foot soak contains warm water and lavender essential oil, and is followed by reflexology treatment with jojoba oil containing lavender for 10 minutes.

c. *Cautions:* Avoid foot reflexology during pregnancy because certain manipulations can lead to premature labor. Those with foot problems, gout, arthritis, and vascular conditions such as varicose veins should be careful using this procedure. Perform a patch test with lavender essential oil prior to foot soak.

d. *Assessments:* Evaluate life satisfaction prior to and after foot reflexology sessions. See http://employees.oneonta.edu/vomsaaw/w/handouts%20-%20happiness/life%20satisfaction%20WvS%20questionnaire.pdf. Evaluate fatigue with the Cancer Fatigue Scale before, 1 hour after, and 4 hours after treatment.

e. *Tips on use:* For foot charts, see http://groups.msn.com/AlternativesToPainandDisease/reflexologyinstructionspg1.msnw

f. *Other considerations:* Quality of life is the most important predictor of survival for advanced cancer clients. See http://groups.msn.com/AlternativesToPainandDisease/reflexologyinstructionspg2.msnw

g. *References/other sources:*

Kesselring, A. (1994). Foot reflex zone massage. *Schweizerische Medizinische Wochenschrift, 62,* 88–93.

National Cancer Institute. (2006). *Immunity and cancer.* Retrieved February 6, 2008, from http://www.nci.nih.gov/cancertopics/understandingcancer/immunesystem/Slide32

2. Massage

a. *Actions/expected responses:* A weak immune system is one of the major factors that promotes cancer metastases after an operation, chemotherapy, or radiation therapy. Fear and stress weaken the immune system. Adequate stress management prior to and after medical treatment may help to prevent metastases. Aromatherapy massage is associated with reducing anxiety and depression in cancer clients, and with promoting sleep.

b. *Routes/dosages/frequencies:* Weekly.

c. *Cautions:* The aged, extremely ill, or dying individuals may require a gentle massage. The head is also a sensitive area; only gentle sweeping motions are used, and energy is not concentrated in that area.

d. *Assessments:* Chart mood and sleep patterns prior to and after massage.

e. *Tips on use:* Go to http://www.ehow.com/how_12801_aromatherapy-with-bodywork.html

f. *Other considerations:* Avoid concentrating energy in any area where cancer may reside.

g. *References/other sources:*

Rho, K. H., Han, S. H., Kim, K. S., & Lee, M. S. (2006). Effects of aromatherapy massage on anxiety and self-esteem in Korean elderly women: A pilot study. *International Journal of Neuroscience, 116*(12), 1447–1555.

Soden, K., Vincent, K., Craske, S., Lucas, C., & Ashley, S. (2004). A randomized controlled trial of aromatherapy massage in a hospice setting. *Palliative Medicine, 18*(2), 87–92.

Wilkinson, S. M., Love, S. B., Westcombe, A. M., Gambles, M. A. Burgess, C. C., Cargill, A., et al. (2007). Effectiveness of aromatherapy massage in the management of anxiety and depression in patients with cancer: A multicenter randomized controlled trail. *Journal of Clinical Oncology, 25*(5), 532–539.

3. Therapeutic touch (TT)

    a. *Actions/expected responses:* A weak immune system is one of the major factors that promotes cancer metastases after an operation, chemotherapy, or radiation therapy. Fear and stress weaken the immune system. Adequate stress management prior to and after medical treatment may help to prevent metastases. Women who received three noncontact therapeutic touch treatments reported increased well-being as opposed to a control group who rested.

    b. *Routes/dosages/frequencies:* 15–20 minutes once a day.

    c. *Cautions:* The aged, extremely ill, or dying should be given a 5 minute (or less) treatment by an experienced practitioner.

    d. *Assessments:* Take a baseline measure of well-being prior to and after administering TT.

    e. *Tips on use:* Center and calm yourself by closing your eyes and focusing on breathing in your abdomen. When relaxed, rub your hands together and feel the tingling sensation as you slowly pull your hands apart until able to feel the energies balancing between the hands. Hold the intent to balance the other person's energy and start with your hands above the woman's head. Keep an inch or so away from the body, bring your hands slowly down, sweeping down the body slowly, ending a few inches past the feet. For more information, go to http://www.healgrief.com/Site/Heal_Grief_in_Your_Body.html

    f. *Other considerations:* Regular TT treatments may enhance the effect achieved.

    g. *References/other sources:*

        Giasson, M. (1998). Effect of therapeutic touch on the well-being of persons with terminal cancer. *Journal of Holistic Nursing, 16*(3), 383–398.

        Tel Aviv University. (2008, February 29). Stress and fear can affect cancer's recurrence. *ScienceDaily.* Retrieved March 9, 2008, from http://www.sciencedaily.com/releases/2008/02/080227142656.htm

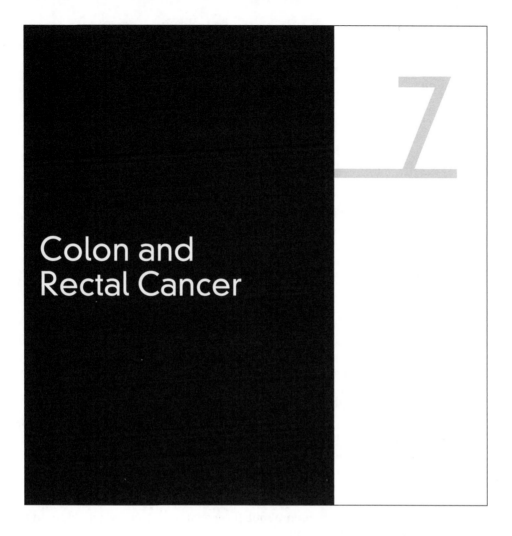

Colon and Rectal Cancer

Surgery is the major medical treatment for colon cancer. Less invasive and effective, evidence-based complementary approaches are available.

Environment

1. Computed Tomography (CT) scans
   a. *Actions/expected responses:* CT scans could be responsible for raising the risk of cancer.
   b. *Routes/dosages/frequencies:* A typical CT scan delivers 50 to 100 times more radiation than a conventional X-ray.
   c. *Cautions:* Brenner and Hall (2007) estimate that one-third of all CT scans might not be necessary.
   d. *Assessments:* Assess number of CT scans.
   e. *Tips on use:* Suggest using the safer options of ultrasound and magnetic resonance imaging, which do not expose women to radiation.
   f. *Other considerations:* An estimated 62 million CT scans were performed in 2006 compared to only 3 million in 1980.

    g. *References/other sources:*

       Brenner, D., & Hall, E. J. (2007). Computed tomography, an increasing source of radiation exposure. *New England Journal of Medicine, 357*(22), 2277–2284.

2. Severe on-the-job aggravation

    a. *Actions/expected responses:* Severe on-the-job aggravation appears to increase the risk of developing colon and rectal cancers. Those who reported a history of workplace problems over the past 10 years faced five and half times the colorectal cancer risk of adults who reported no such problems. Individuals who toil in high-pressure situations while possessing little or no control over workplace decisions face the highest risks.

    b. *Routes/dosages/frequencies:* Anytime over the past 10 years.

    c. *Cautions:* This kind of employment situation may lead to colorectal cancer.

    d. *Assessments:* Assess for severe on-the-job aggravation.

    e. *Tips on use:* Use information gathered to counsel women regarding their work.

    f. *Other considerations:* The study compared 1,079 participants in California and Sweden who answered a series of questions about stressful events.

    g. *References/other sources:*

       Courtney, J. G., Longnecker, M. P., Theorell, T., & deVerdier, M. G. (1993). Stressful life events and the risk of colorectal cancer. *Epidemiology, 4,* 404–411.

3. Smoking

    a. *Actions/expected responses:* Nicotine promotes colon tumor growth.

    b. *Routes/dosages/frequencies:* By mouth.

    c. *Cautions:* Nicotine, an active alkaloid in tobacco, has been implicated in carcinogenesis.

    d. *Assessments:* Assess use of cigarettes or nicotine patches.

    e. *Tips on use:* Caution women about the negative effects of smoking and discuss smoking cessation programs.

    f. *Other considerations:* Introducing women who smoke to a lung cancer victim may provide the motivation to quit smoking.

    g. *References/other sources:*

       Wong, H. P., Yu, L., Lam, E. K., Tai, E. K., Wu, W. K., & Cho, C. H. (2007). Nicotine promotes colon tumor growth and angiogenesis through beta-adrenergic activation. *Toxicology Science, 97*(2), 279–287.

4. Sunlight

    a. *Actions/expected responses:* Studies show a strong correlation between high vitamin D consumption and reduced risk of cancer.

    b. *Routes/dosages/frequencies:* For White women, 10–15 minutes of direct midday sun at least twice a week on the face, arms, hands, or back is sufficient, according to the National Institutes of Health. Darker-skinned women may require three to six times as much exposure.

    c. *Cautions:* More frequent exposure may result in skin cancer. Insufficient exposure to the sun can result in improper absorption of calcium and phosphorus, leading to imperfect skeletal formation as well as bone disorders.

    d. *Assessments:* Assess the amount of time women spend in direct sunlight.

    e. *Tips on use:* Help women to develop a plan for obtaining sufficient sunlight, depending on their lifestyle. Eating lunch outside when weather permits could be one solution. In winter climes, women may need to ingest more cod liver oil, fatty fish and fish oils, and egg yolks.

f. *Other considerations:* Vitamin D2, found in fortified foods, especially breads and cereals, is poorly metabolized by the body. Certain drugs can interfere with vitamin D metabolism, including corticosteroids, phenytoin, heparin, cimetidine, isoniazid, rifampin, phenobarbital, and primidone. Counsel women to find alternate medications whenever possible so they can metabolize vitamin D3.

g. *References/other sources:*

Demgrow, M. (2007, June). High vitamin D: Treatment for cancer prevention? *The Clinical Advisor, 54,* 57.

Jockers, B. S. (2007). Vitamin D sufficiency: An approach to disease prevention. *The American Journal for Nurse Practitioners, 11*(10), 43–50.

5. Water

a. *Actions/expected responses:* Evidence exists of an inverse relationship between glasses of plain water per day and colon cancer risk.

b. *Routes/dosages/frequencies:* Counsel women to drink at least 8, and preferably 10 glasses of water a day to reduce colon cancer risk.

c. *Cautions:* Many tap water systems provide water that contains lead, coliform bacteria, carcinogenic byproducts of chlorination, arsenic, radioactive radon, pesticides, and byproducts of rocket fuel. In addition, many water systems are deteriorating because of old infrastructure and use of out-of-date water treatment technologies.

d. *Assessments:* Assess intake of drinking water.

e. *Tips on use:* Drink distilled or reverse-osmosis filtered water.

f. *Other considerations:* To enhance the taste of water, add several frozen berries or a lemon slice in a glass.

g. *References/other sources:*

NRDC. (2008). *What's on tap? Drinking water in U.S. cities.* Retrieved February 18, 2008 from http://www.nrdc.org/water/drinking/uscities/execsum.asp

Shannon, J., White, E., Shattuck, A. L., & Potter, J. D. (1996). Relationship of foods groups and water intake to colon cancer risk. *Cancer Epidemiology Biomarkers, 5*(7), 495–502.

Exercise/Movement

1. Leisure-time physical activity

a. *Actions/expected responses:* Physical inactivity and high body mass (greater than 29 kg/m²) and increased waist-to-hip ratio have been linked to increased risk of colon cancer, while high physical activity is protective against colon (but not rectal) cancer.

b. *Routes/dosages/frequencies:* 21 hours per week of leisure-time physical activity METs (energy expenditure multiplied by time spent at each activity) reduces risk of colon cancer by 0.54.

c. *Cautions:* To reduce risk of colon cancer, increase physical activity and maintain lean body weight.

d. *Assessments:* Assess leisure-time physical activity and any conditions that might limit exercise.

e. *Tips on use:* Complete a series of warm-up stretches prior to activity and cool-down stretches after physical activity. See http://www.wellness.ma/ adult-fitness/stretching-warmup.htm

f. *Other considerations:* There is evidence for adverse effects of overweight and obesity.

g. *References/other sources:*

Johnson, I. T., & Lund, E. K. (2007). Review article: Nutrition, obesity and colorectal cancer. *Alimentary Pharmacology and Therapy, 26(2)*, 161–181.

Martinez, M. E., Giovannucci, E., Spiegelman, D., Hunter, D. J., Willett, W. C., & Colditz, G. A. (1997). Leisure-time physical activity, body size, and colon cancer in women. Nurses' Health Study Research Group. *Journal of National Cancer Institute, 89*(13), 948–955.

Herbs/Essential Oils

1. Aromatherapy
   a. *Actions/expected responses:* Laboratory and animal studies show that essential oils, such as Roman chamomile, geranium, lavender, and cedarwood can improve the quality of life of women diagnosed with cancer by calming, energizing, and providing antibacterial qualities.
   b. *Routes/dosages/frequencies:* Inhale or apply an essential oil to the skin after first placing several drops in a carrier oil such as jojoba or castor oil.
   c. *Cautions:* Safety testing on essential oils has revealed very few, if any, bad effects.
   d. *Assessments:* Assess for hypersensitivity (skin reactions, nausea, or anorexia). Assess quality of life prior to and after using aromatherapy with essential oils.
   e. *Tips on use:* Keep aromatherapy products in a sealed container, away from heat and moisture. Test reaction to oils by asking the woman to inhale the scent of each oil and to tell which one she likes the best. Besides inhaling or using a diffuser, several drops of essential oil can also be placed in the bath water.
   f. *Other considerations:* Aromatherapy may work by sending chemical messages to the part of the brain that affects mood and emotions.
   g. *References/other sources:*

Atsumi, T., & Tonosaki, K. (2007). Smelling lavender and rosemary increases free radical scavenging activity and decreases cortisol level in saliva. *Psychiatry Research, 150*(1), 89–96.

2. Curcumin
   a. *Actions/expected responses:* This dietary spice possesses anti-inflammatory, antioxidant, antiproliferative and antiangiogenic activities. Effectiveness against cancer has been documented.
   b. *Routes/dosages/frequencies:* Can be used daily as a spice in stews, soups, fish and tofu dishes, and in salad dressings.
   c. *Cautions:* None. Safe in humans, even at high doses of 12 grams a day. In larger quantities it can have strong activity in the common bile duct that

might aggravate the passage of gallstones in women currently suffering from the condition.

    d. *Assessments:* Take a baseline measure for curcumin use.

    e. *Tips on use:* Serve curry or food seasoned with curcumin at least once a week; doing so more often may produce better results.

    f. *Other considerations:* None.

    g. *References/other sources:*

        Anand, P., Kunnumakkara, A. B., Newman, R. A., & Aggarwal, B. B. (2007). Bioavailability of curcumin: Problems and promises. *Molecular Pharmacology, 4*(6), 807–818.

        Corona-Rivera, A., Urbina-Cano, P., Bobadilla-Morales, L., Vargas-Lares, J., Ramirez-Herra, M., Mendoza-Magaua, M. L., et al. (2007). Protective in vivo effect of curcumin on copper genotoxicity evaluated by comet and micronucleus assays. *Journal of Applied Genetics, 48*(4), 389–396.

3. Licorice extract

    a. *Actions/expected responses:* The administration of licorice extract significantly inhibited tumor growth in mice inoculated with colon cancer cells.

    b. *Routes/dosages/frequencies:* 250–500 mg powdered extract three times a day or 2–4 ml (1:1 dilution) three times a day.

    c. *Cautions:* Women undergoing cisplatin therapy should avoid licorice extract. Avoid if lactating, pregnant, or hypertensive. This herb shouldn't be used by women with liver or kidney disease, heart arrhythmias or congestive heart failure, or by those with sensitivity to licorice. Adverse reactions include possible hypertension, edema, headache, weakness, nausea, vomiting, or lack of appetite.

    d. *Assessments:* Assess hypersensitivity to licorice extract.

    e. *Tips on use:* Store licorice in a cool, dry place and to avoid using licorice concurrently with grapefruit juice, diuretics, cardiac glycosides, antihypertensives, antiarrhythmics, and corticosteroids.

    f. *Other considerations:* Women taking licorice extract for extended periods should take additional potassium.

    g. *References/other sources:*

        Lee, C. K., Park, K. K., Lim, S. S., Park, J. H., & Chung, W. Y. (2007). Effects of the licorice extract against tumor growth and cisplatin-induced toxicity in a mouse xenograft model of colon cancer. *Biological Pharmacology Bulletin, 30*(11), 2191–2195.

        Skidmore-Roth, L. (2006). Licorice. In *Handbook of herbs and natural supplements* (pp. 659–665). St. Louis, MO: ElsevierMosby.

Mindset

1. Affirmations

    a. *Actions/expected responses:* Self-affirmation of personal values and beliefs buffers neuroendocrine and psychological stress.

    b. *Routes/dosages/frequencies:* Repeat aloud or write positive affirmations up to 20 times a day such as, "I lovingly forgive and release all of the past," "I choose to fill my world with joy," and "I love and approve of me."

    c. *Cautions:* Ensure affirmations are positive and acceptable.

d. *Assessments:* Assess anxiety prior to and after completing affirmations for a week.

e. *Tips on use:* Write favorite affirmations on 3 by 5 cards and place them where they will be read frequently.

f. *Other considerations:* Find more affirmations information at http://www.successconsciousness.com/index_00000a.htm

g. *References/other sources:*

Hay, L. (2000). *Heal your body.* Carlsbad, CA: Hay House.

Schwarzer, R., Babler, J., Kwiatek, P., Schroder, K., & Zang, J. W. (1997). The assessment of optimistic self-beliefs: Assessment of general perceived self-efficacy in thirteen cultures. *World Psychology, 3*(1–2), 177–190.

Nutrition

1. Almonds
   a. *Actions/expected responses:* Almonds and other nuts may reduce cancer risk and do so via at least one almost lipid-associated component.
   b. *Routes/dosages/frequencies:* One handful of almonds a day.
   c. *Cautions:* Almonds have a high fat content; do not exceed the recommended amount.
   d. *Assessments:* Assess intake of almonds and any sensitivity to the food.
   e. *Tips on use:* Choose unsalted and nonoiled brands.
   f. *Other considerations:* If difficult to digest, eat them in cereal earlier in the day, or crush them and put them in smoothies, stews, soups, sauces, or place them on top of fish and bake.
   g. *References/other sources:*

   Davis, P. A., & Iwahashi, C. K. (2001). Whole almonds and almond fractions reduce aberrant crypt foci in a rat model of colon carcinogenesis. *Cancer Letters, 165*(1), 27–33.

2. Berries
   a. *Actions/expected responses:* Black raspberry and strawberry extracts showed the most significant ability to inhibit the growth of colon cancer cells.
   b. *Routes/dosages/frequencies:* Eat raspberries or strawberries daily.
   c. *Cautions:* Avoid raspberries or strawberries if hypersensitive to them.
   d. *Assessments:* Assess hypersensitivity to raspberries and strawberries.
   e. *Tips on use.* Use local berries in the summer and rely on frozen berries the rest of the year.
   f. *References/other sources:*

   Seeram, N. P., Adams, L. S., Zhang, Y., Lee, R., Sand, D., Scheuller, H. S., et al. (2006). Blackberry, black raspberry, blueberry, cranberry, red raspberry, and strawberry extract inhibit growth and stimulate apoptosis of human cancer cells in vitro. *Journal of Agriculture and Food Chemistry, 54*(25), 9329–9339.

3. Flaxseed
   a. *Actions/expected responses:* Flaxseed contains high levels of omega-3 fatty acids and lignans effective in preventing colon tumor development.

b. *Routes/dosages/frequencies:* 1–6 tbsp a day by mouth as flaxseed meal or ground flaxseeds in cereal, salads, smoothies, or stirred into a glass of water.

c. *Cautions:* Should not be used by women with bowel obstruction, dehydration, or sensitivity to flax. Adverse reactions include nausea, vomiting, anorexia, diarrhea, and flatulence.

d. *Assessments:* Assess use of flax, sensitivity to the seeds, and possible interactions with medications.

e. *Tips with use:* Flaxseeds can be ground at home using a small food processor or coffee grinder right before ingestion.

f. *Other considerations:* Flax may decrease absorption of medications if taken concurrently. Flax may increase (a) the risk of bleeding if taken with anticoagulants/antiplatelets, (b) the action of antidiabetes agents if taken concurrently, or (c) the action of laxatives, resulting in diarrhea.

g. *References/other sources:*

Bommareddy, A., Arasada, B. L., Mathees, D. P., & Dwivedi, C. (2006). Chemopreventive effects of dietary flaxseed on colon tumor development. *Nutrition in Cancer, 54*(2), 216–222.

4. Garlic

a. *Actions/expected responses:* One randomized controlled trial reported a statistically significant (29%) reduction in both size and number of colon adenomas after taking aged garlic extract. Five of eight case control/cohort studies suggested a protective effect of high intake of raw/cooked garlic, and two of eight studies suggested a protective effect for distal colon. A published meta-analysis of seven of these studies confirmed this inverse association, with a 30% reduction in relative risk. Eleven animal studies demonstrated a significant anticarcinogenic effect of garlic and/or its constituents.

b. *Routes/dosages/frequencies:* By mouth daily. As number of portions of garlic rises, risk of colorectal cancer decreases.

c. *Cautions:* Avoid use if sensitive to garlic. May interact with antiplatelet drugs.

d. *Assessments:* Assess use of garlic. Aim to increase amount used.

e. *Tips on use:* Use more garlic in cooking. Odorless garlic is also available. Organically grown garlic contains more cancer-fighting selenium.

f. *Other considerations:* The methyl allyl trisulfide in garlic dilates blood vessel walls and inhibits blood clotting without the side effects of antiplatelet or anticoagulant therapy drugs. It improves circulation, food digestion, stimulates the immune system, is a natural antibiotic that doesn't kill good digestive bacteria, and therefore isn't as disruptive to the body's systems as are antibiotics. Treats fungal and viral infections.

g. *References/other sources:*

Galeone, C., Pelucchi, C., Levi, F., Negri, E., Franceschi, S., Talamin, R., et al. (2006). Onion and garlic use and human cancer. *American Journal of Clinical Nutrition, 84*(5), 1027–1032.

Irion, C. W. (1999). Growing alliums and brassicas in selenium-enriched soils increases their anticarcinogenic potentials. *Medical Hypotheses, 53*(3), 232–235.

Macan, H., Uykimpang, R., Clconcel, M., Takasu, J., Razon, R., Amagase, H., et al. (2006). Aged garlic extract may be safe for patients on warfarin therapy. *Journal of Nutrition, 136*(3 Suppl.), 793S–795S.

Ngo, S. N., Williams, D. B., Cobiac, L., & Head, R. J. (2007). Does garlic reduce risk of colorectal cancer? A systematic review. *Journal of Nutrition, 137*(10), 2264–2269.

5. Green tea

   a. *Actions/expected responses:* Numerous studies have shown the colon cancer preventive activity of green tea.

   b. *Routes/dosages/frequency.* By mouth, 1 tsp tea leaves in 8 oz hot water. Drink two to five cups per day.

   c. *Cautions:* Green tea may decrease iron absorption. Dairy products may decrease the therapeutic effects of green tea. Avoid during kidney inflammation, gastrointestinal ulcers, insomnia, heart and blood vessel disease, or increased intraocular pressure or use decaffeinated form.

   d. *Assessments:* Assess intake of green tea.

   e. *Tips on use:* Decaffeinated green tea may decrease side effects such as hypertension, anxiety, nervousness, or insomnia of the caffeinated version.

   f. *Other considerations:* Green tea may interact with antacids, anticoagulants, beta-adrenergic blockers, benzodiazepines, bronchodilators, and MAOIs and should not be used concurrently. Digestive process affects anticancer activity of tea in gastrointestinal cells; add citrus (such as lemon juice) or take ascorbic acid (vitamin C) to protect the catechins in green tea from digestive degradation.

   g. *References/other sources:*

   American Association for Cancer Research. (2007, August 12). Green tea boosts production of detox enzymes, rendering cancerous chemicals harmless. *ScienceDaily.* Retrieved December 20, 2007, from http://www.sciencedaily.com/releases/2007/08/070810194923.htm

   Coppola, D., & Malafa, M. (2007). Green tea polyphenols in the prevention of colon cancer. *Front Bioscience, 12,* 2309–2315.

   Federation of American Societies for Experimental Biology. (2008, April 10). Digestive process affects anti-cancer activity of tea in gastrointestinal cells. *ScienceDaily.* Retrieved April 20, 2008, from http://www.sciencedaily.com/releases/2008/04/080407172713.htm

   Skidmore-Roth, L. (2006). Green tea. In *Handbook of herbs and natural supplements* (pp. 535–539). St. Louis, MO: ElsevierMosby.

6. Mediterranean diet

   a. *Actions/Responses:* Mediterranean diet is linked with prevention of cancers.

   b. *Routes/dosages/frequencies:* High daily intake of vegetables, legumes, fruits, antioxidants and antiproliferatives, whole grain foods (high fiber), fish, and unsaturated fatty acids such as olive oil; low intake of saturated fatty acids, dairy products, meat, and poultry; and low to moderate intake of alcohol. For more information, go to http://www.mayoclinic.com/health/mediteraneandiet/CL00011

   c. *Cautions/adverse reactions:* Drink only one, 5-ounce glass of red wine a day; drinking more has been linked with health problems including cancers. Excessive dietary intake of sugar, refined carbohydrates, and animal products (meat and dairy products with high content of saturated fat), also known as a traditional Western diet, is linked with cancer. Eat only whole grains and check labels carefully; to ensure whole grains are being ingested, eat brown rice, barley, and oats.

d. *Assessments:* Assess intake of foods listed in "Other considerations." Sixty-eight percent of women do not eat five portions of fruits and vegetables a day.

e. *Tips for use:* Introduce more fruits and vegetables into the diet by eating them as snacks. Polynesian foods often use pineapple and other fruits with fish and chicken. Fruit or vegetable juices as a beverage are another way to introduce more produce into the diet. If sweetener is desired, use stevia. It has no calories or side effects and has been found to repair DNA.

f. *Other considerations:* Eat foods that are especially protective against cancer, including: apples with their peelings, pineapple (bromelain), cranberries, red grapes, strawberries, peaches, citrus fruits (contain limonene, which increases the production of enzymes that help the body dispose of carcinogens), watercress (which reduces risk of cancer via decreased damage to DNA), pears, bananas (contain caffeic acid, which aids the production of an enzyme that makes it easier for the body to get rid of carcinogens, and ferulic acid, which binds to nitrates, possibly preventing them from converting to cancer-causing nitrosamines), carrots (vitamin A, a retinoid), tomatoes, squash, corn, peanuts, oats, and barley. Also counsel women to eat daily servings of leafy green vegetables (like spinach and turnip greens) and soybeans, other dried beans, and peas (high in protective fiber, provide protease inhibitors that suppress enzyme production in cancer cells to slow tumor growth), which are all natural sources of folate, which prevents changes to DNA that can lead to cancer. Encourage women to eat daily portions of brassica vegetables, including broccoli, cauliflower, cabbage, Brussels sprouts and kohlrabi, which contain sulforaphane and other isothiocyantestes that stimulate the production of anticancer enzymes to bolster the body's natural ability to ward off cancer, and indoles that stimulate enzymes that make the hormone estrogen less effective. Also encourage women to eat allium vegetables daily, including garlic, onions, leeks, and chives, which can help block the action of cancer-causing chemicals. Counsel them to buy organic foods. They are grown in selenium-rich soils, giving them greater anticarcinogenic potential. Teach women not to microwave their vegetables and fruits; microwaving broccoli resulted in a loss of 97%, 74%, and 87% of its three major antioxidant compounds, respectively; steaming for 5 minutes resulted in a loss of only 11%, 0%, and 8%, respectively, of the same antioxidants.

g. *References/other sources:*

Aggarwal, B. B., & Ichikawa, H. (2005). Molecular targets and anticancer potential of indole-3-carbinol and its derivatives. *Cell Cyle, 4*(9), 1201–1215.

Ames, B. N. (1998). Micronutrients prevent cancer and delay aging. *Toxicology Letter, 102–103,* 5–18.

Fields, A. L., Soprano, D. R., & Soprano, K. J. (2007). Retinoids in biological control and cancer. *Journal of Cell Biochemistry, 102*(4), 886–898.

Galeone, C., Pelucchi, C., Levi, F., Negri, E., Franceschi, S., Talamini, R., et al. (2006). Onion and garlic use and human cancer. *American Journal of Clinical Nutrition, 84*(5), 1027–1032.

Ghanta, S., Banerjee, A., Poddar, A., & Chattopadhyay, S. (2007). Oxidative DNA damage preventive activity and antioxidant potential of Stevia rebaudiana (Bertoni) Bertoni, a natural sweetener. *55*(26), 10962–10967.

Gill, C. I., Haldar, S., Boyd, L. A., Bennett, R., Whiteford, J., Butler, M., et al. (2007). Watercress supplementation in diet reduces lymphocyte DNA damage and alters blood antioxidant status in healthy adults. *American Journal of Clinical Nutrition, 85*(2), 504–510.

Irion, C. W. (1999). Growing alliums and brassicas in selenium-enriched soils increases their anticarcinogenic potentials. *Medical Hypotheses, 53*(3), 232–235.

Maurer, H. R. (2001). Bromelain: Biochemistry, pharmacology and medical use. *Cell and Molecular Life Science, 58*(9),1234–1245.

Mitrou, P. N., Kipnis, V., Thiebaut, A. C., Reedy, J., Subar, A. F., Wirfalt, E., et al. (2007). Mediterranean dietary pattern and prediction of all-cause mortality in a US population: Results from the NIH-AARP Diet and Health Study. *Archives of Internal Medicine, 167*(22), 2461–2468.

Phytochemicals for cancer protection (1995). *American Institute for Cancer Research Newsletter, 46*, 46.

Sun, J., Chu, Y. F., Wu, X., & Liu, R. H. (2002). Antioxidant and antiproliferative activities of common fruits. *Journal of Agricultural and Food Chemistry, 50*(23), 6910–1916.

Vallejo, F., Tomas-Barberan, F. A., & Garcia-Viguera, C. (2003). Phenolic compounds content in edible parts of broccoli inflorescences after domestic cooking. *Journal of Science and Food Agriculture, 83*(14), 1151–1156.

7. Pomegranate seed oil
   a. *Actions/expected responses:* Pomegranate seed oil in the diet significantly inhibited the incidence of colon adenocarcinomas.
   b. *Routes/dosages/frequencies:* Seven to eight drops a day.
   c. *Cautions:* Avoid during first trimester of pregnancy.
   d. *Assessments:* Assess pregnancy status of women prior to recommending pomegranate seed oil.
   e. *Tips on use:* Keep pomegranate seed oil in a cool, dry place, away from heat and humidity.
   f. *Other considerations:* For more information, go to http://64.233.169.104/search?q=cache:Sx60RjdNpCgJ:www.rimonest.com/doc/faq1.doc+dosage +of+pomegranate+seed+oil&hl=en&ct=clnk&cd=12&gl=us
   g. *References/other sources:*
      Kohno, H., Suzuki, R.,Yasui,Y., Hosokawa, M., Miyashita, K., & Tanaka,T. (2004). Pomegranate seed oil rich in conjugated linolenic acid suppresses chemically induced colon carcinogenesis in rats. *Cancer Science, 95*(6), 481–486.

8. Probiotics
   a. *Actions/expected responses:* Probiotics (lactic acid bacteria or LAB) are present in many foods such as yogurt. Probiotics increase immune cell activity and may suppress the growth of bacteria that convert procarcinogens into carcinogens.
   b. *Routes/dosages/frequencies:* Eat plain yogurt with active organisms daily to reduce the proliferation of cancer cells.
   c. *Cautions:* None unless women are sensitive to yogurt.

d. *Assessments:* Assess intake of plain yogurt with live cultures.

e. *Tips on use:* Obtain plain, nonsweetened yogurt and sweeten it with banana, raisins, or molasses.

f. *Other considerations:* Nonorganic milk products may contain growth hormones. Use organic yogurt.

g. *References/other sources:*

Matar, C., & Perdigon, G. (2007). The application of probiotics in cancer. *British Journal of Nutrition, 98*(1 Suppl.), S105–S110.

9. Selenium

a. *Actions/expected responses:* Selenium is a chemopreventive agent that has shown efficacy in reducing colon cancer incidence.

b. *Routes/dosages/frequencies:* By mouth, no more than 400 mcg per day.

c. *Cautions/adverse reactions:* Rare, but do not exceed suggested dosage. For more information, on how to find selenium in foods, go to http://ods.od.nih.gov/factsheets/selenium.asp

d. *Assessments:* Evaluate symptoms prior to and after increasing dietary selenium.

e. *Tips on use:* If a selenium supplement is taken, factor in the intake of these foods to keep the dosage of selenium under 400 mcg. The highest level of selenium is found in Brazil nuts (275 mcg per three to four nuts), fish (20–68 mcg per 3 oz), and whole wheat spaghetti (36 mcg per cup).

f. *Other considerations:* Selenium may also protect the heart.

g. *References/other sources:*

Decensi, A., & Costa, A. (2000). Recent advances in cancer chemoprevention, with emphasis on breast and colorectal cancer. *European Journal of Cancer, 36*(6), 694–709.

Schrauzer, G. N. (2001). Nutritional selenium supplements: Product types, quality and safety. *Journal of American College of Nutrition, 20*(1), 1–4.

10. Soy

a. *Actions/expected responses:* Risk of colon cancer was reduced in women with an increased soy intake.

b. *Routes/dosages/frequencies:* 1/2 cup of dried soybeans or 1 cup of tofu or 1–3 cups of miso soup a day.

c. *Cautions:* Miso is heavily salted and should not be consumed by women with salt-sensitive hypertension.

d. *Assessments:* Assess intake of soy protein.

e. *Tips on use:* Replace portions of chicken or beef in stir-fry with small chunks of tofu, use soy burgers instead of beef burgers, snack on ¼ cup of soy nuts or 4 ounces of soy milk. Use miso as a base for vegetable soups and stews.

f. *Other considerations:* The fermentation process transforms isoflavones in miso into their active form, which is more easily used by the body.

g. *References/other sources:*

Henkel, J. (2000). Soy: Health claims for soy protein. *FDA Consumer Magazine* (May/June). Retrieved January 24, 2008, from www.fda.gov/Fdac/features/2000/300_soy.html

Oba, S., Nagata, C., Shimizu, N., Shimizu, H., Kametani, M., Takeyama, N., et al. (2007). Soy product consumption and the risk of colon cancer: A prospective study in Takayama, Japan. *Nutrition in Cancer, 57*(2), 151–157.

11. Sugar
    a. *Actions/expected responses:* Dietary sugars (sucrose and dextrin) act as either a coinitiator or promoter of preneoplastic lesions in the colon.
    b. *Routes/dosages/frequencies:* By mouth, daily.
    c. *Cautions:* Eating foods with simple sugars may lead to preneoplastic lesions in the colon.
    d. *Assessment:* Assess use of simple sugar foods: candy, cookies, cake, pies, sugar-sweetened cereals and breads, or sodas.
    e. *Tips on use:* Use safer sweeteners such as stevia or molasses.
    f. *Other considerations:* Stevia, an herb, is an alternative sweetener that prevents DNA damage, can be used by women diagnosed with diabetes or hypoglycemia, and acts like a general tonic. Use this herb in either liquid or powder form.
    g. *References/other sources:*
       Ghanta, S., Banerjee, A., Poddar, A., & Chattopadyay, S. (2007). Oxidative potential of Stevia rebaudiana (Bertoni) Bertoni, a natural sweetener. *Journal of Agricultural and Food Chemistry, 55*(26), 10962–10967.
       Poulsen, M., Molck, A. M., Thorup, I., Breinholt, V., & Meyer, O. (2001). The influence of simple sugars and starch given during pre-or post-initiation on aberrant crypt foci in rat colon. *Cancer Letters, 167*(2), 135–143.
12. Vitamin C
    a. *Actions/expected responses:* Vitamin C intake in foods and supplements is associated with a 30%–70% reduction in colon cancer risk.
    b. *Routes/dosages/frequencies:* By mouth, daily.
    c. *Cautions:* None unless allergic to vitamin C foods or supplements.
    d. *Assessments:* Assess intake of vitamin C and sensitivity to vitamin C foods or supplements.
    e. *Tips on use:* Increase their intake of vitamin C foods (asparagus, avocadoes, beet greens, black currants, broccoli, Brussels sprouts, cantaloupe, collards, dandelion greens, grapefruit, kale, lemons, mangos, mustard greens, onions, oranges, papaya, green peas, sweet peppers, persimmons, pineapple, radishes, spinach, strawberries, Swiss chard, tomatoes, turnip greens, and watercress.
    f. *Other considerations:* Vitamin C aids in the production of interferon, an immune system chemical that kills bacteria and viruses.
    g. *References/other sources:*
       Sandler, R. S. (2003). Associations of micronutrients with colon cancer risk in African Americans and Whites: Results from the North Carolina Colon Cancer Study. *Cancer Epidemiological Biomarkers and Prevention, 12*(8), 747–754.
13. Vitamin E
    a. *Actions/expected responses:* Natural and synthetic analogues of vitamin E can be used effectively as anticancer therapy either alone or in combination to enhance the therapeutic efficacy and reduce toxicity of other anticancer agents.
    b. *Routes/dosages/frequencies:* Daily high vitamin intake through combined foods and supplements was associated with a 70% reduced risk for colon cancer, especially in African Americans.
    c. *Cautions:* Obtain vitamin E from food whenever possible.

d. *Assessments:* Assess vitamin E intake.

e. *Tips on use:* Increase daily intake of leafy green vegetables (collards, mustard greens, kale), legumes, nuts, seeds, whole grains, brown rice, eggs, oatmeal, organ meats, sweet potatoes, and wheat germ.

f. *Other considerations:* African Americans have the highest incidence of colon cancer among all U.S. racial/ethnic groups.

g. *References/other sources:*

Satia-About, J., Galanko, J. A., Martin, C. F., Potter, J., Ammerman, A., & Sandler, R. S. (2003). Associations of micronutrients with colon cancer risk in African Americans and Whites: Results from the North Carolina Colon Cancer Study. *Cancer Epidemiological Biomarkers and Prevention, 12*(8), 747–754.

Sylvester, P. W. (2007). Vitamin E and apoptosis. *Vitamins and Hormones, 76,* 329–356.

Stress Management

1. Mindfulness meditation

a. *Actions/expected responses:* A weak immune system is one of the major factors that promotes cancer metastases after an operation, chemotherapy, or radiation therapy. Fear and stress weaken the immune system. Adequate stress management prior to and after medical treatment may help to prevent metastases. Women who reported high stress had a 1.64-fold higher risk of colon cancer mortality.

b. *Routes/dosages/frequencies:* Stress in daily life. Comments by women that include high or extreme stress warrant intervention.

c. *Cautions:* When stress is assessed, suggest stress reduction methods, including mindfulness meditation (see p. 33 for more information on this approach).

d. *Assessments:* Ask, "Do you feel stress during your daily life?"

e. *Tips on use:* Go to http://www.stjohn.org/innerpage.aspx?PageID=1779 or http://www.mindfulnessmeditationcentre.org/breathingGathas.htm

f. *Other considerations:* None.

g. *References/other sources:*

Kojima, M., Wakai, K., Tokudome, S., Tamakoshi, K., Toyoshima, H., Watanabe, Y., et al. (2005). Perceived psychologic stress and colorectal cancer mortality: Findings from the Japan Collaborative Cohort Study. *Psychosomatic Medicine, 67,* 72–77.

Tel Aviv University. (2008, February 29). Stress and fear can affect cancer's recurrence. *ScienceDaily.* Retrieved March 9, 2008, from http://www.sciencedaily.com/releases/2008/02/080227142656.htm

Supplements

1. Calcium

a. *Actions/expected responses:* Calcium supplementation has been shown to decrease the risk of recurrence of colorectal adenomas in randomized trials and may extend for up to 5 years after cessation of 4 years of treatment.

b. *Routes/dosages/frequencies:* 1200 mg of calcium daily.

c. *Cautions/adverse reactions:* Take calcium supplements with food to prevent the formation of kidney stones.

d. *Assessments:* Evaluate symptoms prior to and after increasing calcium intake.

e. *Tips on use:* Calcium citrate is more absorbable than calcium carbonate.

f. *Other considerations:* None.

g. *References/other sources:*

   Grau, M. V., Baron, J. A., Sandler, R. S., Wallace, K., Haile, R. W., Church, T. R., et al. (2007). Prolonged effect of calcium supplementation on risk of colorectal adenomas in a randomized trial. *Journal of the National Cancer Institute, 99*(2), 129–136.

2. Pycnogenol and ginkgo biloba extract

   a. *Actions/expected responses:* Either pycnogenol or ginkgo biloba extract can protect against antimutagenic activity in animal studies.

   b. *Routes/dosages/frequencies:* 5–100 microgram/mL.

   c. *Cautions:* Until more research is completed, pregnant and lactating women should not use these supplements, nor should they be given to children. Ginkgo should not be taken concurrently with anticoagulants.

   d. *Assessments:* Assess reaction to pycnogenol and ginkgo.

   e. *Tips on use:* Store supplements in a cool, dry place.

   f. *Other considerations:* Pycnogenol has also been found useful in preventing venous thrombosis, thrombophlebitis, gingival bleeding and plaque, inflammatory bowel disease, venous insufficiency, digestive conditions, and menopause symptoms.

   g. *References/other sources:*

      Krizkova, L., Chovanova, Z., Durackova, Z., & Krajcovic, J. (2008). Antimutagenic in vitro activity of plan polyphenols: Pycnogenol and Ginkgo biloba extract. *Phytotherapy Research, 22*(3), 384–388.

Touch

1. Acupressure

   a. *Actions/expected responses:* Acupressure is a safe and effective tool for managing chemotherapy-induced nausea and vomiting.

   b. *Routes/dosages/frequencies:* Stimulating PC6 point for at least 6 hours at the onset of chemotherapy reduced symptoms in 70% of women.

   c. *Cautions:* None.

   d. *Assessments:* Assess for nausea and vomiting.

   e. *Tips on use:* PC6 is situated in the middle of the front of the forearm above the wrist crease.

   f. *Other considerations:* For more information go to http://www.handbag.com/healthfit/complementary/acupressure/

   g. *References/other sources:*

      Gardani, G., Cerrone, R., Biella, C., Mancini, L., Proserpio, E., Casiraghi, M., et al. (2006). Effect of acupressure on nausea and vomiting induced by chemotherapy in cancer patients. *Minerva Medicine, 97*(5), 391–394.

2. Foot reflexology
   a. *Actions/expected responses:* Foot reflexology significantly reduced nausea, vomiting, and fatigue in women with breast cancer undergoing chemotherapy. Self-administered foot reflexology also enhances natural killer cells and IgG, strengthening the immune system against cancer and possibly preventing tumor development.
   b. *Routes/dosages/frequencies:* Four 40-minute treatments.
   c. *Cautions:* None unless the feet have been injured.
   d. *Assessments:* Obtain a baseline for natural killer cells and IgG pre- and post-reflexology.
   e. *Tips on use:* See http://groups.msn.com/AlternativesToPainandDisease/ reflexologyinstructionspg1.msnw and http://groups.msn.com/Alternatives ToPainandDisease/reflexologyinstructionspg2.msnw
   f. *Other considerations:* Foot reflexology has been shown to significantly improve life satisfaction, the most important predictor of survival for women with advanced cancer.
   g. *References/other sources:*
      Fox Chase Cancer Center. (2007, November 1). Quality of life is the most important predictor of survival for advanced cancer patients. *Science-Daily.* Retrieved November 12, 2007, from http://www.sciencedaily. com/releases/2007/10/07/071030170208.htm
      National Cancer Center. (2006). Immunity and cancer. Retrieved February 6, 2008, from http://www.nci.nih.go/cancertopics/understanding cancer/immunesystem/Slide32
3. Therapeutic touch (TT)
   a. *Actions/expected responses:* Women who received three noncontact therapeutic touch treatments reported increased well-being as opposed to a control group who rested.
   b. *Routes/dosages/frequencies:* 15–20 minutes once a day.
   c. *Cautions:* The aged, extremely ill, or dying should be given a 5 minute (or less) treatment by an experienced practitioner.
   d. *Assessments:* Take a baseline measure of well-being prior to and after administering TT.
   e. *Tips on use:* Center and calm yourself by closing your eyes and focusing on breathing in your abdomen. When relaxed, rub your hands together and feel the tingling sensation as you slowly pull your hands apart until able to feel the energies balancing between the hands. Hold the intent to balance the other person's energy and start with your hands above the head. Keep an inch or so away from the body, bring your hands slowly down, sweeping down the body slowly, ending a few inches past the feet. For more information, go to http://www.healgrief.com/Site/Healing_Tools.html
   f. *Other considerations:* Regular TT treatments may enhance the effect achieved.
   g. *References/other sources:*
      Giasson, M. (1998). Effect of therapeutic touch on the well-being of persons with terminal cancer. *Journal of Holistic Nursing, 16*(3), 383–398.

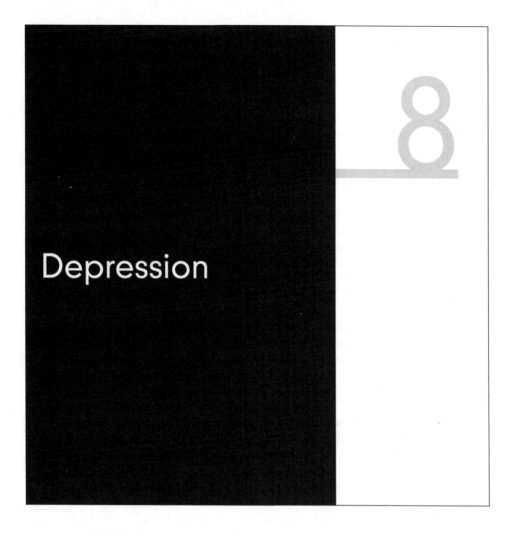

Depression

Medical treatment for depression includes antidepressants, which can have major side effects. Recent research provides support for complementary approaches for depression.

Environment

1. Sunlight
   a. *Actions/expected responses:* Vitamin D deficiency may play a role in depression. Studies show a strong correlation between high vitamin D intake (sunlight) and lower rates of depression.
   b. *Routes/dosages/frequencies:* For light-skinned women, 10–15 minutes of direct midday sun at least twice a week on the face, arms, hands, or back is sufficient, according to the National Institutes of Health. Darker-skinned women may require three to six times as much exposure.
   c. *Cautions:* More frequent exposure to sunlight could result in skin cancer. Insufficient exposure to the sun can result in improper absorption of

calcium and phosphorus, leading to imperfect skeletal formation as well as bone disorders.

d. *Assessments:* Assess the amount of time spent in direct sunlight. For women living in northern climes assess their interest in using short wavelength light. Depression can be assessed using the Hamilton Depression Rating Scale: http://healthnet.umassmed.edu/mhealth/HAMD.pdf.

e. *Tips on use:* Develop a plan for obtaining sufficient sunlight, depending on lifestyle. Eating lunch outside when weather permits could be one solution. In colder climes use short wavelength blue light, take a tablespoon of cod liver oil daily, or eat fatty fish, fish oils, and egg yolks. Supplements of vitamin D3 (calciferol) may be necessary for certain women.

f. *Other considerations:* Vitamin D2, found in fortified foods, especially breads and cereals, is poorly metabolized by the body. Certain drugs can interfere with vitamin D metabolism, including corticosteroids, phenytoin, heparin, cimetidine, isoniazid, rifampin, phenobarbital, and primidone. Counsel women to find alternate medications whenever possible so they can metabolize vitamin D3.

g. *References/other sources:*

Armstrong, D. J., Meenagh, G. K., Bickle, I., Lee, A. S., Curran, E. S., & Finch, M. B. (2007). Vitamin D deficiency is associated with anxiety and depression in fibromyalgia. *Clinical Rheumatology, 26*(4), 551–554.

Berk, M., Sanders, K. M., Pasco, J. A., Jacka, F. N., Williams, L. J., Hayes, A. L., et al. (2007). Vitamin D deficiency may play a role in depression. *Medical Hypothesis, 69*(6), 1316–1319.

Glickman, G., Bynre, B., Pineda, C., Hauck, W. W., & Brainard, G. C. (2006). Light therapy for seasonal affective disorder with blue narrow-band light-emitting diodes (LEDS). *Biological Psychiatry, 59*(6), 502–507.

Jockers, B. S. (2007). Vitamin D sufficiency: An approach to disease prevention. *The American Journal for Nurse Practitioners, 11*(10), 43–50.

Lansdowne, A. T., & Provost, S. C. (1998). Vitamin D3 enhances mood in healthy subjects during winter. *Psychopharmacology, 135*(4), 319–323.

Exercise/Movement

1. Exercise

a. *Actions/expected responses:* Exercise has been used effectively as an alternative or adjunctive treatment. It is one of the determinants for psychological well-being.

b. *Routes/dosages/frequencies:* Any form of exercise is beneficial (even a single workout), although strength training and aerobic activity seem to have the most pronounced effects.

c. *Cautions:* Exercise without adequate warming up and cooling down can lead to injury.

d. *Assessments:* Assess use of exercise and inclination to increase movement.

e. *Tips on use:* For warm-up and cool-down exercises, go to http://www.wellness.ma/adultfitness/stretching-warmup.htm

f. *Other considerations:* Depressed women are more apt to report improvement from exercise than from either counseling or antidepressants (chiefly because of the adverse effects of the latter). Physical activity also boosts self-confidence, improves body image, and provides a sense of self-worth and strength. Study findings support the use of exercise in the acute treatment of, and in ongoing lifestyle management for, individuals with mood disorders. Halting exercise can also bring on depressive symptoms. Computer-generated phone calls may be an effective, low-cost way to encourage sedentary women to exercise.

g. *References/other sources:*

Barbour, K. A., Edenfield, T. M., & Blumenthal, J. A. (2007). Exercise as a treatment for depression and other psychiatric disorders: A review. *Journal of Cardiopulmonary and Rehabilitation Prevention, 27*(6), 359–367.

Beck, M. (2007). Should we be targeting exercise as a routine mental health intervention? *Acta Neuropsychiatric, 19*(3), 217–218.

Benda, B. (2002, September-October). An integrative approach to depression. *Integrative Nursing,* 4.

Stanford University Medical Center (2007, December 5). Computer calls can talk couch potatoes into walking, study finds. *ScienceDaily.* Retrieved December 10, 2007, from http://www.sciencedaily.com/releases/2007/12/071204122000.htm

Tucker, M. E. (2005, September). Halt to exercise = depression. *Clinical Psychiatric News,* 33.

Herbs/Essential Oils

1. Ginkgo biloba
   a. *Actions/expected responses:* Ginkgo biloba therapy can reduce sleep disturbances (increased awakenings and non-REM sleep) associated with antidepressant medication.
   b. *Routes/dosages/frequencies:* 240 mg per day.
   c. *Cautions:* Ginkgo must be carefully coordinated with medications because it can interact with aspirin and antiplatelet drugs, increasing clotting time. Avoid using concurrently with anticonvulsants, buspirone, trazadone, St. John's wort, MAOIs, or fluoexetine, and never exceed suggested dosage. Not to be used during pregnancy, given to children, or used by those with coagulation or platelet disorders, hemophilia, seizures, or hypersensitivity to this herb. Adverse reactions could include transient headache, anxiety, restlessness, vomiting, lack of appetite, diarrhea, flatulence, or rash, but a meta-analysis of unconfounded, randomized, double-blind controlled studies found no significant differences between ginkgo and placebo in the proportion of participants experiencing adverse events.
   d. *Assessments:* Chart changes in depression prior to and after taking ginkgo.
   e. *Tips on use:* Follow bottle directions.
   f. *Other considerations:* Discuss use with a certified or expert herbalist for best results. Ginkgo may take from 1–6 months to achieve full effectiveness.
   g. *References/other sources:*
      Hemmeter, U., Annen, B., Bischof, R., Bruderlin, U., Hatzinger, M., & Holsboer-Trachsler, E. (2001). Polysommographic effects of adjuvant ginkgo biloba therapy. *Pharmacopsychiatry, 34*(2), 50–59.

Skidmore-Roth, L. (2006). Ginkgo biloba. In *Mosby's handbook of herbs and natural supplements* (3rd ed., pp. 487–492). St. Louis, MO: ElsevierMosby.

Stough, C., Clarke, J., Lloyd, J., & Nathan, P. J. (2001). Neuropsychological changes after 30-day ginkgo biloba administration in healthy participants. *International Journal of Neuropsychopharmacology, 4*(2), 131–134.

2. Sage
   a. *Actions/expected responses:* In a double-blind, placebo-controlled crossover study, sage was shown to improve mood in healthy participants.
   b. *Routes/dosages/frequencies:* 600 mg dried sage leaf once a week.
   c. *Cautions:* Sage is a uterine stimulant and should not be used during pregnancy; this herb should not be used during lactation or be given to children. Women with hypersensitivity to sage should not use it, and those diagnosed with diabetes and seizure disorders should be monitored closely. Adverse effects include nausea, vomiting, anorexia, stomatitis, cheilitis, dry mouth, oral irritation, and seizures.
   d. *Assessments:* Assess mood prior to and 4 hours after dose. A depression tool women can use to assess their level of depression appears at http://www.drugdigest.org/DD/HRA/DepressionHRA/0,10630,,00.html
   e. *Tips on use:* Store sage in a cool, dry place. Separate intake by two hours from iron salts.
   f. *Other considerations:* Interactions with sage include anticonvulsants, antidiabetes agents, central nervous system depressants, iron salts, and hypoglycemic and sedative herbs.
   g. *References/other sources:*
      Kennedy, D. O. (2006). Effects of cholinesterase inhibiting sage (Salia officinalis) on mood, anxiety and performance on a psychological stressor battery. *Neuropsychopharmacology, 31*(4), 845–852.

3. St. John's wort
   a. *Actions/expected responses:* For mild-to-moderate depression, St. John's wort is a safe, inexpensive alternative (approximately $15–$30 per month) to prescription medication. Because of inconsistency of clinical trial evidence, more studies are needed to show efficacy for major or severe depression.
   b. *Routes/dosages/frequencies:* 300 mg taken by mouth with food three times a day.
   c. *Cautions:* It causes milder unwanted effects (nausea, vomiting, diarrhea, dizziness, anxiety, dry mouth, confusion, and headache) than most prescription antidepressants. St. John's wort can interfere with many of the antiretrovirals used in HIV therapy, digoxin, warfarin, oral contraceptives, and some antidepressants.
   d. *Assessments:* Assess depression prior to and after taking St. John's wort.
   e. *Tips on use:* Can be taken as capsules, tablets, teas, or concentrated extracts.
   f. *Other considerations:* Women who are lactating or pregnant should avoid St. John's wort, as should women with severe depression, suicidal ideations or plans, and anyone with an allergy to plants and pollen.
   g. *References/other sources:*
      Linde, K., Mulrow, C. D., Berner, M., & Egger, M. (2005). St. John's wort for depression. *Cochrane Database System Review, 18*(2), CD000448.

Sego, S. (2006, July). St. John's wort. *The Clinical Advisor,* 135–137.

Mindset

1. Affirmations
   a. *Actions/expected responses:* Self-affirmation of personal values and beliefs buffers neuroendocrine and psychological stress.
   b. *Routes/dosages/frequencies:* Repeat aloud or write positive affirmations up to 20 times a day such as "I go beyond other peoples' expectations," "I create a life that's right for me," or "Even though I am depressed I fully accept and approve of myself and know that God/the Universe (whichever is preferred) loves and accepts me completely and unconditionally."
   c. *Cautions:* Ensure affirmations are positive and acceptable to the woman.
   d. *Assessments:* Assess depression on a scale of 1 (low) to 10 (high) prior to and after completing affirmations for a week.
   e. *Tips on use:* Write favorite affirmations on 3 by 5 cards and place them in spots in home, car, or work area where they will be read frequently.
   f. *Other considerations:* Find more affirmations information at www.success consciousness.com/index_00000a.htm
   g. *References/other sources:*
      Benor, D. J. (2008, Winter). WHEE: Wholistic Hybrid of EMDR and EFT: A new approach to self-healing and stress relief. *Beginnings*, 12–13.
      Hay, L. (2000). *Heal your body.* Carlsbad, CA: Hay House.
      Schwarzer, R., Babler, J., Kwiatek, P., Schroder, K., & Zang, J. W. (1997). The assessment of optimistic self-beliefs: Assessment of general perceived self-efficacy in thirteen cultures. *World Psychology, 3*(1–2), 177–190.
2. Cognitive-behavioral therapy (CBT)
   a. *Actions/expected responses:* CBT can be as helpful as antidepressants for women with depression and is superior in preventing relapse.
   b. *Routes/dosages/frequencies:* A weekly session for 6 weeks.
   c. *Cautions:* None.
   d. *Assessments:* Assess depression prior to and after CBT sessions.
   e. *Tips on use:* Ask women to keep a diary of depression symptoms during the 6 weeks.
   f. *Other considerations:* Between-session assignments are often given to help women apply concepts learned during sessions.
   g. *References/other sources:*
      DeRubeis, R. J., Hollon, S. D., & Amsterdam, J. D. (2005). Cognitive therapy vs. medications in the treatment of moderate to severe depression. *Archives of General Psychiatry, 62,* 409–416.
      Jancin, B. (2005). CBT improves post-CABG depression in women. *Clinical Psychiatry News,* (July), 57.
      National Association of Cognitive-Behavioral Therapists. (2008). What is cognitive behavior therapy? Retrieved July 30, 2008, from www.nacbt. org/whatiscbt.htm
3. Mindfulness meditation
   a. *Actions/expected responses:* Mindfulness is the ability to live in the present moment. One way to practice this form of meditation is to label emotions by saying, for example, "I'm feeling depressed right now," or "I'm feeling real low right now," or whatever the emotion is. During the labeling of emotions, the right ventrolateral prefrontal cortex of the brain is activated, which turns down activity in the amygdala and enhances mood.

b. *Routes/dosages/frequencies:* Encourage women to label their feelings as a way to enhance mood.

c. *Cautions:* None.

d. *Assessments:* Assess mood prior to and after labeling feelings.

e. *Tips on use:* Provide cue sheets or cards to remind women to label their feelings.

f. *Other considerations:* None.

g. *References/other sources:*

University of California, Los Angeles. (2007, June 22). Putting feelings into words produces therapeutic effects in the brain. *ScienceDaily*. Retrieved February 3, 2008, from http://www.sciencedaily.com/releases/2007/06/070622090727.htm

4. Prayer

a. *Actions/expected responses:* Intercessory prayer offered for the benefit of another person has been shown to have positive effects on depression.

b. *Routes/dosages/frequencies:* As often as possible.

c. *Cautions:* None.

d. *Assessments:* Assess depression prior to and after intercessory prayer.

e. *Tips on use:* None.

f. *Other considerations:* Prayer should be combined with other methods of care.

g. *References/other sources:*

Arizona State University. (2007, March 15). Does God answer prayer? Researcher says 'Yes.' *ScienceDaily*. Retrieved January 29, 2007 from http://www.sciencedaily.com/releases/2007/03/070314195638.htm

Nutrition

1. Folate

a. *Actions/expected responses:* Nearly 40% of depressed women have low folate levels. Folic acid (the synthetic form of folate) is metabolized in the liver, while folate is metabolized in the gut, an easily saturated system. Fortification can lead to significant unmetabolized folic acid entering the blood stream, with the potential to cause a number of health problems. Undigested folic acid accelerates cognitive decline in older adults with low vitamin B12 status. For sources of folate, ask women to go to http://ohioline.osu.edu/hyg-fact/5000/5553.html. Vitamin B12 can be found in liver, fish, milk, eggs, tempeh, and B-50 supplements.

b. *Routes/dosages/frequencies:* None.

c. *Cautions:* Avoid foods fortified with folic acid and eat foods high in folate instead.

d. *Assessments:* Take a baseline measure for depression and then take a measure after increasing vitamin B12 and folate.

e. *Tips on use:* Calcium supplementation can improve B12 absorption. Good sources of vitamin B12 and folate appear in "Actions/Expected Responses": include them in daily menus.

f. *Other considerations:* Serotonin plays a role in the regulation of mood and depression. Decreased serotonin can be reversed by the administration of folate. The following medications can lead to B12 deficiencies and a need for more foods high in folate: H2 blockers (such as ranitidine), proton pump inhibitors (e.g., omeprazole), colchicines, zicovudine, nitrous oxide anesthesia, metformin, phenformin, and potassium supplements.

g. *References/other sources:*

Chambers, K. H. (2003). *Health benefits of folic acid.* New York: Medical Education Collaboration.

Wright, J., Dainty, J., & Fingles, P. (2007). Folic acid metabolism in human subjects: Potential implications for proposed mandatory folic acid fortification in the UK. *British Journal of Nutrition, 98,* 667–675.

2. Omega-3 fatty acids

a. *Actions/expected responses:* Epidemiological and animal studies have suggested that dietary fish or fish oil rich in omega-3 fatty acids have positive effects on depressive symptoms. The level of omega-3 fatty acids in participants' blood is correlated with their score on three accepted tests for depression. In another study, omega-3 fatty acids, found in fatty fish like salmon, were associated with increased gray matter volume in the areas of the brain commonly linked to mood and behavior.

b. *Routes/ dosages/frequencies:* The higher the dietary intake of fatty fish, the higher the level of omega-3 fatty acids in portions of the brain regulating mood. Daily intake of 1.7 grams DHA and 0.6 grams EPA (omega 3 group) showed positive effects on depressive symptoms.

c. *Cautions:* Farmed fish contains more PCBs, and 11 other environmental toxins are present at higher levels than in wild fish. Farmed fish may also be less nutritious.

d. *Assessments:* Assess depression levels prior to and after eating fatty fish.

e. *Tips on use:* The following fish contain the most omega-3 fatty acids and are the least tainted: 6 ounces of wild Atlantic salmon, 3 ounces of sardines in sardine oil, 6 ounces of wild rainbow trout, 3 ounces of mackerel, 6 ounces of specialty or gourmet Pacific Albacore tuna canned in water.

f. *Other considerations:* Smaller, family-owned tuna fisheries fresh-freeze their fish and only cook it once, preserving their natural juices and fats. The larger commercial canneries cook their fish twice, during which time natural juices and fats are lost.

g. *References/other sources:*

Indiana University. (2004, January 9). Farmed salmon more toxic than wild salmon, study finds. *ScienceDaily.* Retrieved February 3, 2008, from http://www.sciencedaily.com/releases/2004/01/040109072244.htm

Norwegian School of Veterinary Science. (2008, February 28). Farmed fish fed cheap food may be less nutritious for humans. *ScienceDaily.* Retrieved March 9, 2008, from http://www.sciencedaily.com/releases/2008/02/080226164105.htm

University of Pittsburgh Medical Center. (2006, March 4). Omega 3 fatty acids influence mood, impulsivity and personality, study indicates. *ScienceDaily.* Retrieved February 3, 2008, from http://www.sciencedaily.com/releases/2006/03//060303205050.htm

USDA Nutrient Composition Database. USDA food composition data (2005). Retrieved from http://www.nal.usda.gov/fnic/foodcomp/Data/index.html

3. Sulfur
   a. *Actions/expected responses:* Sulfur foods have clinical applications in the treatment of depression.
   b. *Routes/dosages/frequencies:* Counsel women to eat several sulfur foods daily.
   c. *Cautions:* None unless women are sensitive to the food.
   d. *Assessments:* Assess use of sulfur foods.
   e. *Tips on us:* Foods to focus on include cabbage, peas, beans, cauliflower, Brussels sprouts, eggs, horseradish, shrimp, chestnuts, mustard greens, onions, and asparagus.
   f. *Other considerations:* None
   g. *References/other sources:*
      Parcell, S. (2002). Sulfur in human nutrition and applications in medicine. *Alternative Medicine Review, 7*(1), 22–44.
4. Walnuts, fish, molasses
   a. *Actions/expected responses:* Food choices can have a tremendous influence on how women feel and act. Walnuts, molasses, and fish high in omega-3 fatty acids and uridine have the same effect as antidepressants.
   b. *Routes/dosages/frequencies:* By mouth, 1 tbsp of molasses daily and a handful of walnuts can be eaten daily to raise mood. Three to four ounces of fatty fish (mackerel, tuna, salmon) can be eaten three times a week.
   c. *Cautions:* None unless sensitive to specific foods.
   d. *Assessments:* Assess intake of walnuts, fish, and molasses.
   e. *Tips on use:* Choose walnuts that are unsalted and without added oil, ocean-grown fish, and blackstrap molasses.
   f. *Other considerations:* Omega-3 fatty acids and uridine, two naturally occurring substances in fish, walnuts, and molasses, prevent the development of signs of depression.
   g. *References/other sources:*
      Neves, L. (2005). *Food ingredients may be as effective as antidepressants: Researchers discover "mood foods" relieve signs of depression.* Press release, February 10, McLean Hospital, Public Affairs, Belmont, MA. Retrieved April 7, 2008, from http://www.mclean.harvard.edu/news/press/current.php?id=72

Stress Management

1. Relaxation breathing exercises
   a. *Actions/expected responses:* Breathing retraining, with or without physical exercise, can decrease depression.
   b. *Routes/dosages/frequencies:* 30 minutes a day for 6–12 weeks can retrain fast shallow breathing to slower, less frequent breathing.
   c. *Cautions:* None. Abdominal breathing is preferable to shallow chest breathing.
   d. *Assessments:* Assess depression level prior to and after breathing retraining.
   e. *Tips on use:* Focus on letting breathing slowly move down toward the abdomen.
   f. *Other considerations:* For more information go to http://www.citytech.cuny.edu/files/students/counseling/stresshb.pdf

g. *References/other sources:*

Kim, S., & Kim, H. A. (2005). Effects of relaxation breathing exercises on anxiety, depression and leukocytes in hemopoietic stem cell transplantation patients. *Cancer Nursing, 28*(1), 79–83.

Supplements

1. Chromium picolinate
   a. *Actions/expected responses:* Chromium is an essential trace element required for proper metabolic functioning, especially the metabolism of glucose. It is available from dietary sources such as brown rice, brewer's yeast, molasses, tea, cheese, meat, chicken, corn, dairy products, eggs, mushrooms, potatoes, and some wines and beers. Taking a chromium picolinate supplement can improve symptoms of appetite increase, increased eating, carbohydrate cravings, and diurnal variation in feelings, such as depression.
   b. *Routes/dosages/frequencies*: 600 mcg per day.
   c. *Cautions:* Avoid chromium supplements containing ma huang, a powerful stimulant that boosts metabolism, steps up heart rate, heightens alertness, and may increase muscle strength. Chromium should not be used during pregnancy or lactation. Adverse reactions may include headache, insomnia, mood change, restlessness, and irritability. High doses (above the recommended amount) can lead to anemia, thrombocytopenia, hemolysis, renal failure, and hepatic dysfunction.
   d. *Assessments:* Assess depression from 1 (no depression) to 10 (extreme depression) prior to and after taking chromium.
   e. *Tips on use:* Store chromium supplements in a cool, dry place, away from heat and moisture; avoid taking this supplement with zinc, iron, or calcium supplements, which decrease absorption of chromium; and take chromium with complex carbohydrates (fruits, vegetables, and whole grain products) for increased absorption.
   f. *Other considerations:* This supplement may be especially useful for women diagnosed with diabetes; chromium enhances the potency of insulin, allowing the body to get by with a lowered insulin output.
   g. *References/other sources:*

   Docherty, J. P., Sack, D. A., Roffman, M., Finch, M., & Komorowski, J. R. (2005). A double-blind, placebo-controlled, exploratory trial of chromium picolinate in atypical depression: Effect on carbohydrate craving. *Journal of Psychiatric Practice, 11*(5), 302–314.

   Skidmore-Roth, L. (2006). Chromium. In *Mosby's handbook of herbs and natural supplements* (pp. 298–301). St. Louis, MO: ElsevierMosby.
2. Vitamin B6
   a. *Actions/expected responses:* Lack of vitamin B6 is related to increases in depression. Vitamin B6 is a building block for serotonin; decreased levels of serotonin have been associated with increased depression.
   b. *Routes/dosages/frequencies:* 1.6 mg per day for most women. Pregnant women require an additional 0.1 mg per day, and those who are lactating require an additional 0.7–0.8 mg daily. For food sources of vitamin B6, go

to   http://dietary-supplements.info.nih.gov/factsheets/vitaminb6.asp#h2 or http://lpi.oregonstate.edu/infocenter/vitamins/vitaminB6

c. *Cautions:* If taken as a supplement, vitamin B6 can cause neurological disorders, such as loss of sensation in legs and imbalance, when taken in high doses (200 mg or more per day) over a long period of time. Vitamin B6 toxicity can damage sensory nerves, leading to numbness in the hands and feet as well as difficulty walking, which recedes when the vitamin supplement is withdrawn.

d. *Assessments:* On a scale from 0 (no depression) to 10 (extreme depression) ask women to assess anxiety prior to and 1 and 4 hours after eating more vitamin B3-rich foods.

e. *Tips on use:* It is safer to take a multivitamin and even safer to eat foods rich in vitamin B6. This vitamin is sensitive to ultraviolet light and heat, so large amounts of this nutrient are lost during the cooking process. Raw fruits and vegetables are preferable. Store multivitamin bottles in a cool dry place and keep their covers tightly closed.

f. *Other considerations:* Several surveys have found that more than half of all women over age 60 consume less than the current recommended daily allowance of vitamin B3 (1.5 mg per day).

g. *References/other sources:*

University of Miami School of Medicine. (1995, June 6). Researchers at UM School of Medicine link Vitamin B6 deficiency to stress. *Vital Signs,* 19.

Touch

1. Acupressure with massage

    a. *Actions/expected responses:* Women in an acupressure group showed significantly greater improvement in depression than a control group who received routine care.

    b. *Routes/dosages/frequencies:* 12 minutes per day, three days a week, for four weeks.

    c. *Cautions:* Only gentle acupressure should be used in injured or sore areas.

    d. *Assessments:* Ask women to rate their depression symptoms before and after treatment.

    e. *Tips on use:* For more information on using acupressure, go to http://www.eclecticenergies.com/acupressure/howto.php

    f. *Other considerations:* Changes in mood may begin to occur immediately and continue for several days.

    g. *References/other sources:*

    Cho, Y. C., & Tsay, S. L. (2004). The effect of acupressure with massage on fatigue and depression in patients with end-stage renal disease. *Journal of Nursing Research, 12*(1), 51–59.

    Dayton, B. R. (1987). *Caregiver's introduction to High Touch acupressure.* Friday Harbor, WA: High Touch Network.

2. Massage therapy

    a. *Actions/expected responses:* Depressed pregnant women who received massage therapy reported lower levels of anxiety and depression and less pain than women participating in either progressive muscle relaxation or a control group that received standard prenatal care.

   b. *Routes/dosages/frequencies:* Weekly 20-minute massage therapy sessions administered by a woman's significant other.

   c. *Cautions:* No adverse effects were reported.

   d. *Assessments:* Ask women to rate their depression symptoms prior to and after treatment.

   e. *Tips on use:* Stroking, squeezing, and stretching techniques are used on the head, arms, legs, feet, and back. For techniques to use, go to www.videojug.com/film/how-to-do-a-relaxing-hand-and-arm-massage, http://www.ifilm.com/video/28622378, http://www.ifilm.com/video/2797488, or http://www.drfoot.co.uk/foot_massage.htm

   f. *Other considerations:* The offspring of pregnant women can benefit from massage therapy as demonstrated by reduced fetal activity and better neonatal outcome for the massage group.

   g. *References/other sources:*

     Field, T., Diego, M. A., Hernandez-Reif, M., Schanberg, S., & Kuhn, C. (2004). Massage therapy effects on depressed pregnant women. *Journal of Psychosomatic Obstetrical Gynecology, 25*(2), 115–122.

3. Reflexology

   a. *Action/expected response:* Middle-aged women who gave themselves a foot reflexology massage reduced their depression and strengthened their immune system.

   b. *Routes/dosages/frequencies:* 40–60 minutes daily self-foot massage or as tolerated for 6 weeks.

   c. *Cautions:* Pregnant women should avoid foot reflexology because certain manipulations can lead to premature labor. Those with foot problems, gout, arthritis, and vascular conditions such as varicose veins should be careful using this procedure.

   d. *Assessments:* Evaluate depression symptoms prior to and after foot reflexology sessions.

   e. *Tips on use:* Focus on massaging the whole foot. For foot charts, see http://groups.msn.com/AlternativesToPainandDisease/reflexologyinstructionspg1.msnw

   f. *Other considerations:* See http://groups.msn.com/AlternativesToPainandDisease/reflexologyinstructionspg2.msnw

   g. *References/other sources:*

     Kesselring, A. (1994). Foot reflex zone massage. *Schweizerische Medizinische Wochenschrift, 62,* 88–93.

     Lee, Y. M. (2006). Effects of self-foot reflexology massage on depression, stress responses and immune functions of middle aged women. *Taehan Kanho Hakhoe Chi, 36*(1), 179–188.

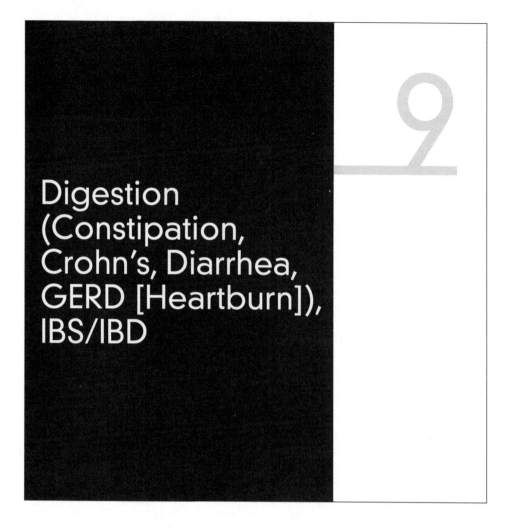

Digestion (Constipation, Crohn's, Diarrhea, GERD [Heartburn]), IBS/IBD

Many digestive complaints are treated with medications, most of which have negative side effects. Evidence shows complementary approaches can be effective and safe, with none or relatively few side effects.

Environment

1. Handwashing
   a. *Actions/expected responses:* Hand washing can reduce the incidence of diarrhea by up to 30%.
   b. *Routes/dosages/frequencies:* Before eating.
   c. *Cautions:* Infection by the germs that cause diarrhea occur by consuming contaminated food and drink, by person-to-person contact, or by direct contact with feces.
   d. *Assessments:* Assess hand washing prior to eating.
   e. *Tips on use:* Good hand washing technique includes washing with soap and water or an alcohol-based sanitizer. Antimicrobial cleaners are as good as soap and water, but not as effective as alcohol-based sanitizers.

   f. *Other considerations:* Hand contact with ready-to-eat food consumed without further washing or cooking can transmit more germs than food that is prepared and cooked at home.
   g. *References/other sources:*
      Center for the Advancement of Health. (2008, January 25). Hand washing can reduce diarrhea episodes by about one third. *ScienceDaily.* Retrieved January 30, 2008, from http://www.sciencedaily.com/releases/2008/01/080122203221.htm
      Mayo Clinic. (2008). *Hand washing: An easy way to prevent infection.* Retrieved July 30, 2008, from http://www.mayoclinic.com/health/hand-washing/HQ00407
2. Power-frequency fields and wireless communications
   a. *Actions/expected responses:* Allergic and inflammatory responses are associated electromagnetic fields (EMFs).
   b. *Routes/dosages/frequencies:* Current levels of long-term exposure to some kinds of electromagnetic fields are not protective of public health.
   c. *Cautions:* Scientific evidence raises concerns about the health impacts of mobile or cell phone radiation, power lines, interior wiring and grounding of buildings, and appliances such as microwaves, wireless technologies, and electric blankets.
   d. *Assessments:* Assess exposure to EMFs listed in item c.
   e. *Tips on use:* Until new public safety limits and limits on further deployment of risky technologies are warranted, avoid exposure to EMFs whenever possible. Also counsel women to limit the duration and number of cell phone calls, stay away from cell phone antennas, use a headset, and keep cell phones away from the body. Avoid high tension electrical wires and new or upgraded power lines.
   f. *Other considerations:* An international working group of renowned scientists, researchers, and public health policy professionals (The Bioinitiative Working Group) has released its report on electromagnetic fields and health. It raises serious concerns about the safety of existing public limits that regulate how much EMF is allowable from power lines, cell phones, and many other EMF sources of exposure in daily life.
   g. *References/other sources:*
      Hardell, L., & Sage, C. (2007). Biological effects from electromagnetic field exposure and public exposure standards. *Biomedical Pharmacotherapy, 62*(2), 104–109.

Exercise/Movement

1. Exercise
   a. *Actions/expected responses:* Regular physical exercise, such as walking or swimming can be effective against constipation.
   b. *Routes/dosages/frequencies:* Daily.
   c. *Cautions:* Avoid overdoing it. Nonstrenuous exercise is best.
   d. *Assessments:* Assess amount of daily exercise.
   e. *Tips on use:* For warm-up and cool-down exercises, go to http://www.wellness.ma/adult-fitness/stretching-warmup.htm
   f. *Other considerations:* Use in combination with adequate hydration and dedicated bathroom time for best results.

g. *References/other sources:*

National Digestive Diseases Information Clearinghouse. (2007). *Constipation.* Retrieved July 30, 2008, from http://digestive.niddk.nih.gov/ddiseases/pubs/constipation/

Herbs/Essential Oils

1. Aloe vera
   a. *Actions/expected responses:* Anti-inflammatory, antibacterial, antifungal, protective against liver conditions and inhibits growth of tumors.
   b. *Routes/dosages/frequencies:* 1–3 ounces three times a day after meals.
   c. *Cautions:* Caution women not to use aloe vera if they're sensitive to it.
   d. *Assessments:* Assess digestive inflammation prior to and after taking aloe vera.
   e. *Tips on use:* Only buy aloe vera gel from a health food store, buy the herb in a glass container if possible, never drink the juice or gel from home aloe plants (this can lead to diarrhea), and store aloe vera gel in the refrigerator once opened.
   f. *Other Considerations:* Aloe contains vitamins A, B-complex, E, carboxypeptidase (anti-inflammatory enzyme), magnesium, potassium, calcium, magnesium, manganese, copper, zinc, chromium, iron, glucomannans (immunomodulator), saponins (antiseptic), anthraquinone (aids absorption in the gastrointestinal tract), salicylic acid (anti-inflammatory), and amino acids (protein building blocks).
   g. *References/other sources:*

   Kametani, S., Oikawa, T., Kojima-Yuasa, A., Kennedy, D. O., Norikura, T., Honzawa, M., & Matsui-Yusa, I. (2008). Mechanism of growth inhibitory effect of cape aloe extract in ehrlich ascites tumor cells. *Journal of Nutrition Science and Vitaminology, 53*(6), 540–546.

   Skidmore-Roth, L. (2006). Aloe. In *Mosby's handbook of herbs and natural supplements* (pp. 30–35). St. Louis, MO: ElsevierMosby.

2. Chamomile
   a. *Actions/expected responses:* Anti-inflammatory and antispasmotic. Used to treat digestive conditions such as irritable bowel syndrome, indigestion, colitis, and Crohn's disease.
   b. *Routes/dosages/frequencies:* 2–4 ounces of tea as needed.
   c. *Cautions:* Should not be used during pregnancy or lactation or taken by women sensitive to sunflowers, ragweed, echinacea, feverfew, or milk thistle. Do not take concurrently with other sedatives or alcohol.
   d. *Assessments:* Assess for gastrointestinal symptoms prior to and after drinking tea.
   e. *Tips on use:* Store chamomile in a cool, dry place.
   f. *Other considerations:* Chamomile may also enhance sleep and can reduce anxiety.
   g. *References/other sources:*

   McKay, D. L., & Blumberg, J. B. (2006). A review of the bioactivity and potential health benefits of chamomile tea. *Phytotherapy Research, 20*(7), 519–530.

   Skidmore-Roth, L. (2006). Chamomile. In *Mosby's handbook of herbs and natural supplements* (pp. 264–268). St. Louis, MO:ElsevierMosby.

3. Fenugreek
   a. *Actions/expected responses:* Treats gastrointestinal complaints, including constipation, dyspepsia and gastritis, and inflammatory bowel disease.
   b. *Routes/dosages/frequencies:* One cup of tea, one to three times a day.
   c. *Cautions:* Can cause premature labor. Because of the rapid rate at which this herb moves through the bowel and coats the gastrointestinal tract, fenugreek can reduce the absorption of all medications, foods, and supplements taken concurrently. There may be an increased risk of bleeding if taken with anticoagulants. Because fenugreek lowers blood glucose levels, hypoglycemia is a possibility when used concurrently with oral antidiabetes agents.
   d. *Assessments:* Assess gastrointestinal complaints prior to and after drinking fenugreek tea.
   e. *Tips on use:* Keep tea in a tightly covered glass jar in a cool, dry spot.
   f. *Other considerations:* Fenugreek may decrease LDL (the "bad" cholesterol) and total cholesterol, reduce pain, and protect against ulcers.
   g. *References/other sources:*
      Langmead, L., Dawson, C., Hawkins, C., Banna, N., Loo, S., & Rampton, D. S. (2002). Antioxidant effects of herbal therapies used by patients with inflammatory bowel disease. *Alimentary Pharmacology Therapy, 16*(2), 197–205.
      Skidmore-Roth, L. (2006). Fenugreek. In *Mosby's handbook of herbs and natural supplements* (pp. 435–439). St. Louis MO: ElsevierMosby.
4. Ginger
   a. *Actions/expected responses:* Treats gastrointestinal complaints, including stomach upset, nausea, and dyspepsia.
   b. *Routes/dosages/frequencies:* 500–1,000 mg of powdered root or 1,000 mg of fresh root in divided doses daily. The fresh root can be used in stir fry or other dishes.
   c. *Cautions:* Increased bleeding time is possible when ginger is used by women taking oral anticoagulants.
   d. *Assessments:* Assess gastrointestinal complaints prior to and after ginger intake.
   e. *Tips on use:* Keep ginger in a tightly covered glass jar in a cool, dry spot.
   f. *Other considerations:* Ginger allergies aren't common, but they do occur, including eye reactions. Contact rashes have occurred, but primarily in individuals who work with ginger or who have a positive allergy test for balsam of Peru.
   g. *References/other sources:*
      Sego, S. (2007, April). Ginger. *The Clinical Advisor,* 159–160.
      Skidmore-Roth, L. (2006). Ginger. In *Mosby's handbook of herbs and natural supplements* (pp. 480–486). St. Louis, MO: ElsevierMosby.
5. Milk thistle
   a. *Actions/expected responses:* Can help normalize liver functions.
   b. *Routes/dosages/frequencies:* Standard capsule doses are 420–800 mg orally per day and may be divided into two to three doses.
   c. *Cautions:* Though generally well-tolerated, milk thistle can have a mild laxative effect and could worsen menstrual cramping. Pregnant women or women planning to become pregnant, lactating women, and children

should not use milk thistle. Women sensitive to pollen-bearing plants should avoid milk thistle.

d. *Assessments:* Assess digestive function prior to and after taking milk thistle.

e. *Tips on use:* Store milk thistle products in a cool, dry place.

f. *Other considerations:* Milk thistle has been used to treat hepatotoxicity due to poisonous mushrooms, cirrhosis of the liver, chronic candidiasis, hepatitis C, exposure to toxic chemicals, and liver transplantation.

g. *References/other sources:*

Sego, S. (2007, June). Milk thistle. *The Clinical Advisor,* 136–137.

Tamayo, C., & Diamond, S. (2007). Review of clinical trials evaluating safety and efficacy of milk thistle. *Integrative Cancer Therapies, 6*(2), 146–157.

6. Peppermint tea

a. *Actions/expected responses:* Animal studies demonstrate a relaxation effect on gastrointestinal (GI) tissue.

b. *Routes/dosages/frequencies:* Leaves are used to make tea. Counsel women to drink one to three cups of tea a day.

c. *Cautions:* Adverse reactions to peppermint tea have not been reported.

d. *Assessments:* Assess digestion symptoms prior to and after drinking peppermint tea.

e. *Tips on use:* Counsel women to store tea in a cool, dry place.

f. *Other considerations:* Peppermint tea has also shown analgesic and anesthetic effects in the central and peripheral nervous system, immunomodulating actions, and chemopreventive potential.

g. *References/other sources:*

McKay, D. L., & Blumberg, J. B. (2006). A review of the bioactivity and potential health benefits of peppermint tea. *Phytotherapy Research, 20*(8), 619–633.

Mindset

1. Affirmations

a. *Actions/expected responses:* Self-affirmation of personal values and beliefs buffers neuroendocrine and psychological stress.

b. *Routes/dosages/frequencies:* Ask women to repeat aloud or write positive affirmations up to 20 times a day such as, "I take in the new and lovingly assimilate it," "Life is sweet and full of joy," and "I release the past at a rate that is right for me."

c. *Cautions:* Ensure affirmations are positive and acceptable to the woman.

d. *Assessments:* Assess anxiety prior to and after completing affirmations for a week.

e. *Tips on use:* Ask women to write their favorite affirmations on 3 by 5 cards and place them in places where they will be read frequently.

f. *Other considerations:* Find more affirmations information at www.success consciousness.com/index_00000a.htm

g. *References/other sources:*

Hay, L. (2000). *Heal your body.* Carlsbad, CA: Hay House.

Schwarzer, R., Babler, J., Kwiatek, P., Schroder, K., & Zang, J. W. (1997). The assessment of optimistic self-beliefs: Assessment of general perceived self-efficacy in thirteen cultures. *World Psychology, 3*(1–2), 177–190.

2. Cognitive-behavioral therapy (CBT)
   a. *Actions/expected responses:* CBT works as well as standard care for irritable bowel syndrome (IBS).
   b. *Routes/dosages/frequencies:* 6 weeks of group CBT.
   c. *Cautions:* None.
   d. *Assessments:* Assess IBS symptoms prior to and after taking part in CBT.
   e. *Tips on use:* For more information, go to http://www.mind.org.uk/Information/Booklets/Making+sense/MakingSenseCBT.htm
   f. *Other Considerations:* Routine clinical care may have adverse effects, while CBT does not.
   g. *References/other sources:*
      Boyce, P. M., Talley, N. J., Balsam, B., Koloski, N. A., & Truman, G. (2003). A randomized controlled trial of cognitive behavior therapy, relaxation training and routine clinical care for the irritable bowel syndrome. *American Journal of Gastroenterology, 98*(10), 2209–2218.

3. Hypnosis
   a. *Actions/expected responses:* Hypnosis can provide a relaxed state for women with IBS, thereby modulating gastrointestinal physiology, perceived rectal distension, and improved mood. Some results lasted up to 6 years following treatment.
   b. *Routes/dosages/frequencies:* Women can listen to a hypnosis tape or to a practitioner who follows a specific protocol for IBS.
   c. *Cautions:* While the majority (71%) show improvement in response to treatment initially, 19% reported slight worsening of symptoms.
   d. *Assessments:* Assess IBS symptoms prior to and after hypnosis.
   e. *Tips on use:* Direct women to http://www.ibshypnosis.com/ for information about hypnosis.
   f. *Other considerations:* None.
   g. *References/other sources:*
      Gonsalkorale, W. M., Miller, V., Afzal, A., & Whorwell, P. J. (2003). Long term benefits of hypnotherapy for irritable bowel syndrome. *Gut, 52*(11), 1623–1629.
      Houghton, L. A., Calvert, E. L., Jackson, N. A., Cooper, P., & Whorwell, P. J. (2002). Visceral sensation and emotion: A study using hypnosis. *Gut, 51*(5), 701–704.
      Simren, M. (2006). Hypnosis for irritable bowel syndrome: The quest for the mechanism of action. *International Journal of Clinical Experimental Hypnosis, 54*(1), 65–84.

Nutrition

1. Cinnamon
   a. *Actions/expected responses:* Cinnamon contains antiulcerogenic compounds and gastric cytoprotection factors.
   b. *Routes/dosages/frequencies:* Add 1–2 tsp of cinnamon to food as a spice.
   c. *Cautions:* Until more research is conducted, avoid during pregnancy and lactation in large doses. Can be used safely as a spice.

d. *Assessments:* Assess use of cinnamon and hypersensitivity, including wheezing or rash.

e. *Tips on use:* Store cinnamon in a cool, dry place.

f. *Other considerations:* Sprinkle cinnamon on oatmeal, rice, or pears and to try it on other foods such as stews, prunes, cereals, and soups.

g. *References/other sources:*

Skidmore-Roth, L. (2006). Cinnamon. In *Mosby's handbook of herbs and natural supplements* (pp. 302–305). St. Louis, MO: ElsevierMosby.

Tanaka, S., Yoon, Y. H., Fukui, H., Tabata, M., Akira, T., Okano, K., et al. (1989). Antiulcerogenic compounds isolated from Chinese cinnamon. *Planta Medica, 55*(3), 245–248.

2. Cow's milk (avoid)

a. *Actions/expected responses:* E. coli is known to be present during Crohn's disease in increased numbers and may be due to ingesting milk and milk products.

b. *Routes/dosages/frequencies:* Milk and milk products can harbor the bacterium called Mycobacterium paratuberculosis that can make their way into the body's system.

c. *Cautions:* This bacterium is a likely trigger for a circulating antibody protein (ASCA) that is found in about two-thirds of women with Crohn's disease, suggesting these women may have been infected by the Mycobacterium.

d. *Assessments:* Assess intake of milk or dairy products.

e. *Tips on use:* Avoid milk and dairy products.

f. *Other considerations:* These Mycobacterium release a complex molecule containing a sugar called mannose. These molecules prevent a type of white blood cells, called macrophages, from killing internalized E. coli.

g. *References/other sources:*

University of Liverpool. (2007, December 13). How bacteria in cows' milk may cause Crohn's disease. *ScienceDaily.* Retrieved December 23, 2007, from http://www.sciencedaily.com/releases/2007/12/071210104002.htm

3. Curcumin (turmeric)

a. *Actions/Expected responses:* Curcumin is a natural dietary produce spice shown to significantly attenuate colitis and treat Crohn's disease.

b. *Routes/dosage/frequencies:* Orally in or on foods one to two times a day.

c. *Cautions:* Turmeric is considered safe for most adults. High doses or long-term use of turmeric may cause indigestion. Women with gallbladder disease should avoid using turmeric as a dietary supplement, as it may worsen the condition.

d. *Assessments:* Assess digestive complaints prior to and after using curcumin. Assess sensitivity to the herb.

e. *Tips on use:* The spice may be sprinkled on salads, baked potatoes, stews, soups, curries, rice, poultry, or fish and may be used in cooking.

f. *Other considerations:* None.

g. *References/other sources:*

Deguchi, Y., Andoh, A., Inatomi, O., Yagi, Y., Bamba, S., Araki, Y., et al. (2007). Curcumin prevents the development of dextran sulfate sodium (DSS)-induced experimental colitis. *Digestive Diseases and Sciences, 52*(11), 2993–2998.

4. Fasting
   a. *Actions/expected responses:* Fasting has a protective effect on the progression of colitis.
   b. *Routes/dosages/frequencies:* Consuming only water for 2 days.
   c. *Cautions:* Women diagnosed with diabetes or hypoglycemia may not do well fasting.
   d. *Assessments:* Assess interest in fasting to reduce colitis symptoms.
   e. *Tips on use:* Fasting can also mean drinking only fruit and vegetable juices and eating no solid food. This method is a healthier approach.
   f. *Other considerations:* Some soothing juices include carrot, apple, papaya, aloe vera, and banana. For more information on fasting, go to http://www.healingdaily.com/juicing-for-health/how-to-fast.htm
   g. *References/other sources:*
      Savendahl, L., Underwood, L. E., Haldeman, K. M., Ulshen, M. H., & Lund, P. K. (1997). Fasting prevents experimental murine colitis produced by dextran sulfate sodium and decrease interleukin-1 beta and insuline-like growth factor I messenger ribonucleic acid. *Endocrinology, 138*(2), 734–740.

5. Fat, spices, and reflux
   a. *Actions/expected responses:* Meals high in fat can provoke reflux, possibly through delayed gastric emptying. Additional spices, such as curry, do not increase reflux.
   b. *Routes/dosages/frequencies:* Any fat meals can provoke reflux.
   c. *Cautions:* To protect against reflux, avoid fatty meals.
   d. *Assessments:* Assess intake of fatty meals.
   e. *Tips on use:* Reduce or eliminate fatty animal products and concentrate their meals on fruits, vegetables, grains, and fish.
   f. *Other considerations:* None.
   g. *References/other sources:*
      Schonfeld, J., & Evans, D. F. (2007). Fat, spices and gastro-esophageal reflux. *Zeitschrift fur Gastroenterologie, 45*(2), 171–175.

6. Low carbohydrate diets
   a. *Actions/expected responses:* Very low carbohydrate diets (such as the Atkins-type diets) interfere with gut health by reducing butyrate production (important for preventing colorectal cancer cell development).
   b. *Routes/dosages/frequencies:* Butyrate is a short chain fatty acid and is produced in the gut when the bacteria ferment the carbohydrate present in food.
   c. *Cautions:* If insufficient butyrate is produced, risk of colorectal cancer may increase.
   d. *Assessments:* Assess intake of carbohydrate. A normal maintenance diet should be composed of 13% protein, 52% carbohydrate, and 35% fat.
   e. *Tips on use:* When eating low carbohydrate diets, eat plenty of sources of fiber such as fruit and vegetables.
   f. *Other considerations:* Butyrate is used by intestinal bacteria as a source of energy and also is used by the cells that line the gut wall.
   g. *References/other sources:*
      Rowett Research Institute. (2007, June 20). Very low carbohydrate diets may disrupt long-term gut health. *ScienceDaily.* Retrieved April 2, 2008, from http://www.sciencedaily.com/releases/2007/06/070619173537.htm

7. Overweight and gastro-esophageal reflux disease (GERD)
   a. *Actions/expected responses:* In a meta-analysis of studies, six showed a statistically significant association between obesity and GERD. Overweight and obesity increase the risk of GERD and complications such as erosive esophagitis.
   b. *Routes/dosages/frequencies:* Weight loss may help improve symptoms.
   c. *Cautions:* Postmenopausal hormone therapy in women strengthened the association between GERD symptoms and high body mass index, or BMI (overweight = 25 to 30; obese = greater than 30).
   d. *Assessments:* Assess BMI and need for weight loss.
   e. *Tips on use:* See pp. 287–298 for weight loss ideas.
   f. *Other considerations:* The odds ratio of developing erosive esophagitis is 1.7 times greater in women with a BMI of 25 or higher than among women who weigh less.
   g. *References/other sources:*
      Hamphel, H., Abraham, N. S., & El-Serag, H. B. (2005). Meta-analysis of obesity and the risk of gastroesophageal reflux disease and its complications. *Annals of Internal Medicine, 143,* 199–211.
8. Water
   a. *Actions/expected responses:* Water replaces lost fluids while caffeinated beverages or alcohol increase fluid output, leeching out needed liquids, minerals, and vitamins. Constipation can be a sign of inadequate fluid intake.
   b. *Routes/dosages/frequencies:* At least 8–10 glasses a day.
   c. *Cautions:* Tap water and even bottled water can contain parasites, weed killers, nitrates (correlated with spontaneous miscarriage and so-called blue-baby syndrome), salmonella, E. coli, chlorine, fluoride, and other potentially dangerous substances.
   d. *Assessments:* Assess type and quantity of water women drink.
   e. *Tips on use:* Drink (and cook with) only distilled water or reverse-osmosis filtered water.
   f. *Other considerations:* Fluid intake is probably adequate when thirst is rarely experienced and when urine is colorless or slightly yellow. As women age, they may experience less thirst. Drink water before thirst sets in, because by that time dehydration may already have taken over.
   g. *References/other sources:*
      Mayo Clinic. (2007, August 13). *How much water should you drink? It depends.* Retrieved February 16, 2008, from http://www.mayoclinic.com/health/water/NU00283

Stress Management

1. Cognitive-behavioral therapy (CBT)
   a. *Actions/expected responses:* Women with irritable bowel syndrome (IBS) who used CBT in combination with mebeverine saw their symptoms improve more than those who received the antispasmodic drug alone.
   b. *Routes/dosages/frequencies:* Keep a daily log of thought and perception problems that could lead to IBS, such as believing external events cause

symptoms; feeling helpless and fragile/lacking control over what is experienced or felt; believing there is a perfect love and relationship, that anger is bad and destructive, that the past determines the present, that adults must have love and approval to survive, that worth is determined by achievement, that it's possible to be perfect and competent at all times, and that it's important to always please other people and never go after what you want. Read *How to Stubbornly Refuse to Make Yourself Miserable About Anything* by Albert Ellis.

  c. *Cautions:* Women in acute stress may not find this approach helpful.

  d. *Assessments:* Assess IBS symptoms prior to and after cognitive behavioral work.

  e. *Tips on use:* Question any beliefs that lead to IBS symptoms.

  f. *Other considerations:* See CBT information at http://www.mind.org.uk/ Information/Booklets/Making+sense/MakingSenseCBT.htm

  g. *References/other sources:*

British Association for the Advancement of Science. (2007, September 14). Counselling conquers constipation. *ScienceDaily*. Retrieved September 14, 2007, from http://www.sciencedaily.com/releases/2007/09/070912160935.htm

Bryant, R. A., Sackville, T., Dang, S. T., Moulds, M., & Guthrie, R. (1999). On treating acute stress disorder: Evaluation of cognitive behavior therapy and supportive counseling techniques. *American Journal of Psychiatry, 156*(11), 1780–1786.

National Association of Cognitive Behavioral Therapists Organization. (2007). *What is Cognitive Behavioral Therapy*. Retrieved July 30, 2008, from http://nacbt.org/whatiscbt.htm

Supplements

1. Probiotics

  a. *Actions/expected responses:* Probiotics, the so-called good bacteria, render the digestive tract unfavorable for more aggressive bacteria. Probiotics have also been shown to induce intestinal production of anti-inflammatory cytokines, all while reducing the production of proinflammatory cytokines.

  b. *Routes/dosages/frequencies:* Probiotics (e.g., Multidophilus) are available in health food stores. Follow directions on bottle, usually two capsules a day with meals or a large glass of water.

  c. *Cautions:* Do not use concurrently with antibiotics; separate by 2 hours. Should not be used concurrently with immunosuppressants. May decrease the action of warfarin. May decrease the absorption of garlic; separate by 2 hours.

  d. *Assessments:* Assess for antibiotic, immunosuppressant, warfarin, and garlic use.

  e. *Tips on use:* Keep probiotics refrigerated or they will lose their potency.

  f. *Other considerations:* This supplement also inhibits the growth of vaginal microorganisms. Multidophilus treats a variety of gastrointestinal conditions.

g. *References/other sources:*

Fedorak, R., & Madsen, K. (2004). Probiotics and the management of inflammatory bowel disease. *Inflammatory Bowel Disease, 10,* 286–299.

2. Pycnogenol
   a. *Actions/expected responses:* Within 12 hours, pycnogenol significantly ameliorated inflammation by radical scavenging activity in rats with inflammatory bowel disease
   b. *Routes/dosages/frequencies:* By gavage as part of enteral nutrition or by mouth as a capsule (50 mg three times a day).
   c. *Cautions:* Theoretically, pycnogenol may interact with immunosuppressants and cause reduced blood platelet aggregation. No other adverse reactions are known.
   d. *Assessments:* Assess level of inflammation prior to and 12 hours after ingesting pycnogenol.
   e. *Tips on use:* Keep bottle in a cool, dry place. Take with a full glass of water.
   f. *Other considerations:* Avoid using pycnogenol when lactating or giving the supplement to children. Pycnogenol is a mixture of bioflavonoids from pine bark that also has antitumor properties, prevents venous thrombosis and thrombophlebitis, reduces menopause symptoms, and is superior for venous insufficiency and microangiopathy compared to diosmin and hesperidin.
   g. *References/other sources:*

Mochizuki, M., & Hasegawa, N. (2004). Therapeutic efficacy of pycnogenol in experimental inflammatory bowel diseases. *Phytotherapy Research, 18*(12), 1027–1028.

Touch

1. Acupressure
   a. *Actions/Expected responses:* Pressing on stomach meridians can affect gastric action by activating a singling pathway, providing evidence for traditional Chinese medicine approaches such as acupressure/acupuncture.
   b. *Routes/dosages/frequencies:* On the ridge of the cavity directly below the pupil of eye, press for 5 seconds and release for 5 second up to five times.
   c. *Cautions:* This acupressure point may not be suitable for women with eye or nearby facial wounds.
   d. *Assessments:* Assess response of symptoms to acupressure.
   e. *Tips to use:* Use a light but firm pressure.
   f. *Other considerations:* For more information on using acupressure, go to http://www.eclecticenergies.com/acupressure/howto.php
   g. *References/other sources:*

Yan, J., Yang, Z. B., Chang, X. R., Yi, S. X., Lin, Y. P., & Zhong, Y. (2007). Expressions of epidermal growth factor receptor signaling substances in gastric mucosal cells influenced by serum derived from rats treated with electroacupuncture at stomach meridian acupoints. *Zong Xi Yi Jie He Xue Bao, 5*(3), 338–342.

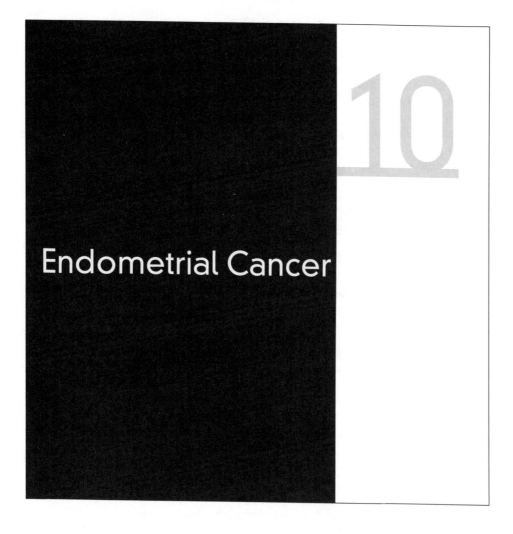

Endometrial Cancer

Medical treatments for endometrial cancer include drugs and surgery. Many complementary approaches offer safe and effective alternatives.

Environment

1. Alcohol
   a. *Actions/expected responses:* Alcohol can increase the risk of endometrial cancer in postmenopausal women.
   b. *Routes/dosages/frequencies:* Consuming two or more alcohol beverages a day may double a woman's risk of endometrial cancer.
   c. *Cautions:* Previous studies have shown that alcohol consumption has been associated with higher levels of estrogens in postmenopausal women, which could be the mechanism by which daily alcohol intake increases risk of endometrial cancer.
   d. *Assessments:* Assess intake of alcohol.
   e. *Tips on use:* Limit intake of alcoholic beverages to one a day.

    f. *Other considerations:* Lean women may be more sensitive to modest elevations in hormone levels from alcohol than are obese women who already have levels of estrogen that can mask alcohol as an independent risk factor.

    g. *References/other sources:*

        University of Southern California. (2007, September 8). Frequent alcohol consumption increases cancer risk in older women. *ScienceDaily.* Retrieved. February 23, 2008, from http://www.sciencedaily.com/releases/2007/09/070907150936.htm

2. Computed Tomography (CT) scans

    a. *Actions/expected responses:* CT scans could be responsible for raising the risk of cancer.

    b. *Routes/dosages/frequencies:* A typical CT scan delivers 50 to 100 times more radiation than a conventional X-ray.

    c. *Cautions:* Brenner and Hall (2007) estimate that one-third of all CT scans might not be necessary.

    d. *Assessments:* Assess number of CT scans.

    e. *Tips on use:* Suggest using the safer options of ultrasound and magnetic resonance imaging, which do not expose women to radiation.

    f. *Other considerations:* An estimated 62 million CT scans were performed in 2006 compared to only 3 million in 1980.

    g. *References/other sources:*

        Brenner, D., & Hall, E. J. (2007). Computed tomography, an increasing source of radiation exposure. *New England Journal of Medicine, 357*(22), 2277–2284.

3. Overweight/obesity

    a. *Actions/expected responses:* Half of all cases of endometrial cancer are attributable to overweight or obesity.

    b. *Routes/dosages/frequencies:* Women with a body mass index (BMI) of 25–29.9 are defined as overweight, and women with a BMI of 30 or more are defined as obese, according to the World Health Organization's criteria.

    c. *Cautions:* Menopausal status is a key factor in the relation between BMI and risk of endometrial cancer among women.

    d. *Assessments:* Assess overweight status.

    e. *Tips on use.* See pp. 187–298.

    f. *Other considerations:* None.

    g. *References/other sources:*

        British Medical Journal. (2007, November 10). Overweight and obesity cause 6,000 cancers a year in UK. *ScienceDaily.* Retrieved November 29, 2007, from http://www.sciencedaily.com/releases/2007/11/071106174207.htm

4. Sunlight

    a. *Actions/expected responses:* Researchers at the Moores Cancer Center at University of California, San Diego have shown a clear association between deficiency in exposure to sunlight, especially ultraviolet B (UVB), and endometrial cancer.

    b. *Routes/dosages/frequencies:* For light-skinned women, 10–15 minutes of direct midday sun at least twice a week on the face, arms, hands, or back is sufficient, according to the National Institutes of Health. Darker-skinned women may require three to six times as much exposure.

c. *Cautions:* More frequent exposure could result in skin cancer. Insufficient exposure to the sun can result in improper absorption of calcium and phosphorus, leading to imperfect skeletal formation as well as bone disorders. Vitamin D supplements can suppress the immune system.

d. *Assessments:* Assess the amount of time spent in direct sunlight.

e. *Tips on use:* Develop a plan for obtaining sufficient sunlight, depending on lifestyle. Eating lunch outside when weather permits could be one solution. In colder climes, take a tablespoon of cod liver oil daily, eat fatty fish and fish oils, and egg yolks. Supplements of vitamin D3 (calciferol) may be necessary for certain women, but should never be taken if a chronic illness has been diagnosed; sunlight and identified foods are preferable.

f. *Other considerations:* Vitamin D2, found in fortified foods, especially breads and cereals, is poorly metabolized by the body. Certain drugs can interfere with vitamin D metabolism, including corticosteroids, phenytoin, heparin, cimetidine, isoniazid, rifampin, phenobarbital, and primidone. Counsel women to find alternate medications whenever possible so they can metabolize vitamin D3.

g. *References/other sources:*

Autoimmunity Research Foundation. (2008, January 27). Vitamin D deficiency study raises new questions about disease and supplements. *ScienceDaily*. Retrieved February 13, 2008, from http://www.sciencedaily.com/releases/2008/01/080125223302.htm

University of California–San Diego. (2007, November 16). Deficiency in exposure to sunlight linked to endometrial cancer. *ScienceDaily*. Retrieved November 29, 2007, from http://www.sciencedaily.com/releases/2007/11/071114162728.htm

Exercise/Movement

1. Exercise

a. *Actions/expected responses:* Epidemiological and biologic evidence shows that vigorous activity, as well as light and moderate intensity activities, such as housework, gardening, or walking for transportation, may reduce risk for endometrial cancer, with the strongest evidence found for household activities.

b. *Routes/dosages/frequencies:* Inactive premenopausal women have the highest risk of endometrial cancer.

c. *Cautions:* None for light and moderate intensity activities.

d. *Assessments:* Assess level of activity.

e. *Tips on use:* Encourage premenopausal women to increase their household activity if they're inactive.

f. *Other considerations:* Fourteen of 18 studies of physical activity and endometrial cancer show a convincing or possible protective effect of physical activity on endometrial cancer risk.

g. *References/other sources:*

Cust, A. E., Armstrong, B. K., Friedenreich, C. M., Slimani, N., & Bauman, A. (2007). Physical activity and endometrial cancer risk: A review of the current evidence, biologic mechanisms and the quality of physical activity assessment methods. *Cancer Causes Control, 18*(3), 243–258.

Friedenreich, C., Cust, A., Lahmann, P. H., Steindorf, K., Boutron-Rualt, M. C., Clavel-Chapelon, F., et al. (2007). Physical activity and risk of endometrial cancer: The European prospective investigation into cancer and nutrition. *International Journal of Cancer, 121*(2), 347–355.

Herbs/Essential Oils

1. Aromatherapy
   a. *Actions/expected responses:* Laboratory and animal studies show that essential oils, such as Roman chamomile, geranium, lavender, and cedarwood can improve the quality of life of women diagnosed with cancer by calming, energizing, and providing antibacterial qualities.
   b. *Routes/dosages/frequencies:* Inhale or apply an essential oil to the skin after first placing several drops in a carrier oil such as jojoba or castor oil.
   c. *Cautions:* Safety testing on essential oils has revealed very few, if any, bad effects.
   d. *Assessments:* Assess for hypersensitivity (skin reactions, nausea, or anorexia). Assess quality of life prior to and after using aromatherapy with essential oils.
   e. *Tips on use:* Keep aromatherapy products in a sealed container, away from heat and moisture. Test reaction to oils by asking the woman to inhale the scent of the each oil and to tell which one she likes the best. Besides inhaling or using a diffuser, several drops of essential oil can also be placed in the bath water.
   f. *Other considerations:* Aromatherapy may work by sending chemical messages to the part of the brain that affects mood and emotions.
   g. *References/other sources:*
      Atsumi, T., & Tonosaki, K. (2007). Smelling lavender and rosemary increases free radical scavenging activity and decreases cortisol level in saliva. *Psychiatry Research, 150*(1), 89–96.
2. Glycyrrhizin (licorice)
   a. *Actions/expected responses:* Glycyrrhizin generated a significant decrease in the incidence of endometrial adenocarcinoma.
   b. *Routes/dosages/frequencies:* By mouth, 250–500 mg three times a day.
   c. *Cautions:* Should not be used by pregnant or lactating women, given to children, or used by anyone diagnosed with liver or kidney disease, hypertension, arrhythmias, congestive heart failure, or if hypersensitive to the herb.
   d. *Assessments:* Assess for all the conditions listed under "Cautions." Assess for medications and herbs that may interact with licorice: cardiac glycosides, antihypertensives, antiarrhythmias, and corticosteroids.
   e. *Tips on use:* Store licorice products in a cool, dry place.
   f. *Other considerations:* Increase potassium intake if using licorice for extended periods.
   g. *References/other sources:*
      Niwa, K., Lian, Z., Onogi, K., Yan, W., Tang, L., Mori, H., et al. (2007). Preventive effects of glycyrrhizin on estrogen-related endometrial carcinogenesis in mice. *Oncology and Reproduction, 17*(3), 617–622.

3. Milk thistle
   a. *Actions/expected responses:* Silymarin, the active substance in milk thistle, stimulates detoxification pathways, inhibits the growth of certain cancer cell lines, exerts direct cytotoxic activity toward certain cancer cell lines, and may increase the efficacy of certain chemotherapy agents.
   b. *Routes/dosages/frequencies:* 200 to 400 mg milk thistle per day.
   c. *Cautions:* Adverse effects are rare, but may include stomach pain, nausea, vomiting, diarrhea, headache, rash, joint pain, and anaphylaxis in allergic women. Pregnant and lactating women or those who are hypersensitive (have a known sensitivity to ragweed, marigolds, or chrysanthemums) should avoid milk thistle.
   d. *Assessments:* Assess hypersensitivity to milk thistle.
   e. *Tips on use:* Milk thistle may protect against liver damage from chemotherapy and radiation.
   f. *Other considerations:* Preliminary research suggests that silibinin (an ingredient of milk thistle) may enhance the tumor-fighting effects of cisplatin and doxorubicin.
   g. *References/other sources:*

   Bokemeyer, C., Fells, L. M., & Dunn, T. (1996). Silibinin protects against cisplatin-induced nephrotoxicity without compromising cisplatin on isofamide anti-tumor activity. *British Journal of Cancer, 74,* 2036–2041.

   National Cancer Institute. (2007). *Milk thistle.* Retrieved February 18, 2008, from http://www.cancer.gov/cancertopics/pdq/cam/milkthistle

   Zi, X., Mukhtar, H., & Agarwal, R. (1997). Novel cancer chemopreventive effects of a flavonoid antioxidant silymarin: Inhibition of mRNA expression of an endogenous tumor promoter TNF-alpha. *Biochemical Biophysical Research Communication, 239,* 334–339.

Mindset

1. Affirmations
   a. *Actions/expected responses:* Self-affirmation of personal values and beliefs buffers neuroendocrine and psychological stress.
   b. *Routes/dosages/frequencies:* Repeat aloud or write positive affirmations up to 20 times a day such as, "I release all secrets and all of the past" and "I fill my present with peace and joy."
   c. *Cautions:* Ensure affirmations are positive and acceptable.
   d. *Assessments:* Assess anxiety prior to and after completing affirmations for a week.
   e. *Tips on use:* Write favorite affirmations on 3 by 5 cards and place them where they will be read frequently.
   f. *Other considerations:* Find more affirmations information at www.success consciousness.com/index_00000a.htm
   g. *References/other sources:*

   Hay, L. (2000). *Heal your body.* Carlsbad, CA: Hay House.

   Schwarzer, R., Babler, J., Kwiatek, P., Schroder, K., & Zang, J. W. (1997). The assessment of optimistic self-beliefs: Assessment of general perceived self-efficacy in thirteen cultures. *World Psychology, 3*(1–2), 177–190.

Nutrition

1. Animal fat and animal protein
   a. *Actions/expected responses:* High consumption of meat, eggs, and fresh fish is associated with elevated risk for endometrial cancer.
   b. *Routes/dosages/frequencies:* The higher the intake of animal fat and animal protein, the higher the risk. A significant 50% excess risk of endometrial cancer was found among women with the highest intake of processed meat and fish, compared to women in the lowest quartile of intake.
   c. *Cautions:* Reduce intake of animal fat and animal protein to reduce their risk of endometrial cancer.
   d. *Assessments:* Assess daily intake of animal fat and animal protein.
   e. *Tips on use:* Start replacing animal protein with plant protein such as tofu (crumble it in with chopped beef or eggs), soy cheese, soy meat, soy burgers, soy milk (in place of regular milk), and so forth.
   f. *Other considerations:* Animal protein can also be replaced by beans and rice or stir fried vegetables and rice.
   g. *References/other sources:*
      Shu, X. O., Zheng, W., Potischman, N., Brinton, L. A., Hatch, M. C., Gao, Y.T., et al. (1993). A population-based case-control study of dietary factors and endometrial cancer in Shanghai, People's Republic of China. *American Journal of Epidemiology, 137*(2), 155–165.
      Zheng, W., Kushi, L. H., Potter, J. D., Sellers, T. A., Doyle, T. J., Bostick, R. M., et al. (1995). Dietary intake of energy and animal foods and endometrial cancer incidence. The Iowa Women's Health Study. *American Journal of Epidemiology, 142*(4), 388–394.
2. Curcumin (turmeric)
   a. *Action/expected responses:* Curcumin has been demonstrated to have an antitumor effect in endometrial cancer cells.
   b. *Routes/dosages/frequencies:* 400–600 mg by mouth three times a day (standardized to curcumin content).
   c. *Cautions:* Avoid using if diagnosed with bile duct obstruction, peptic ulcer, hyperacidity, gallstones, bleeding disorders, or hypersensitivity to the herb. Adverse effects include nausea, vomiting, anorexia, and hypersensitivity reactions.
   d. *Assessments:* Assess for hypersensitivity reactions including contact dermatitis. If found, discontinue use of curcumin. Assess for use of anticoagulants, NSAIDS, and immunosuppressants.
   e. *Tips on use:* Counsel women to store curcumin in a cool, dry place, away from heat and moisture and take curcumin on an empty stomach.
   f. *Other considerations:* May interact with heparin, salicylates, warfarin, cyclosporine, and NAIDSs.
   g. *References/other sources:*
      Yu, Z., & Shah, D. M. (2007). Curcumin down-regulates Ets-1 and Bcl-2 expression in human endometrial carcinoma HEC-1-A cells. *Gynecology Oncology, 106*(3), 541–548.
3. Folate
   a. *Actions/expected responses:* Folate intake may decrease the risk of endometrial cancer and modify genotype risk.

b. *Routes/dosages/frequencies:* Leafy green vegetables (like spinach and turnip greens), fruits (citrus fruits and juices), and dried beans and peas are all natural sources of folate that can help meet the suggested amount of 1,000 micrograms (mcg) a day. Women on diets who do not eat breads, cereals, or pasta, who abuse alcohol, or who take medications that interfere with folate absorption may not receive sufficient amounts of the nutrient and may need additional amounts.

c. *Cautions:* Medications and medical conditions that increase the need for folate or result in an increased excretion of folate include: anticonvulsant medications, metformin, sulfasalazine, triamterene, methotrexate, barbiturates, pregnancy and lactation, alcohol abuse, malabsorption, kidney dialysis, liver disease, and certain anemias. Because folate is a water-soluble B-vitamin, unneeded amounts will be eliminated in the urine.

d. *Assessments:* Assess for signs of folate deficiency: anemia, diarrhea, loss of appetite, weight loss, weakness, sore tongue, headaches, heart palpitations, irritability, forgetfulness, behavioral disorders, and an elevated level of homocysteine.

e. *Tips on use:* Avoid flour-fortified foods as a source of folic acid; new research has shown the introduction of flour fortified with folic acid into common foods has been linked to colon cancer.

f. *Other considerations:* Exceeding 1,000 mcg per day of folate may trigger vitamin B12 deficiency. To compensate, women can take a multivitamin that contains B12 or eat at least one food daily that contains B12: nutritional yeast (unless susceptible to candida), clams, eggs, herring, kidney, liver, mackerel, seafood, milk, or dairy products.

g. *References/other sources:*

Blackwell Publishing Ltd. (2007, November 5). Folic acid linked to increased cancer rate, historical review suggests. *ScienceDaily.* Retrieved November 29, 2007, from http://www.sciencedaily.com/releases/2007/11/07/071102111956.htm

Office of Dietary Supplements. (2005). *Dietary supplement fact sheet: Folate.* Bethesda, MD: NIH Clinical Center, National Institutes of Health. Retrieved November 25, 2007, from http://ods.od.nih.gov

Xu, W. H., Shrubsole, M. J., Xiang, Y. B., Cai, Q., Zhao, G. M., Ruan, Z. X., et al. (2007). Dietary folate intake, MTHFR genetic polymorphisms, and the risk of endometrial cancer among Chinese women. *Cancer Epidemiology Biomarkers Prevention, 16*(2), 281–287.

4. Garlic and brassica vegetables

a. *Actions/expected responses:* Garlic and brassica vegetables readily uptake inorganic and anticarcinogenic selenium from soil and incorporate it into bioactive organic chemicals. Cruciferous vegetables are associated with a reduced risk of cancer.

b. *Routes/dosages/frequencies:* Eat garlic and brassica vegetables daily as a cancer-preventive measure.

c. *Cautions:* None unless sensitive to these vegetables. Avoid microwaving vegetables; this method destroys most of their helpful antioxidants.

d. *Assessments:* Assess use of garlic and brassica vegetables.

e. *Tips on use:* Garlic can be baked in its skin or chopped and used in tomato sauce, stews, fish, tofu, and other foods. Cut into small pieces and lightly steam brassica vegetables for 5 minutes in a small amount of water to release all amino acids and antioxidants. If any liquids remain, cool and drink them later or use in cooking.

f. *Other considerations:* Brassica vegetables include: broccoli, cauliflower, Brussels sprouts, collards, kohlrabi, and kale, as well as more than 350 other plants, such as arugula, mustard, radish, daikon, watercress, horseradish, and wasabi.

g. *References/other sources:*

Gill, C. I., Haldar, S., Boyd, L. A., Bennett, R., Whiteford, J., Butler, M., et al. (2007). Watercress supplementation in diet reduces lymphocyte DNA damage and alters blood antioxidant status in healthy adults. *American Journal of Clinical Nutrition, 85*(2), 504–510.

Irion, C. W. (1999). Growing alliums and brassicas in selenium-enriched soils increases their anticarcinogenic potentials. *Medical Hypothesis, 53*(3), 232–235.

Vallejo, F., Tomas-Barberan, F. A., & Garcia-Viguera, C. (2003). Phenolic compounds content in edible parts of broccoli inflorescences after domestic cooking. *Journal of Science and Food Agriculture, 83*(14), 1151–1156.

5. Soy and fiber consumption

a. *Actions/expected responses:* Regular intake of soy foods is associated with a reduced risk of endometrial cancer, as is increased fiber from whole grains, vegetables, fruits, and seaweeds.

b. *Routes/dosages/frequencies:* Eat tofu, soybeans, tempeh, soy cheese, and/or drink soy milk and 8–10 servings (1/2 cup each) of vegetables and fruits daily. Use seaweeds as a source of minerals and taste for stews, salads, soups, and other dishes.

c. *Cautions:* No absolute contraindications are known. Hypersensitivity can arise to soy. Adverse reactions include nausea, bloating, diarrhea, and abdominal pain.

d. *Assessments:* Assess for hypersensitivity to soy.

e. *Tips on use:* Store soy products, whole grains, fresh fruits, and vegetables in a cool, dry place.

f. *Other considerations:* Soy food intake is especially beneficial to women with a high body mass index and waist-hip ratio. Among nonusers of supplements, a diet composed of sugar and sugary foods, refined carbohydrates, and animal products was associated with increased risk of endometrial cancer, regardless of fruit and vegetable consumption. Stevia is a safe sweetener that can repair DNA damage.

g. *References/other sources:*

Dalvi, T. B., Canchola, A. J., & Horn-Ross, P. L. (2007). Dietary patterns, Mediterranean diet, and endometrial cancer risk. *Cancer Causes Control, 18*(9), 957–966.

Ghanta, S., Banerjee, A., Poddar, A., & Chattopadhyay, S. (2007). Oxidative DNA damage preventive activity and antioxidant potential of Stevia rebaudiana (Bertoni) Bertoni, a natural sweetener, *55*(26), 10962–10967.

Goodman, M. T., Wilkens, L. R., Hankin, J. H., Lyu, L. C., Wu, A. H., & Kolonel, L. N. (1997). Association of soy and fiber consumption with the risk of endometrial cancer. *American Journal of Epidemiology, 146*(4), 294–306.

Xu, W. H., Zheng, W., Xiang, Y. B., Ruan, Z. X., Cheng, J. R., Dai, Q., et al. (2004). Soya food intake and risk of endometrial cancer among Chinese women in Shanghai population based case-control. *British Medical Journal, 328*(7451), 1285.

6. Sulfur foods
   a. *Actions/expected responses:* Sulfur foods have clinical applications in the treatment of cancer.
   b. *Routes/dosages/frequencies:* Counsel women to eat several sulfur foods daily.
   c. *Cautions:* None unless women are sensitive to the food.
   d. *Assessments:* Assess use of sulfur foods.
   e. *Tips on use:* Foods to focus on include cabbage, peas, beans, cauliflower, Brussels sprouts, eggs, horseradish, shrimp, chestnuts, mustard greens, onions, and asparagus.
   f. *Other considerations:* None.
   g. *References/other sources:*
      Parcell, S. (2002). Sulfur in human nutrition and applications in medicine. *Alternative Medicine Review, 7*(1), 22–44.

7. Tea
   a. *Actions/expected responses:* Tea is inversely associated with endometrial cancer.
   b. *Routes/dosages/frequencies:* Drink tea daily.
   c. *Cautions:* None unless sensitive to caffeine.
   d. *Assessments:* Assess sensitivity to tea.
   e. *Tips on use:* Choose decaffeinated teas. Digestive process affects anticancer activity of tea in gastrointestinal cells; add citrus (such as lemon juice) or take ascorbic acid (vitamin C) to protect the catechins in green tea from digestive degradation.
   f. *Other considerations:* None.
   g. *References/other sources:*
      American Association for Cancer Research. (2007, August 12). Green tea boosts production of detox enzymes, rendering cancerous chemicals harmless. *ScienceDaily.* Retrieved December 20, 2007, from http://www.sciencedaily.com/releases/2007/08/070810194923.htm
      Federation of American Societies for Experimental Biology. (2008, April 10). Digestive process affects anti-cancer activity of tea in gastrointestinal cells. *ScienceDaily.* Retrieved April 20, 2008, from http://www.sciencedaily.com/releases/2008/04/080407172713.htm
      Xu, W. H., Dai, Q., Xiang, Y. B., Long, J. R., Ruan, Z. X., Cheng, J. R., et al. (2007). Interaction of soy food and tea consumption with CYP19A1 genetic polymorphisms in the development of endometrial cancer. *American Journal of Epidemiology, 166*(12), 1420–1430.

Stress Management

1. Stress management
   a. *Actions/expected responses:* A weak immune system is one of the major factors that promotes cancer metastases after an operation, chemotherapy or radiation therapy.

b. *Routes/dosages/frequencies:* Adequate stress management prior to and after medical treatment may help to prevent metastases.

c. *Cautions:* Fear and stress weaken the immune system.

d. *Assessments:* Assess knowledge of stress management techniques.

e. *Tips on use:* Learn stress-management procedures.

f. *Other considerations:* For teaching/learning materials, go to: http://www.mindfulnessmeditationcentre.org/breathingGathas.htm, http://www.santosha.com/asanas/asana.html, and http://www.healgrief.com/Site/Heal_Grief_in_Your_Body.html

g. *References/other sources:*

Tel Aviv University. (2008, February 29). Stress and fear can affect cancer's recurrence. *ScienceDaily.* Retrieved March 9, 2008, from http://www.sciencedaily.com/releases/2008/02/080227142656.htm

Supplements

1. Pycnogenol and ginkgo biloba extract

   a. *Actions/expected responses:* Either pycnogenol or ginkgo biloba extract can protect against antimutagenic activity in animal studies.

   b. *Routes/dosages/frequencies:* 5–100 microgram/mL.

   c. *Cautions:* Until more research is completed, pregnant and lactating women should not use these supplements, nor should they be given to children. Ginkgo should not be taken concurrently with anticoagulants.

   d. *Assessments:* Assess reaction to pycnogenol and ginkgo.

   e. *Tips on use:* Store supplements in a cool, dry place.

   f. *Other considerations:* Pycnogenol has also been found useful in preventing venous thrombosis, thrombophlebitis, gingival (gum) bleeding and plaque, inflammatory bowel disease, venous insufficiency, digestive conditions, and menopause symptoms.

   g. *References/other sources:*

   Krizkova, L., Chovanova, Z., Durackova, Z., & Krajcovic, J. (2008). Antimutagenic in vitro activity of plan polyphenols: Pycnogenol and Ginkgo biloba extract. *Phytotherapy Research, 22*(3), 384–388.

2. Vitamins A, C, and E

   a. *Actions/expected responses:* Dietary intake of foods high in vitamins A, C, and E and/or vitamin supplementation may decrease the risk of endometrial cancer. When derived from plant sources, all three vitamins show an inverse relationship to this type of cancer. Dietary intake of animal origin nutrients was correlated with a high risk for endometrial cancer.

   b. *Routes/dosages/frequencies:* By mouth. The best way to obtain vitamins is via food. See "Assessments" section for food sources. If women are extremely ill, stressed, or can't or don't eat well, a multivitamin or juices made from fresh vegetables and fruits may be the best approach.

   c. *Cautions:* If supplements are chosen, choose brands that do not contain additional herbs, fillers, dyes, and so forth. Strive for the least processed form available. Vitamin C should not be taken when fat resides in the stomach because at this time it can promote, rather than prevent, the formation of certain cancer-causing chemicals.

d. *Assessments:* Assess intake of vitamin A foods (animal livers, apricots, asparagus, beet greens, broccoli, cantaloupe, carrots, collards, dandelion greens, papaya, peaches, red peppers, spinach, sweet potatoes, Swiss chard, turnip greens, watercress, yellow squash), vitamin C foods (asparagus, avocadoes, beet greens, black currants, broccoli, Brussels sprouts, cantaloupe, collards, dandelion greens, grapefruit, kale, lemons, mangos, mustard greens, onions, oranges, papayas, green peas, sweet peppers, persimmons, pineapple, radishes, spinach, strawberries, Swiss chard, tomatoes, turnip greens, and watercress), and vitamin E foods (brown rice, cold-pressed vegetable oils, cornmeal, dark green leafy vegetables, eggs, legumes, nuts, oatmeal, organ meats, seeds, soybeans, wheat germ, and whole grains).

e. *Tips on use:* Store supplements in a cool, dry place. Follow directions on the bottle.

f. *Other considerations:* Juicers are available online and at health food stores. Making juices may be especially useful for women who have lost their appetite or have digestion issues.

g. *References/other sources:*

Balch, J. F., & Balch, P. A. (1997). *Prescription for nutritional healing.* Garden City Park, NY: Avery Publishing Group.

Combet, E., Paterson, S., Iijama, K., Winter, J., Mullen, W., Crozier, A., et al. (2007). Fat transforms ascorbic acid from inhibiting to promoting acid-catylsed N. nitrosation. *Gut, 56,* 1678–1684.

Sylvester, P. W. (2007). Vitamin E and apoptosis. *Vitamins and Hormones, 76,* 329–356.

Xu, W. H., Dai, Q., Xiang, Y. B., Zhao, G. M., Ruan, Z. X., Cheng, J. R., et al. (2007). Nutritional factors in relation to endometrial cancer: A report from a population-based case-control study in Shanghai. *International Journal of Cancer, 120*(8), 1776–1881.

Touch

1. Acupressure

a. *Actions/expected responses:* Acupressure is a safe and effective tool for managing chemotherapy-induced nausea and vomiting.

b. *Routes/dosages/frequencies:* Stimulating the PC6 point for at least 6 hours at the onset of chemotherapy reduced symptoms in 70% of women.

c. *Cautions:* None.

d. *Assessments:* Assess for nausea and vomiting.

e. *Tips on use:* PC6 is situated in the middle of the front of the forearm above the wrist crease.

f. *Other considerations:* For more information go to http://www.handbag.com/healthfit/complementary/acupressure/.

g. *References/other sources:*

Gardani, G., Cerrone, R., Biella, C., Mancini, L., Proserpio, E., Casiraghi, M., et al. (2006). Effect of acupressure on nausea and vomiting induced by chemotherapy in cancer patients. *Minerva Medicine, 97*(5), 391–394.

2. Reflexology, aromatherapy, and foot soak
   a. *Actions/expected responses:* A combined reflexology, aromatherapy, and foot soak significantly improved fatigue in women with advanced cancer.
   b. *Routes/dosages/frequencies:* 3 minutes of a foot soak in warm water containing lavender essential oil, followed by a 10 minute reflexology treatment with jojoba oil containing lavender for up to eight treatments.
   c. *Cautions:* Complete a patch test for sensitivity to lavender.
   d. *Assessments:* Assess for fatigue. A multidimensional self-assessment of fatigue appears at: http://www.son.washington.edu/research/maf/
   e. *Tips on use:* For foot charts, scroll down at http://www.footreflexology.blogspot.com
   f. *Other considerations:* For more information go to http://www.drfoot.co.uk/foot_massage.htm and http://www.etherealescape.co.uk/reflexology.php
   g. *References/other sources:*
      Kohara, H., Miyauchi, T., Suehiro, Y., Ueoka, H., Takeyama, H., & Morita, T. (2004). Combined modality treatment of aromatherapy, footsoak, and reflexology relieves fatigue in patients with cancer. *Journal of Palliative Medicine, 7*(6), 791–796.

3. Therapeutic touch (TT)
   a. *Actions/expected responses:* Women who received three noncontact therapeutic touch treatments reported increased well-being as opposed to a control group who rested.
   b. *Routes/dosages/frequencies:* 15–20 minutes once a day.
   c. *Cautions:* The aged, extremely ill, or dying should be given a 5-minute (or less) treatment by an experienced practitioner.
   d. *Assessments:* Take a baseline measure of well-being prior to and after administering TT.
   e. *Tips on use:* Center and calm yourself by closing your eyes and focusing on breathing in your abdomen. When relaxed, rub your hands together and feel the tingling sensation as you slowly pull your hands apart until you are able to feel the energies balancing between the hands. Hold the intent to balance the other person's energy and start with your hands above the woman's head. Keep an inch or so away from the body, bring your hands slowly down, sweeping down the body slowly, ending a few inches past the feet. For more information, go to http://www.healgrief.com/Site/Heal_Grief_in_Your_Body.html and scroll down to Therapeutic Touch.
   f. *Other considerations:* Regular TT treatments may enhance the effect achieved.
   g. *References/other sources:*
      Giasson, M. (1998). Effect of therapeutic touch on the well-being of persons with terminal cancer. *Journal of Holistic Nursing, 16*(3), 383–398.

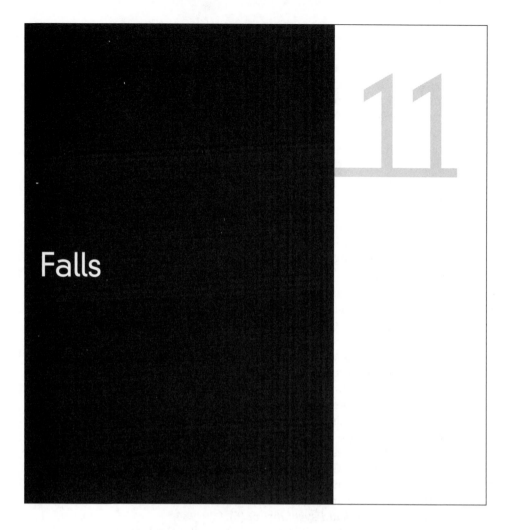

Falls

Falls can be dangerous and may require medical treatment. Complementary approaches have been shown to reduce incidence of falls.

Environment

1. Fall prevention
   a. *Actions/expected responses:* Environmental actions women can take to prevent falls include: using nonpharmacological approaches instead of medications associated with dizziness (benzodiazepines and sleeping pills that increase risk of daytime sedation, falls, and cognitive and psychomotor impairment), using adequate daytime lighting, wearing nonslip footwear (lightweight tie shoe with a hard rubber sole is best), sitting on the edge of the bed and assessing strength prior to standing or walking (gently massaging the arms, chest, and head can bring needed oxygen to the brain), obtaining assistance when getting out of bed or walking as needed (having a bell by the bedside to call for help).

b. *Routes/dosages/frequencies:* Prepare for walking by using a walker, cane, or assistance as needed.

c. *Cautions:* Antipsychotics should not be used as they are linked with increased risk of hospitalization for femur fracture.

d. *Assessments:* Assess for sleep-promoting medications, nonslip footwear, bedside bell and flashlight, walker, cane, and ability to stand and walk.

e. *Tips on use:* Provide bell, flashlight, walker, nonslip footwear, and/or assistance when needed.

f. *Other considerations:* Encourage women to carry small loads and avoid laundry baskets and large boxes, concentrate on walking, arrange furniture to accommodate wide walking areas, keep clutter and tripping hazards off the floor, anchor all rugs and carpeting and remove throw rugs without nonskid backing, install mounted handrails on indoor and outdoor steps and teach women to use them, and keep a phone next to the bed.

g. *References/other sources:*

Conn, D. K., & Madan, R. (2006). Use of sleep-promoting medications in nursing home residents: Risks versus benefits. *Drugs and Aging, 23* 271–287.

Cooper, J. W., Freeman, M. H., Cook, C. L., & Burfield, A. H. (2007). Assessment of psychotropic and psychoactive drug loads and falls in nursing facility residents. *Consulting Pharmacist, 22*(6), 483–489.

De Lepeire, J., Bouwen, A., De Coninck, L., & Buntinx, F. (2003). Insufficient lighting in nursing homes. *Journal of the American Medical Directors Association, 8*(5), 314–317.

Gerber, L. (2007). Keeping clients fall-free. *The Nursing Spectrum FL, 7,* 19.

Liperoti, R., Onder, G., Lapane, K. L., Mor, V., Friedman, J. H., Bernabei, R., et al. (2007). Conventional and atypical antipsychotics and the risk of femur fracture among elderly patients: Results of a case-control study. *Journal of Clinical Psychiatry, 68*(6), 929–934.

Rubenstein, L. A. (2006). Falls in older people: Epidemiology, risk factors and strategies for prevention. *Age and Ageing, 35*(2 Suppl.), ii37–ii41.

Exercise/Movement

1. Supervised group exercise

a. *Actions/expected responses:* Supervised group exercise is more effective at reducing the risk factors related to falling among older women living in a nursing home than is unsupervised home exercise. Although education and home safety assessment improved quality of life in older women, only exercise training led to improvements in functional reach, balance, and fear of falling. Even a modest amount of gentle exercise can improve balance.

b. *Routes/dosages/frequencies:* 30–45 minutes three times a week for 8 to 16 weeks.

c. *Cautions:* Clear exercise area and monitor participants for falls or other adverse reactions.

d. *Assessments:* Assess balance prior to and after engaging in an exercise program using one leg and tandem standing.

e. *Tips on use:* Exercises include a set of stretching exercises to promote flexibility, simple leg raises, marching, lifting two pound weights or less, and using sensing exercises to promote balance such as dimming the room and asking participants to walk slowly on a treadmill or bend over and pick up a lit flashlight.

f. *Other considerations:* For questions to use to assess exercise and how to begin physical activity, go to http://firststeptoactivehealth.com/providers/. For a sample active health kit, go to http://firststeptoactivehealth.com/samplekit/index.htm

g. *References/other sources:*

Blackwell Publishing Ltd. (2007, July 10). Exercise in elderly improves quality of life. *ScienceDaily.* Retrieved February 26, 2008, from http://www.sciencedaily.com/releases/2007/07/070705123157.htm

Donat, H., & Ozcan, A. (2007). Comparison of the effectiveness of two programmes on older adults at risk of falling: Unsupervised home exercise and supervised group exercise. *Clinical Rehabilitation, 21*(3), 272–283.

Gerber, L. (2007). Keeping clients fall-free. *www.nurse.com,* 7, 19.

Sullivan, M. G. (2005). Gentle exercises can lead to improved balance. *Clinical Psychiatry News, 33*(9), 48.

2. Yoga

a. *Actions/expected responses:* An Iyengar yoga program specifically designed for those over 65 increased the gait (faster stride) and postural stability (increased flexibility of lower extremities) of older women.

b. *Routes/dosages/frequencies:* 9-week program using props allowed women to gradually master the poses while building their confidence level.

c. *Cautions:* Go to http://yoga.lifetips.com/cat/56770/yoga-cautions/

d. *Assessments:* Assess gait and flexibility and number of falls prior to and after yoga participation.

e. *Tips on use:* Go to http://www.santosha.com/asanas/asana.html

f. *Other considerations:* None.

g. *References/other sources:*

Temple University. (2008, April 8). Yoga poses can prevent falls in women over 65, study suggests. *ScienceDaily.* Retrieved April 20, 2008, from http://www.sciencedaily.com/releases/2008/04/080404114445.htm

Mindset

1. Affirmations

a. *Actions/expected responses:* Self-affirmation of personal values and beliefs buffers neuroendocrine and psychological stress.

b. *Routes/dosages/frequencies:* Repeat aloud or write positive affirmations up to 20 times a day such as, "I stand and walk strong and balanced" and "I have the power and strength to maneuver in my life."

c. *Cautions:* Ensure affirmations are positive and acceptable.

d. *Assessments:* Assess anxiety prior to and after completing affirmations for a week.

e. *Tips on use:* Write favorite affirmations on 3 by 5 cards and place them where they will be read frequently.

f. *Other considerations:* Find more affirmations information at www.success consciousness.com/index_00000a.htm

g. *References/other sources:*

Hay, L. (2000). *Heal your body.* Carlsbad, CA: Hay House.

Schwarzer, R., Babler, J., Kwiatek, P., Schroder, K., & Zang, J. W. (1997). The assessment of optimistic self-beliefs: Assessment of general perceived self-efficacy in thirteen cultures. *World Psychology, 3*(1–2), 177–190.

Nutrition

1. Blueberries

a. *Actions/expected responses:* Many fruits and vegetables have been studied for their antioxidants, which protect the body against oxidative stress. Only blueberries came out on top in tests of balance and coordination.

b. *Routes/dosages/frequencies:* 1 cup a day of fresh or frozen blueberries.

c. *Cautions:* None, unless sensitive to this fruit.

d. *Assessments:* Assess balance and coordination after eating blueberries.

e. *Tips on use:* It may take up to 8 weeks to see a change in balance.

f. *Other considerations:* The phytochemicals present in blueberries, strawberries, and spinach may have properties that increase cell membrane fluidity, allowing important nutrients and chemical signals to pass in and out of the cell, thereby reducing inflammatory processes in tissues.

g. *References/other sources:*

Joseph, J. A., Shukitt-Halle, B., Denisova, N. A., Bielinksi, D., Martin, A., McEwen, J. J., et al. (1999). Reversals of age-related declines in neuronal signal transduction, cognitive, and motor behavioral deficits with blueberry, spinach, or strawberry dietary supplementation. *Journal of Neuroscience, 19*(18), 8114–8121.

2. Omega-3 fatty acids

a. *Actions/expected responses:* A high intake of omega-3s appears to preserve bone density, keeping bones stronger and protecting against falls and fractures.

b. *Routes/dosages/frequencies:* Consume ocean-grown salmon, tuna, and Spanish mackerel up to 12 ounces a week in 3–4 ounce servings (about the size of the palm of the hand when cooked). Dip fish in soy flour or drink soy milk to make bone tissue even stronger and protect against falls. Use olive oil for salads and cooking. Eat beans and rice several times a week, along with a serving of winter squash (orange or yellow). Use flaxseeds in water, drinks, soups, salads or as a coating on food or tofu prior to baking, broiling, or sautéing.

c. *Cautions:* Steer clear of large fish such as shark, swordfish, and tilefish, which contain more mercury. Also resist farm-fed fish, which may be less nutritious.

d. *Assessments:* Assess balance prior to and after intake of fish and other omega-3 sources.

e. *Tips on use:* Other sources of omega-3s are winter squash, walnuts, olive oil, beans (pinto, black, baked, etc.), and flaxseeds.

f. *Other considerations:* Grind flaxseeds in a food processor or coffee grinder.

g. *References/other sources:*

Longley, R. (2008). FDA warns women of seafood dangers: Mercury in fish may harm unborn children. FDA Food Safet Retrieved July 31, 3008 from: http://usgovinfo.about.com/cs/consumer/a/fdaonfish.htm (For more information, call 1-888SAFEFOOD 24 hours a day.)

Norwegian School of Veterinary Science. (2008, February 28). Farmed fish fed cheap food may be less nutritious for humans. *Science-Daily*. Retrieved March 9, 2008, from http://www.sciencedaily.com/releases/2008/02/080226164105.htm

Ward, W. E., & Fonseca, D. (2007). Soy isoflavones and fatty acids: Effects on bone tissue postovariectomy in mice. *Molecular Nutrition and Food Research, 51*(7), 824–831.

3. Tea
   a. *Actions/expected responses:* While drinking tea is associated with increased bone mineral density, protecting against falls and fractures, coffee is negatively associated with bone strength.
   b. *Routes/dosages/frequencies:* No trend in number of cups, so women can drink one to six cups a day.
   c. *Cautions:* Caffeinated tea can lead to jitteriness and insomnia in susceptible women.
   d. *Assessments:* Assess intake of coffee and tea.
   e. *Tips on use:* Use decaffeinated tea.
   f. *Other considerations:* The findings about tea strengthening bones is irrespective of smoking status, use of hormone replacement therapy, coffee drinking, and whether milk was added to tea.
   g. *References/other sources:*

Hegarty, V. M., May, H. M., & Khaw, K-T. (2000). Tea drinking and bone mineral density in older women. *American Journal of Clinical Nutrition, 71*(4), 1003–1007.

Muraki, S., Yamamoto, S., Ishibashi, H., Oka, H., Yoshimura, N., Kawaguchi, H., et al. (2007). Diet and lifestyle associated with increased bone mineral density: Cross-sectional study of Japanese elderly women at an osteoporosis outpatient clinic. *Journal of Orthopaedic Science, 12*(4), 317–320.

Supplements

1. Vitamin D
   a. *Actions/expected responses:* Nursing home residents who received high amounts of vitamin D had a lower number of falls and a lower incidence rate of falls over 5 months than those taking lower amounts.
   b. *Routes/dosages/frequencies:* 800 IU by mouth, daily.
   c. *Cautions:* It is not known what effect taking this amount of vitamin D may have on specific women. At least one study has shown that taking additional vitamin D can depress the immune system.
   d. *Assessments:* Assess rate of falls prior to and after taking supplemental vitamin D.
   e. *Tips on use:* Because of the potential for depressing the immune system, for light-skinned women, spending 5 minutes outside at noontime,

exposing the face and hands to sunshine three times a week provides sufficient vitamin D. (Darker-skinned women may need up to 40 minutes in the sun.)

f. *Other considerations:* None.

g. *References/other sources:*

Autoimmunity Research Foundation. (2008, January 27). Vitamin D deficiency study raises new questions about disease and supplements. *ScienceDaily.* Retrieved February 13, 2008, from http://www.science daily.com/releases/2008/01/080125223302.htm

Broe, K. E., Chen, T. C., Weinberg, J., Bischoff-Ferrari, H. A., Holick, M. F., & Kiel, D. P. (2007). A higher dose of vitamin D reduces the risk of falls in nursing home residents: A randomized, multiple-dose study. *Journal of the American Geriatrics Society, 55*(2), 234–239.

JAMA and Archives Journals. (2008, January 15). Vitamin D2 supplements may help prevent falls among high-risk older women. *ScienceDaily.* Retrieved January 22, 2008, from http://www.sciencedaily.com/releases/2008/01/080114162516.htm

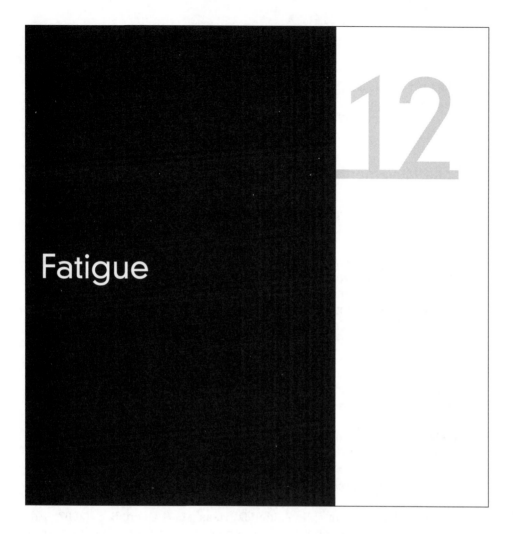

Fatigue

12

Fatigue, and symptoms vary considerably over time. Recent evidence supports the idea that complementary approaches may be effective.

Environment

1. Blue light
   a. *Actions/expected responses:* Blue light exposure may be a countermeasure for fatigue, particularly during the night. Women exposed to blue light were able to sustain a high level of alertness during the night.
   b. *Routes/dosages/frequencies:* 6 hours at night.
   c. *Cautions:* Blue light, if misused, can cause damage to the eye and exposures need to be carefully monitored.
   d. *Assessments:* Assess fatigue levels prior to and after using blue light.
   e. *Tips on use:* Blue light for shift workers could improve safety in potentially dangerous situations that may arise because of sleepiness on the job.
   f. *Other considerations:* The eye detects light to reset the body clock to the 24-hour day.

g. *References/other sources:*

Harvard Medical School. (2006). Blue light may fight fatigue. Division of Sleep Medicine. Retrieved July 31, 2008, from http://sleep.med.harvard.edu/news/28/Blue+Light+May+Fight+Fatigue

Exercise/Movement

1. Exercise
   a. *Actions/expected responses:* Exercise improves fatigue, physical functioning, and appears to be safe. It is more effective at combating fatigue than usual care.
   b. *Routes/dosages/frequencies:* Progressive walking, simple strength training movements, and stretching activities work for women. Yoga can be effective for older women between the ages of 65 and 85.
   c. *Cautions:* Work your way into an exercise program, always using warm-ups prior to and after exercising. For more information on warm-ups go to http://www.mydr.com.au/default.asp?article=2339
   d. *Assessments:* Assess fatigue prior to and after exercising.
   e. *Tips on use:* See http://yoga.lifetips.com/cat/56770/yoga-cautions/ and http://www.santosha.com/asanas/asana.html
   f. *Other considerations:* for more information on exercise, go to http://exercise.lifetips.com
   g. *References/other sources:*

Center for the Advancement of Health. (2008, April 17). Exercise combats cancer-related fatigue, review shows. *ScienceDaily*. Retrieved April 24, 2008, from http://www.sciencedaily.com/releases/2008/04/080415194430.htm

Flegal, K. E., Kishiyama, S., Zajdel, D., Haas, M., & Oken, B. S. (2007). Adherence to yoga and exercise intervention in a 6-month clinical trial. *BMC Complementary and Alternative Medicine, 9,* 37.

Ingram, C., & Visovsky, C. (2007). Exercise intervention to modify physiologic risk factors in cancer survivors. *Seminars in Oncology Nursing, 23*(4), 275–284.

Rooks, D. S., Gautam, S., Romeling, M., Cross, M. L., Stratigakis, D., Evans, B., et al. (2007). Group exercise, education, and combination self-management in women with fibromyalgia: A randomized trial. *Archives of Internal Medicine, 167*(20), 2192–2000.

Herbs/Essential Oils

1. Garlic
   a. *Actions/expected responses:* Garlic produces symptomatic improvement in women with fatigue, systematic fatigue due to cold, or lassitude of indefinite cause.
   b. *Routes/dosages/frequencies:* Raw garlic by mouth, one clove daily.
   c. *Cautions:* Garlic can stimulate labor, so it should be avoided by pregnant women. Garlic can also increase clotting time and irritate stomach

inflammation. The herb should not be used by women hypersensitive to garlic. Drugs that may interact with garlic include anticoagulants (although aged garlic extract is relatively safe and poses no serious hemorrhagic risk when closely monitored during warfarin therapy), insulin, oral antidiabetes agents, and oral contraceptives. Acidophilus can decrease the absorption of garlic. Separate the two by 3 hours for best absorption.

d. *Assessments:* Assess hypersensitivity to garlic.

e. *Tips on use:* Store garlic in a sealed container away from heat and moisture.

f. *Other considerations:* Discontinue use of garlic before undergoing any invasive procedure in which bleeding may occur.

g. *References/other sources:*

Macan, H., Uykimpang, R., Alconcel, M., Takasu, J., Razon, R., Amagase, H., et al. (2006). Aged garlic extract may be safe for patients on warfarin therapy. *Journal of Nutrition, 136*(3 Suppl.), 793S–795S.

Morihara, N., Nishihama, T., Ushijima, M., Ide, N., Takeda, H., & Hayama, M. (2007). Garlic as an anti-fatigue agent. *Molecular Nutrition and Food Research, 51*(11), 1329–1334.

Skidmore-Roth, L. (2006). Garlic. In *Mosby's handbook of herbs and natural supplements* (pp. 471–477). St. Louis, MO: ElsevierMosby.

2. Ginseng

a. *Actions/expected responses:* Lessens fatigue; energizes.

b. *Routes/dosages/frequencies:* Capsules of 200–500 mg extract daily.

c. *Cautions:* Should not be used during pregnancy or lactation or by women with hypertension, cardiac disorders, breast cancer, other estrogen-dependent conditions, or hypersensitivity to it. Adverse reactions include anxiety, restlessness, palpitations, hypertension, chest pain, nausea, vomiting, anorexia, diarrhea, and rash.

d. *Assessments:* Assess for pregnancy or lactation prior to using of ginseng. Assess level of fatigue prior to and after taking ginseng. Assess for adverse reactions.

e. *Tips on use:* Use other stimulants and antidiabetes agents carefully if taking concurrently with ginseng. Warning: Panax ginseng and Siberian ginseng are not the same thing.

f. *Other considerations:* Ginseng may interact with anticoagulants, immuno-suppressants, insulin, and MAOIs.

g. *References/other sources:*

Mayo Clinic. (2007, June 4). Ginseng shows potential reducing cancer-related fatigue. *Mayo Clinic Women's Healthsource, 11*(11), 3.

Skidmore-Roth, L. (2006). Ginseng. In *Mosby's handbook of herbs and natural supplements* (pp. 92–498). St. Louis: ElsevierMosby.

Mindset

1. Affirmations

a. *Actions/expected responses:* Self-affirmation of personal values and beliefs buffers neuroendocrine and psychological stress.

b. *Routes/dosages/frequencies:* Repeat aloud or write positive affirmations up to 20 times a day such as, "I am filled with energy and enthusiasm" and "I love my life and love what I do."

c. *Cautions:* Ensure affirmations are positive and acceptable to the woman.

d. *Assessments:* Assess anxiety prior to and after completing affirmations for a week.

e. *Tips on use:* Write favorite affirmations on 3 by 5 cards and place them where they will be read frequently.

f. *Other considerations:* Find more affirmations information at www.success consciousness.com/index_00000a.htm

g. *References/other sources:*

Hay, L. (2000). *Heal your body.* Carlsbad, CA: Hay House.

Schwarzer, R., Babler, J., Kwiatek, P., Schroder, K., & Zang, J. W. (1997). The assessment of optimistic self-beliefs: Assessment of general perceived self-efficacy in thirteen cultures. *World Psychology, 3*(1–2), 177–190.

2. Cognitive-behavioral therapy (CBT)

a. *Actions/expected responses:* CBT is a clinically effective treatment for fatigue.

b. *Routes/dosages/frequencies:* Eight weekly sessions.

c. *Cautions:* None known.

d. *Assessments:* Assess fatigue before and after CBT therapy.

e. *Tips on use:* For more information, go to http://www.mind.org.uk/Informa tion/Booklets/Making+Sense/MakingSenseCBT.htm

f. *Other considerations:* Both CBT and relaxation training (RT) are clinically effective treatments, although the effects for CBT are greater than those for RT. Even after 6 months, both treatment groups reported levels of fatigue equivalent to those of the healthy comparison group. For more information on RT, go to http://www.alternateheals.com/relaxation-therapy/home-relaxation-treatments.htm

g. *References/other sources:*

Van Kessel, K., Moss-Morris R., Wiloughby, E., Chalder, T., Johnson, M. H., & Robinson, E. (2008). A randomized controlled trial of cognitive behavior therapy for multiple sclerosis fatigue. *Psychosomatic Medicine, 70*(2), 205–213.

Nutrition

1. Micronutrients

a. *Actions/expected responses:* Inadequate intake of micronutrients, especially for women, are often the cause of fatigue.

b. *Routes/dosages/frequencies:* Eating a healthy diet of 10 servings (1/2 cup) of fruits and vegetables and omega-3 and omega-6 fatty acids can provide needed vitamins and minerals and reduce fatigue.

c. *Cautions:* Older women, pregnant women, and young adult women with demanding lifestyles who are physically active and whose dietary behavior is characterized by poor choices and/or regular dieting are at special risk for fatigue.

   d. *Assessments:* Assess fatigue prior to and after changing to a more healthy regimen.
   e. *Tips on use:* Keep a food/mood diary of everything ingested and track patterns. Once you identify how your food intake affects mood, the more apt you will be to change to a healthier way.
   f. *Other considerations:* For information on how to use telephone counseling, newsletters, and recipes to help change eating habits, go to http://www.healthyeatingucsd.org/pages/whelStudy.htm. For a discussion and listing of fatty acids, go to http://www.ific.org/publications/factsheets/omega3fs.cfm
   g. *References/other sources:*
      Huskisson, E., Maggini, S., & Ruf, M. (2007). The role of vitamins and minerals in energy metabolism and well-being. *Journal of International Medical Research, 35*(3), 277–289.
      Yehuda, S., Rabinovitz, S., & Mostofsky, D. I. (2005). Mixture of essential fatty acids lowers test anxiety. *Nutrition and Neuroscience, 8*(4), 265–267.
2. Reduce sugary foods
   a. *Actions/expected response:* Sugary foods can result in fatigue.
   b. *Routes/dosages/frequencies:* Avoid sugary foods.
   c. *Cautions:* Sugary foods usually replace needed micronutrients in the diet.
   d. *Assessments:* Assess use of sugary foods by keeping a food diary.
   e. *Tips on use:* Use alternative sweetners such as bananas, pineapple juice, raisins.
   f. *Other considerations:* If sweeteners are needed, use stevia; it has no calories or side effects and has been shown to repair DNA.
   g. *References/other sources:*
      Ghanta, S., Banerjee, A., Poddar, A., & Chattopadhyay, S. (2007). Oxidative DNA damage preventive activity and antioxidant potential of Stevia rebaudiana (Bertoni) Bertoni, a natural sweetener. *55*(26), 10962–10967.
      Osako, M., Takayama, T., & Kira, S. (2005). Dietary habits, attitudes toward weight control and subjectives symptoms of fatigue in young women. *Nippon Koshu Eisei Zasshi, 51*(5), 387–398.

Touch

1. Acupressure with massage
   a. *Actions/Expected responses:* Women who received acupressure with massage showed significantly greater improvement in reducing fatigue than women who didn't receive the treatment.
   b. *Routes/dosages/frequencies:* 12 minutes per day, 3 days per week, for 4 weeks.
   c. *Cautions:* Go to http://www.healthphone.com/consump_chinese/a_understanding_chineseourself/about_acupressure/about_acupressure.htm
   d. *Assessments:* Assess openness to massage and acupressure and response to treatment.
   e. *Tips on use:* Go to http://www.healthphone.com/consump_chinese/a_understanding_chineseourself/about_acupressure/about_acupressure.htm

    f. *Other considerations:* Evaluate fatigue levels from 1 (none) to 10 (extreme fatigue) after treatment.

    g. *References/other sources:*

        Cho., Y. C., & Tsay, S. L. (2004). The effect of acupressure with massage on fatigue and depression in patients with end-stage renal disease. *Journal of Nursing Research, 12*(1), 51–59.

2. Foot reflexology

    a. *Actions/expected responses:* Life satisfaction was significantly improved in the experimental group after foot reflexology. Combined with aromatherapy and foot soak, reflexology also relieves fatigue in clients with cancer. Foot reflexology or self-administered foot reflexology also significantly enhance and strengthen the immune system so it can catch and eliminate cancer cells and prevent tumors from developing.

    b. *Routes/dosages/frequencies:* Twice a week for 4 weeks. Three-minute foot soak contains warm water and lavender essential oil, and is followed by reflexology treatment with jojoba oil containing lavender for 10 minutes.

    c. *Cautions:* Pregnant women should avoid foot reflexology because certain manipulations can lead to premature labor. Those with foot problems, gout, arthritis, and vascular conditions such as varicose veins should be careful using this procedure. Perform a patch test with lavender essential oil prior to foot soak.

    d. *Assessments:* Evaluate life satisfaction prior to and after foot reflexology sessions. See http://employees.oneonta.edu/vomsaaw/w/handouts%20-%20happiness/life%20satisfaction%20WvS%20questionnaire.pdf. Evaluate fatigue with the Cancer Fatigue Scale before, 1 hour after, and 4 hours after treatment.

    e. *Tips on use:* For foot charts, see http://groups.msn.com/Alternatives ToPainandDisease/reflexologyinstructionspg1.msnw

    f. *Other considerations:* Quality of life is the most important predictor of survival for advanced cancer clients. See http://groups.msn.com/Alterna tivesToPainandDisease/reflexologyinstructionspg2.msnw

    g. *References/other sources:*

        Kesselring, A. (1994). Foot reflex zone massage. *Schweizerische Medizinische Wochenschrift, 62,* 88–93.

        National Cancer Institute. (2006). *Immunity and cancer.* Retrieved February 6, 2008, from http://www.nci.nih.gov/cancertopics/understanding cancer/immunesystem/Slide32

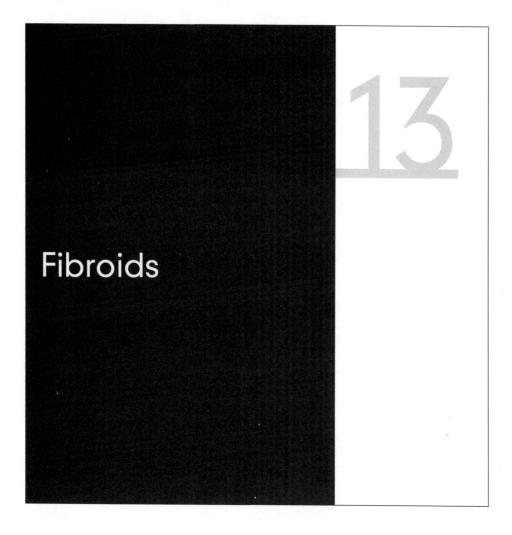

Fibroids

Medical treatment for uterine fibroids includes invasive surgery. Complementary approaches have shown to be effective without being invasive.

Environment

1. Perineal talc
   a. *Actions/expected response:* Researchers conclude that nonhormonal factors influence risk of uterine fibroids, including use of talc powder on the perineum.
   b. *Routes/dosages/frequencies:* Risk of uterine leiomyoma (fibroids) is associated in a graded fashion with the frequency of perineal talc use. No use is best.
   c. *Cautions:* Avoid using talc powder on the perineum to reduce risk for fibroids.
   d. *Assessments:* Assess use of talc on the perineum.
   e. *Tips on use:* Corn starch is a good alternative to using talc.

f. *Other considerations:* Fibroids are linked to hypertension. See pp. 45–64 for ways to reduce blood pressure.

g. *References/other sources:*

Faerstein, E., Szklo, M., & Rosenshein, N. B. (2001). Risk factors for uterine leiomyoma: A practice-based case-control study. II. *American Journal of Epidemiology, 153*(1), 11–19.

Exercise/Movment

1. Exercise

a. *Actions/expected responses:* Exercise may help prevent fibroids.

b. *Routes/dosages/frequencies:* Regular exercise, daily if possible.

c. *Cautions:* Injury can occur without warm-ups and cool downs.

d. *Assessments:* Assess regular exercise.

e. *Tips on use:* See http://yoga.lifetips.com/cat/56770/yoga-cautions/ and http://www.ronjones.org/Coach&Train/BodyXerciseLibrary/index.html

f. *Other considerations:* For more information on exercise, go to http://exercise.lifetips.com

g. *References/other sources:*

Baird, D. D., Dunson, D. B., Hill, M. C., Cousins, D., & Schectman, J. M. (2007). Association of physical activity with development of uterine leiomyoma. *American Journal of Epidemiology, 165*(2), 157–163.

Flegal, K. E., Kishiyama, S., Zajdel, D., Haas, M., & Oken, B. S. (2007). Adherence to yoga and exercise intervention in a 6-month clinical trial. *BMC Complementary and Alternative Medicine, 9,* 37.

Mindset

1. Affirmations

a. *Actions/expected responses:* Self-affirmation of personal values and beliefs buffers neuroendocrine and psychological stress.

b. *Routes/dosages/frequencies:* Repeat aloud or write positive affirmations up to 20 times a day, such as "I release old hurts," "I let go of my patterns that attracted this experience," and "I create positives in my life."

c. *Cautions:* Wait until anxiety has lessened before trying affirmations. Ask women to consider just thinking about affirmations until they are ready to act.

d. *Assessments:* Assess blood pressure prior to and after saying affirmations 20 times for several days.

e. *Tips on use:* Assess beliefs about their fibroids and use them to develop positive affirmations (e.g., "My body is healthy" or "I let go of ideas that upset me").

f. *Other considerations:* For more information go to www.successconsciousness.com/index_00000a.htm.

g. *References/other sources:*

Hay, L. (2000). *Heal your body.* Carlsbad, CA: Hay House.

Kolea, S. L., & van Knippenberg, A. (2006). Controlling your mind without ironic consequences: Self-affirmation eliminates rebound effects after thought suppression. *Journal of Experimental Social Psychology, 43*(4), 671–677.

Mann, T. (2005). Affirmation of personal values buffers neuroendocrine and psychological stress responses. *Psychological Science, 16*, 946–951.

Schwarzer, R., Babler, J., Kwiatek, P., Schroder, K., & Zang, J. W. (1997). The assessment of optimistic self-beliefs: Assessment of general perceived self-efficacy in thirteen cultures. *World Psychology, 3*(1–2), 177–190.

Nutrition

1. Beef, red meat, and ham
   a. *Actions/expected responses:* Women with uterine myomas reported more frequent consumption of beef, other red meat, and ham and less frequent consumption of green vegetables, fruit, and fish.
   b. *Routes/dosages/frequencies:* Reduce or eliminate beef, red meat, and ham, and eat green vegetables, fruit, and fish.
   c. *Cautions:* Meat is also correlated with cancer and heart disease.
   d. *Assessments:* Assess type and frequency of ingestion of red meat and ham.
   e. *Tips on use:* Introduce more green vegetables, fruit, and fish into their meals. Reduce or eliminate beef, red meat, and ham from meals.
   f. *Other considerations:* For ideas about eating more healthy, go to http://www.cooks.com/rec/ch/vegetables.html, http://www.getrichslowly.org/blog/2006/05/10/learning-to-eat-more-meals-at-home/, http://www.msnbc.msn.com/id/14958715/, http://www.ahealthyme.com/topic/fruitvegkids (useful for adults, too), and http://www.bellybytes.com/recipe/
   g. *References/other sources:*
      Chiaffarino, F., Parazzini, F., La Vecchia, C., Chatenoud, L., Di Cintio, E., & Marsico, S. (1999). Diet and uterine myomas. *Obstetrics and Gynecology, 94*(3), 395–398.
2. Soy
   a. *Actions/expected responses:* Soy (genistein) effectively blocks leiomyoma (fibroid) cell growth.
   b. *Routes/dosages/frequencies:* Eat one to two servings of soy a day, preferably fermented for easier digestion, including tempeh (follow the serving size on the package) and miso.
   c. *Cautions:* Avoid eating overprocessed forms or excessive amounts of soy on a regular basis.
   d. *Assessments:* Assess intake of soy and any sensitivity to the food.
   e. *Tips on use:* Stir-fry tempeh with fresh or frozen vegetables or use miso to make a nourishing soup.
   f. *Other considerations:* Tempeh and miso are the most digestible forms of soy.

g. *References/other sources:*

Lee, J. O., Park, M. H., Choi, Y. H., Ha, Y. L., & Ryu, C. H. (2007). New fermentation technique for complete digestion of soybean protein. *Journal of Microbiology and Biotechnology, 17*(11), 1904–1907.

Shushan, A., Ben-Bassat, H., Mishani, E., Laufer, N., & Klein, B. Y. (2007). Inhibition of leiomyoma cell proliferation in vitro by genistein and the protein tyrosine kinase inhibitor TKS050. *Fertility and Sterilization, 87*(1), 127–135.

Touch

1. Chinese approaches
   a. *Actions/expected responses:* 22 of 37 women with symptomatic fibroids treated with acupuncture, Chinese herbs, nutritional therapy, pelvic bodywork, meditation, and guided imagery saw their fibroids disappear, shrink, or stay stable compared with only 32 in 37 in the conventional hormonal manipulation and nonsteroidal anti-inflammatory medication.
   b. *Routes/dosages/frequencies:* Weekly treatments over 6 months.
   c. *Cautions:* Check for adverse reactions to Chinese herbs and acupuncture prior to undergoing treatment.
   d. *Assessments:* Assess knowledge of Chinese approaches and answer any questions. Assess fibroids prior to and after Chinese treatments.
   e. *Tips on use:* Ensure acupuncture needles have been sterilized or are new prior to undergoing a treatment.
   f. *Other considerations:* Both groups had an equal decrease in symptoms of abnormal bleeding and cramping.
   g. *References/others sources:*

   Mehl-Madrona, L. (2002). Complementary medicine treatment of uterine fibroids: A pilot study. *Alternative Therapies in Health and Medicine, 8*(2), 38–40, 44–46.

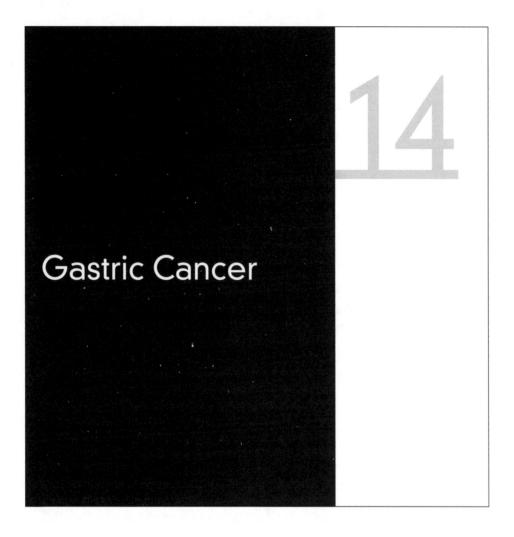

Gastric Cancer

Medical treatment for gastric cancer includes surgical removal of the stomach (gastrectomy) and is the only curative treatment. Radiation therapy and chemotherapy may also be used. Evidence exists that complementary procedures, which are less invasive, may be effective for some women.

Environment

1. Agricultural exposures
   a. *Actions/expected responses:* Gastric cancer in Californian Hispanic farm workers is associated with work in the citrus fruit industry and among those who work in fields treated with 2,4-D, chlordane, propargite, and trifluin.
   b. *Routes/dosages/frequencies:* Working in areas with high use of the phenoxyacetic acid herbicide 2,4-D.
   c. *Cautions:* 2,4-D, chlordane, propargite, and trifluin are linked with gastric cancer.

    d. *Assessments:* Assess agricultural exposure.

    e. *Tips on use:* Avoid pesticides.

    f. *Other considerations:* These findings may have larger public health implications especially in those areas of the country where these pesticides are heavily used and where they may be found in the ambient atmosphere.

    g. *References/other sources:*

        Mills, P. K., & Yang, R. C. (2007). Agricultural exposures and gastric cancer risk in Hispanic farm workers in California. *Environmental Research, 104*(2), 282–289.

2. Computed Tomography (CT) scans

    a. *Actions/expected responses:* CT scans could be responsible for raising the risk of cancer.

    b. *Routes/dosages/frequencies:* A typical CT scan delivers 50 to 100 times more radiation than a conventional X-ray.

    c. *Cautions:* Brenner and Hall (2007) estimate that one-third of all CT scans might not be necessary.

    d. *Assessments:* Assess number of CT scans.

    e. *Tips on use:* Use the safer options of ultrasound and magnetic resonance imaging, which do not expose women to radiation.

    f. *Other considerations:* An estimated 62 million CT scans were performed in 2006 compared to only 3 million in 1980.

    g. *References/other sources:*

        Brenner, D., & Hall, E. J. (2007). Computed tomography, an increasing source of radiation exposure. *New England Journal of Medicine, 357*(22), 2277–2284.

3. Hexavalent chromium (Cr+6) in drinking water

    a. *Actions/expected responses:* Stomach cancer and all cancers are linked in human and animal studies with Cr+6-contaminated drinking water.

    b. *Routes/dosages/frequencies:* By drinking Cr+6-contaminated water, risk of stomach cancer increases.

    c. *Cautions:* Have drinking water checked by a reliable source.

    d. *Assessments:* Assess drinking water for the presence of Cr+6.

    e. *Tips on use:* As a preventive measure, drink and use either distilled water or water that has passed through a reverse-osmosis water filter.

    f. *Other considerations:* Cr+6 has been found in 38% of municipal sources of drinking water in California and is widely used in electroplating, stainless steel production, leather tanning, textile manufacturing, and wood preservation in the United States, the greatest producer of chromium compounds.

    g. *References/other sources:*

        Beaumont, J. J., Sedman, R. M., Reynolds, S. D., Sherman, C. D., Li, L. H., Howd, R. A., et al. (2008). Cancer mortality in a Chinese population exposed to hexavalent chromium in drinking water. *Epidemiology, 19*(1), 12–23.

        Sedman, R. M., Beaumont, J., McDonald, T. A., Reynolds, S., Krowech, G., & Howd, R. (2006). Review of the evidence regarding the carcinogenicity of hexavalent chromium in drinking water. *Journal of Environmental Science and Health Part C, 24*(1), 155–182.

Herbs/Essential Oils

1. Aloe vera (cape aloe)
   a. *Actions/expected responses:* Anti-inflammatory, antibacterial, antifungal, protective against the liver, and inhibits growth of tumors.
   b. *Routes/dosages/frequencies:* 1–3 ounces three times a day after meals.
   c. *Cautions:* Avoid using aloe vera if sensitive to it.
   d. *Assessments:* Assess digestive inflammation prior to and after taking aloe vera.
   e. *Tips on use:* Buy aloe vera gel from a health food store, buy the herb in a glass container if possible, never drink the juice or gel from home aloe plants (this can lead to diarrhea), and store aloe vera gel in the refrigerator once opened.
   f. *Other considerations:* Aloe contains vitamins A, B-complex, E, carboxypeptidase (anti-inflammatory enzyme), magnesium, potassium, calcium, magnesium, manganese, copper, zinc, chromium, iron, glucomannans (immunomodulator), saponins (antiseptic), anthraquinone (aids absorption in the gastrointestinal tract), salicylic acid (anti-inflammatory), and amino acids (protein building blocks).
   g. *References/other sources:*
      Kametani, S., Oikawa, T., Kojima-Yuasa, A., Kennedy, D. O., Norikura, T., Honzawa, M., et al. (2008). Mechanism of growth inhibitory effect of cape aloe extract in ehrlich ascites tumor cells. *Journal of Nutrition Science and Vitaminology, 53*(6), 540–546.
      Skidmore-Roth, L. (2006). Aloe. In *Mosby's handbook of herbs and natural supplements* (pp. 30–35). St. Louis, MO: ElsevierMosby.
2. Aromatherapy
   a. *Actions/expected responses:* Laboratory and clinical research with women has shown that the use of essential oils from plants (typically chamomile, geranium, and lavender) support and balance the mind, body, and spirit and can enhance quality of life.
   b. *Routes/dosages/frequencies:* Inhalation or skin application as requested after initial treatment.
   c. *Cautions:* None known. Safety testing on essential oils has found very few, if any, bad effects.
   d. *Assessments:* Assess for stress prior to and after using aromatherapy.
   e. *Tips on use:* Choose the oils or combinations that work best for them.
   f. *Other considerations:* Inhale a specific essential oil(s) or add a few drops to bath oil or pillow.
   g. *References/other sources:*
      National Cancer Institute. (2008). *Aromatherapy and essential oils.* Retrieved July 31, 2008, from www.cancer.gov/cancertopics/pdq/cam/aromatherapy/patient
      Wilkinson, S. M., Love, S. B., Westcombe, A. M., Gambles, M. A., Burgess, C. C., & Cargill, A. (2007). Effectiveness of aromatherapy massage in the management of anxiety and depression in patients with cancer: A multicenter randomized controlled trail. *Journal of Clinical Oncology, 25*(5), 532–539.

3. Basil leaf
   a. *Actions/expected responses:* Basil leaf extract has tumor inhibition and immune stimulant characteristics.
   b. *Routes/dosages/frequencies:* By mouth, either fresh as a spice in food, or powdered on food.
   c. *Cautions:* When pregnant, avoid basil in large amounts; dietary uses are safe. Basil can have mutagenic effects on fetuses. Women diagnosed with diabetes should use basil cautiously; it can increase the hypoglycemic effects of insulin and oral antidiabetes agents; do not use concurrently.
   d. *Assessments:* Assess use of insulin and oral antidiabetes agents.
   e. *Tips on use:* Cut leaves and place in salads, soups, sauces and stews. Use dried leaves as a tea in half a cup of boiling water; strain and drink half a cup twice a day.
   f. *Other considerations:* Because of its mutagen ability, avoid using large amounts of basil for long periods of time.
   g. *References/other sources:*
      Dasgupta, T., Rao, A. R., & Yadava, P. K. (2004). Chemomodulatory efficacy of basil leaf on drug metabolizing and antioxidant enzymes, and on carcinogen-induced skin and forestomach papillomagenesis. *Phytomedicine, 11*(2–3), 139–151.
      Skidmore-Roth, L. (2006). Basil. In *Mosby's handbook of herbs and natural supplements* (pp. 84–88). St. Louis, MO: ElsevierMosby.

Mindset

1. Affirmations
   a. *Actions/expected responses:* Self-affirmation of personal values and beliefs buffers neuroendocrine and psychological stress.
   b. *Routes/dosages/frequencies:* Repeat aloud or write positive affirmations up to 20 times a day such as, "Life agrees with me" and "I release all hurts and resentments."
   c. *Cautions:* Ensure affirmations are positive and acceptable.
   d. *Assessments:* Assess anxiety prior to and after completing affirmations for a week.
   e. *Tips on use:* Write favorite affirmations on 3 by 5 cards and place them where they will be read frequently.
   f. *Other considerations:* Find more affirmations information at www.success consciousness.com/index_00000a.htm
   g. *References/other sources:*
      Hay, L. (2000). *Heal your body.* Carlsbad, CA: Hay House.
      Schwarzer, R., Babler, J., Kwiatek, P., Schroder, K., & Zang, J. W. (1997). The assessment of optimistic self-beliefs: Assessment of general perceived self-efficacy in thirteen cultures. *World Psychology, 3*(1–2), 177–190.

Nutrition

1. Folate
   a. *Actions/expected responses:* Dietary folates are protective against cancer, but folic acid fortification is associated with cancer. Because national

surveys revealed most women did not consume adequate folate, a grain fortification program is in place.

b. *Routes/dosages/frequencies:* Leafy green vegetables (like spinach and turnip greens), broccoli, fruits (citrus fruits and juices), and dried beans and peas are all natural sources of folate that can help meet the suggested amount of 1,000 micrograms (mcg) a day. Women on diets who do not eat breads, cereals, or pasta, who abuse alcohol, or who take medications that interfere with folate absorption may not receive sufficient amounts of the nutrient and may need additional amounts.

c. *Cautions:* Medications and medical conditions that increase the need for folate or result in an increased excretion of folate include: anticonvulsant medications, metformin, sulfasalazine, triamterene, methotrexate, barbiturates, pregnancy and lactation, alcohol abuse, malabsorption, kidney dialysis, liver disease, and certain anemias. Because folate is a water-soluble B-vitamin, unneeded amounts will be eliminated in the urine.

d. *Assessments:* Assess for signs of folate deficiency: anemia, diarrhea, loss of appetite, weight loss, weakness, sore tongue, headaches, heart palpitations, irritability, forgetfulness, behavioral disorders, and an elevated level of homocysteine.

e. *Tips on use:* Avoid flour-fortified foods as a source of folic acid; new research has shown the introduction of flour fortified with folic acid into common foods has been linked to cancer.

f. *Other considerations:* Exceeding 1,000 mcg per day of folate may trigger vitamin B12 deficiency. To compensate, women can take a multivitamin that contains B12 or eat at least one food daily that contains B12: nutritional yeast (unless susceptible to candida), clams, eggs, herring, kidney, liver, mackerel, seafood, milk, or dairy products.

g. *References/other sources:*

Blackwell Publishing Ltd. (2007, November 5). Folic acid linked to increased cancer rate, historical review suggests. *ScienceDaily.* Retrieved November 29, 2007, from http://www.sciencedaily.com-/releases/2007/11/07/071102111956.htm

Office of Dietary Supplements. (2005). *Dietary supplement fact sheet: Folate.* Bethesda, MD: NIH Clinical Center, National Institutes of Health. Retrieved November 25, 2007, from http://ods.od.nih.gov

2. Fruits, vegetables, and whole grains

a. *Actions/expected responses:* The consumption of fruits and vegetables and whole grains are linked to a decreased risk for cancers. Tomatoes are especially helpful. Tomatoes show a consistent pattern of protection when eaten raw and often. Consuming one serving of raw tomatoes per week reduced the risk of all cancers by 50% for older women. Watercress is linked to a reduced risk of cancer via decreased damage to DNA.

b. *Routes/dosages/frequencies:* Encourage women to eat 5–10 servings (1/2 cup) of fruits and vegetables daily, and 5 servings of whole grains (barley, buckwheat, bulgur/cracked wheat, millet, oatmeal, popcorn, whole-wheat bread and pasta, and/or wild rice).

c. *Cautions:* Some women may be sensitive to certain fruits, vegetables, or grains (especially wheat).

d. *Assessments:* Assess for sensitivity to and affinity for various fruits, vegetables, and grains.

e. *Tips on use:* Go to http://www.cooks.com/rec/ch/vegetables.html and http://www.ahealthyme.com/topic/fruitvegkids (useful for adults, too).

f. *Other considerations:* Fruits and vegetables contain a plethora of anticarcinogenic substances including carotenoids, vitamins C and E, selenium, dietary fiber, flavonoids, polyphenols, and many other health-producing compounds. Grains to avoid: corn flakes, enriched macaroni or spaghetti, couscous, grits, pretzels, white bread, rye bread, white rice.

g. *References/other sources:*

Franceschi, S., Bidoli, E., La Vecchia, C., Talamini, R., D'Avanzo, B., & Negri, E. (1994). Tomatoes and risk of digestive-tract cancers. *International Journal of Cancer, 59*(2), 181–184.

Gill, C. I., Haldar, S., Boyd, L. A., Bennett, R., Whiteford, J., Butler, M., et al. (2007). Watercress supplementation in diet reduces lymphocyte DNA damage and alters blood antioxidant status in healthy adults. *American Journal of Clinical Nutrition, 85*(2), 504–510.

Hord, N. G. (2005). The role of dietary factors in cancer prevention: Beyond fruits and vegetables. *Nutrition in Clinical Practice, 20*(4), 451–459.

3. Green tea

a. *Actions/expected responses:* Green tea is protective against cancer before disease occurs and after onset, possibly by creating a detoxifying effect.

b. *Routes/dosages/frequencies:* Two to five cups of decaffeinated tea daily (1 tsp tea leaves in 8 ounces of hot water).

c. *Cautions:* May decrease iron absorption, so separate iron-rich foods or iron pills by at least 2 hours from green tea ingestion.

d. *Assessments:* Assess for hypersensitivity reactions. Also assess for cardiovascular (increased blood pressure, palpitations, and irregular heartbeat), central nervous system (anxiety, nervousness, insomnia), and gastrointestinal (nausea, heartburn, increased stomach acid) effects.

e. *Tips on use:* Caffeinated green tea can interact with MAOIs and lead to a hypertensive crisis. Avoid taking green tea with anticoagulants/antiplatelets (may increase risk of bleeding), beta-adrenergic blockers (can lead to increased inotropic effects), or benzodiazepines (may increase sedation). Teach women to store green tea in a cool, dry place.

f. *Other considerations:* Dairy products may decrease the therapeutic effects of green tea, so separate their intake by several hours. Digestive process affects anticancer activity of tea in gastrointestinal cells; add citrus (such as lemon juice) or take ascorbic acid (vitamin C) to protect the catechins in green tea from digestive degradation.

g. *References/other sources:*

American Association for Cancer Research. (2007, August 12). Green tea boosts production of detox enzymes, rendering cancerous chemicals harmless. *ScienceDaily.* Retrieved December 20, 2007, from http://www.sciencedaily.com/releases/2007/08/070810194923.htm

Federation of American Societies for Experimental Biology. (2008, April 10). Digestive process affects anti-cancer activity of tea in gastrointestinal cells. *ScienceDaily.* Retrieved April 20, 2008, from http://www.sciencedaily.com/releases/2008/04/080407172713.htm

Pettit, J. L. (2001). Green tea. *Clinician Reviews, 11*(1), 71–72.

Skidmore-Roth, L. (2006). Green tea. In *Mosby's handbook of herbs and natural supplements* (pp. 535–539). St. Louis, MO: ElsevierMosby.

4. Maitake mushrooms

a. *Actions/expected responses:* Animal and human studies have supported the use of maitake for cancer. This mushroom is an immune modulator that helps to normalize the immune system. It exerts an anticancer action by activating interleukin-1 and increasing T-cells.

b. *Routes/dosages/frequencies:* Eat as part of a healthy diet to enhance the immune system.

c. *Cautions:* Avoid if sensitive to this food. May interact with immunosuppressants and antidiabetes agents.

d. *Assessments:* Assess sensitivity to maitake and use of immunosuppressants and antidiabetes agents.

e. *Tips on use.* Store maitake in a clean, dry place, away from heat. For recipes and ways to use maitake, go to http://theforagerpress.com/fieldguide/maitake/maitake-recipes.htm

f. *Other considerations:* Maitake and other mushrooms have been used for thousands of years in Asia for many purposes. Maitake is also available in capsules or as an extract.

g. *References/other sources:*

Kodama, N., Komuta, K., & Nanba, H. (2002). Can maitake MD-fraction aid cancer patients? *Alternative Medicine Review, 7*(3), 236–239.

5. Red and processed meat, onions and garlic

a. *Actions/Expected responses:* Consumption of red and processed meat is positively associated with non-cardiac stomach cancer, while onions and garlic reduce the risk of stomach cancer.

b. *Routes/dosages/frequencies:* Eliminate red and processed meat from the diet. Eat onions and garlic daily.

c. *Cautions:* Red and processed meat is linked with stomach cancer.

d. *Assessments:* Assess intake of red and processed meat, and onions and garlic.

e. *Tips on use:* Add powdered or fresh garlic and onions to salads, stews, sauces, soups, sandwiches, fish, tofu, and other foods.

f. *Other considerations:* Garlic and onions are toxic for many animals. Keep garlic and onions away from pets.

g. *References/other sources:*

Dorant, E., van den Brandt, P. A., Goldbohm, R. A., & Sturmans, F. (1996). Consumption of onions and a reduced risk of stomach carcinoma. *Gastroenterology, 110*(1), 12–20.

Gonzalez, C. A., & Riboli, E. (2006). Diet and cancer prevention: Where we are, where we are going. *Nutrition in Cancer, 56*(2), 225–231.

Stress Management

1. Stress management procedures

a. *Actions/expected responses:* A weak immune system is one of the major factors that promotes cancer metastases after an operation, chemotherapy, or radiation therapy. Fear and stress weaken the immune system. Adequate stress management prior to and after medical treatment may help to prevent metastases.

b. *Routes/dosages/frequencies:* Adequate stress management prior to and after medical treatment may help to prevent metastases.

c. *Cautions:* Use stress management procedures to enhance immune system and protect against metastases.

d. *Assessments:* Assess knowledge of stress management techniques.

e. *Tips on use:* Learn stress management procedures.

f. *Other considerations:* For teaching materials, go to http://www.mindful nessmeditationcentre.org/breathingGathas.htm, http://www.santosha.com/asanas/asana.html, and http://www.alternateheals.com/relaxationtherapy/home.relaxation.treatments.htm

g. *References/other sources:*

Tel Aviv University. (2008, February 29). Stress and fear can affect cancer's recurrence. *ScienceDaily.* Retrieved March 9, 2008, from http://www.sciencedaily.com/releases/2008/02/080227142656.htm

Supplements

1. Beta-carotene, vitamin E, and selenium

   a. *Actions/expected responses:* Supplementation with beta-carotene, vitamin E, and selenium reduced gastric cancer incidence, mortality, and overall cancer mortality in poorly nourished women.

   b. *Routes/dosages/frequencies:* Daily intake of supplements.

   c. *Cautions/adverse reactions:* Take no more than 400 micrograms (mcg) per day of selenium. Reactions are rare, but do not exceed suggested dosage.

   d. *Assessments:* Assess for poor nourishment.

   e. *Tips on use:* Store supplements in a cool, dry place.

   f. *Other considerations:* It's usually safer to obtain vitamins and minerals from food. Food sources of beta-carotene include: sweet potatoes, carrots, kale, spinach, turnip greens, winter squash, collard greens, cilantro, and fresh thyme. Food sources of vitamin E include: sunflower seeds, almonds, filberts, turnip greens, tomato paste, pine nuts, peanut butter, wheat germ, avocado, carrot juice, olive oil, spinach, dandelion greens, sardines, blue crab, Brazil nuts, and pickled herring. For food sources of selenium go to http://ods.od.nih.gov/factsheets/selenium.asp.

   g. *References/other sources:*

   Huang, H. Y., Caballero, B., Chang, S., Alberg, A., Semba, R., Schneyer, C., et al. (2006). Multivitamin/mineral supplements and prevention of chronic disease. *Evidence Reports and Technology Assessments, 139,* 1–117.

2. Pycnogenol and ginkgo biloba extract

   a. *Actions/expected responses:* Either pycnogenol or ginkgo biloba extract can protect against antimutagenic activity in animal studies.

   b. *Routes/dosages/frequencies:* 5–100 microgram/mL.

   c. *Cautions:* Until more research is completed, pregnant and lactating women should not use these supplements, nor should they be given to children. Ginkgo should not be taken concurrently with anticoagulants.

d. *Assessments:* Assess reaction to pycnogenol and ginkgo.

e. *Tips on use:* Store supplements in a cool, dry place.

f. *Other considerations:* Pycnogenol has also been found useful in preventing venous thrombosis, thrombophlebitis, gingival bleeding and plaque, inflammatory bowel disease, venous insufficiency, digestive conditions, and menopause symptoms.

g. *References/other sources:*

Krizkova, L., Chovanova, Z., Durackova, Z., & Krajcovic, J. (2008). Antimutagenic in vitro activity of plan polyphenols: Pycnogenol and Ginkgo biloba extract. *Phytotherapy Research, 22*(3), 384–388.

3. Vitamins A, C, and E

a. *Actions/expected responses:* Dietary intake of foods high in vitamins A, C, and E may decrease the risk of gastric cancer. When derived from plant sources, all three vitamins show an inverse relationship to this type of cancer.

b. *Routes/dosages/frequencies:* By mouth. The best way to obtain vitamins is via food. See "Assessments" section for food sources. If extremely ill, stressed, or can't or don't eat well, a multivitamin or juices made from fresh vegetables and fruits may be the best approach for this population.

c. *Cautions:* If supplements are chosen, choose brands that do not contain additional herbs, fillers, dyes, and so forth. Strive for the least processed form available. Vitamin C should not be taken when fat resides in the stomach because at this time it can promote, rather than prevent, the formation of certain cancer-causing chemicals.

d. *Assessments:* Assess intake of vitamin A foods (animal livers, apricots, asparagus, beet greens, broccoli, cantaloupe, carrots, collards, dandelion greens, papaya, peaches, red peppers, spinach, sweet potatoes, Swiss chard, turnip greens, watercress, yellow squash), vitamin C foods (asparagus, avocadoes, beet greens, black currants, broccoli, Brussels sprouts, cantaloupe, collards, dandelion greens, grapefruit, kale, lemons, mangos, mustard greens, onions, oranges, papayas, green peas, sweet peppers, persimmons, pineapple, radishes, spinach, strawberries, Swiss chard, tomatoes, turnip greens, and watercress), and vitamin E foods (brown rice, cold-pressed vegetable oils, cornmeal, dark green leafy vegetables, eggs, legumes, nuts, oatmeal, organ meats, seeds, soybeans, wheat germ, and whole grains).

e. *Tips on use:* Store supplements in a cool, dry place. Follow directions on the bottle.

f. *Other considerations:* Juicers are available online and at health food stores. Making juices may be especially useful for women who have lost their appetite or have digestion issues.

g. *References/other sources:*

Balch, J. F., & Balch, P. A. (1997). *Prescription for nutritional healing.* Garden City Park, NY: Avery Publishing Group.

Combet, E., Paterson, S., Iijama, K., Winter, J., Mullen, W., Crozier, A., et al. (2007). Fat transforms ascorbic acid from inhibiting to promoting acid-catylsed N. nitrosation. *Gut, 56,* 1678–1684.

Sylvester, P. W. (2007). Vitamin E and apoptosis. *Vitamins and Hormones, 76,* 329–356.

Touch

1. Acupressure
   a. *Actions/expected responses:* Acupressure can reduce nausea and vomiting induced by chemotherapy.
   b. *Routes/dosages/frequencies:* Stimulate the PC6 point for at least 6 hours per day at the onset of chemotherapy. The PC6 point is situated in the middle of the front of the forearm above the wrist crease. Wristbands are available to stimulate this point. The point can be stimulated every 2–3 hours or as needed.
   c. *Cautions:* Avoid using this point if wrists have been injured.
   d. *Assessments:* Assess nausea and vomiting prior to and after stimulating the PC6 point.
   e. *Tips on use:* Wristbands may be easier to use because they can be placed on the wrists and do not require constant self-stimulation.
   f. *Other considerations:* None.
   g. *References/other sources:*
      Klein, J., & Griffiths, P. (2004). Acupressure for nausea and vomiting in cancer patients receiving chemotherapy. *British Journal of Community Nursing, 9*(9), 383–388.
2. Foot reflexology
   a. *Actions/expected responses:* Life satisfaction was significantly improved in the experimental group after foot reflexology. Combined with aromatherapy and foot soak, reflexology also relieves fatigue in clients with cancer. Foot reflexology or self-administered foot reflexology also significantly enhances and strengthens the immune system so that it can catch and eliminate cancer cells and prevent tumors from developing.
   b. *Routes/dosages/frequencies:* Twice a week for 4 weeks. Three-minute foot soak contains warm water and lavender essential oil, and is followed by reflexology treatment with jojoba oil containing lavender for 10 minutes. Four 40-minute self-administered foot reflexology treatments can also be of benefit. See http://www.handbag.com/healthfit/complementary/acupressure.
   c. *Cautions:* Avoid foot reflexology when pregnant because certain manipulations can lead to premature labor. Women with foot problems, gout, arthritis, and vascular conditions such as varicose veins should be careful using this procedure. Perform a patch test with lavender essential oil prior to foot soak.
   d. *Assessments:* Evaluate life satisfaction, fatigue, and or life satisfaction prior to and after foot reflexology sessions. See http://employees.oneonta.edu/vomsaaw/w/handouts%20-%20happiness/life%20satisfaction%20WvS%20questionnaire.pdf. Evaluate fatigue with the Cancer Fatigue Scale before, 1 hour after, and 4 hours after treatment.
   e. *Tips on use:* For foot charts, see http://groups.msn.com/AlternativesToPainandDisease/reflexologyinstructionspg1.msnw
   f. *Other considerations:* Quality of life is the most important predictor of survival for advanced cancer clients. See http://groups.msn.com/AlternativesToPainandDisease/reflexologyinstructionspg2.msnw

g. *References/other sources:*

Fox Chase Cancer Center. (2007, November 1). Quality of life is the most important predictor of survival for advanced cancer patients. *Science-Daily.* Retrieved November 12, 2007, from http://www.sciencedaily.com/releases/2007/10/071030170208.htm

Kesselring, A. (1994). Foot reflex zone massage. *Schweizerische Medizinische Wochenschrift, 62,* 88–93.

3. Therapeutic touch (TT)

a. *Actions/expected responses:* Women who received three noncontact therapeutic touch treatments reported increased well-being as opposed to a control group who rested.

b. *Routes/dosages/frequencies:* 15–20 minutes once a day.

c. *Cautions:* The aged, extremely ill, or dying should be given a 5-minute (or less) treatment by an experienced practitioner.

d. *Assessments:* Take a baseline measure of well-being prior to and after administering TT.

e. *Tips on use:* Center and calm yourself by closing your eyes and focusing on breathing in your abdomen. When relaxed, rub your hands together and feel the tingling sensation as you slowly pull your hands apart until you are able to feel the energies balancing between the hands. Hold the intent to balance the other person's energy and start with your hands above the woman's head. Keep an inch or so away from the body, bring your hands slowly down, sweeping down the body slowly, ending a few inches past the feet. For more information, go to http://www.healgrief.com/Site/Heal_Grief_in_Your_Body.html

f. *Other considerations:* Regular TT treatments may enhance the effect achieved.

g. *References/other sources:*

Giasson, M. (1998). Effect of therapeutic touch on the well-being of persons with terminal cancer. *Journal of Holistic Nursing, 16*(3), 383–398.

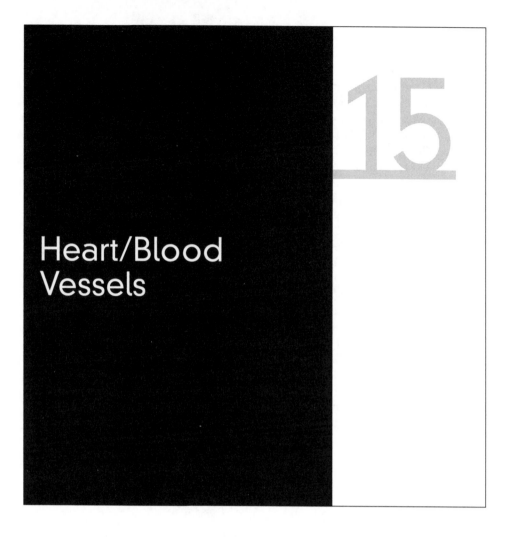

Heart/Blood Vessels

Drugs (that can have negative side effects) and surgery are the medical treatments for heart and blood vessel conditions. Complementary procedures are not invasive and can be quite effective.

Environment

1. Aspirin
   a. *Actions/expected responses:* Randomized clinical trials testing aspirin in relatively low-risk middle-aged women have consistently shown small increases in stroke associated with aspirin use.
   b. *Routes/dosages/frequencies:* Frequent aspirin use is associated with an increased rate of ischemic stroke compared with nonusers.
   c. *Cautions:* Even low doses of aspirin may result in cardiovascular events.
   d. *Assessments:* Assess cardiovascular risk. For more information, go to http://www.med.yale.edu/library/heartbk/3.pdf
   e. *Tips on use:* Discuss the pros and cons of this issue with prescribing health care practitioner.

f. *Other considerations:* Because of increased risk of stroke with aspirin, dietary and lifestyle counseling should remain the most important primary prophylaxis in women with cardiovascular risk factors.

g. *References/other sources:*

Eikelboom, J. W., Hirsh, J., Weitz, J. I., Johnston, M., Qilong, Y., & Yusuf, S. (2002). Aspirin-resistant thromboxane biosynthesis and the risk of myocardial infarction, stroke, or cardiovascular death in patients at high risk for cardiovascular events. *Circulation, 105,* 1650.

Follath, F. (1994). Primary prevention of coronary heart disease with drugs: Wishful thinking or reality? *Therapeutische Umschau, 10,* 677–682.

Kronmal, R. A., Hart, R. G., Manolio, T. A., Talbert, R. L., Beauchamp, A., & Newman, A. (1998). Aspirin use and incident stroke in the cardiovascular health study. *Stroke, 29,* 887–894.

2. C-reactive protein (CRP)

a. *Actions/expected responses:* Studies suggest that CRP is an inflammatory marker that can predict recurrent cardiovascular disease, such as heart attack and stroke. Weight loss reduces CRP.

b. *Routes/dosages/frequencies:* The higher the CRP level, the higher the risk for cardiovascular disease, stroke, and death.

c. *Cautions:* High CRP levels are associated with low survival rates.

d. *Assessments:* Assess weight.

e. *Tips on use:* Stop smoking, lose weight, reduce high blood pressure, and consume less sugar to reduce cardiovascular risks.

f. *Other considerations:* For information on smoking cessation, go to http://www.helpguide.org/mental/quit_smoking_cessation.htm. For information on cardiovascular risk assessment, go to http://hp2010.nhlbihin.net/atpiii/calculator.asp?usertype=prof. For information on weight loss, see pp. 287–298.

g. *References/other sources:*

American Heart Association. (2008). *Inflammation, heart disease and stroke: The role of C-reactive protein.* Retrieved September 2, 2008 from http://www.americanheart.org/presenter.jhtml?identifier=4648

Selvin, E., Paynter, N. P., & Erlinger, T. P. (2007). The effect of weight loss on C-reactive protein: A systematic review. *Archives of Internal Medicine, 167*(1), 31–39.

3. Drinking water

a. *Actions/expected responses:* Water replaces lost fluids, while caffeinated beverages or alcohol increase fluid output, leeching out needed liquids, minerals, and vitamins. Dehydration can lead to fatal coronary heart disease, venous thromboembolism, and mitral valve prolapse.

b. *Routes/dosages/frequencies:* At least 8–10 glasses a day.

c. *Cautions:* Tap water and even bottled water can contain parasites, weed killers, nitrates (correlated with spontaneous miscarriage and so-called blue-baby syndrome), salmonella, E. coli, chlorine, fluoride, and other potentially dangerous substances.

d. *Assessments:* Assess type and quantity of water women drink.

e. *Tips on use:* Drink (and cook with) only distilled water or reverse-osmosis filtered water.

f. *Other considerations:* Fluid intake is probably adequate when thirst is rarely experienced and when urine is colorless or slightly yellow. As women age, they may experience less thirst. Counsel older women to drink water before thirst sets in, because by that time dehydration may already have taken over.

g. *References/other sources:*

Doull, J., Boekelheide, K., Farishian, B. G., Isaacson, R. L., Klotz, J. B., Limeback, H., et al. (2006). *Committee on Fluoride in Drinking Water Board on Environmental Studies and Toxicology, Division of Earth and Life Sciences, National Research Council of the National Academies. Fluoride in drinking water: A scientific review of EPA's standards.* Washington, DC: National Academies Press.

Manz, F. (2007). Hydration and disease. *Journal of American College of Nutrition, 26*(5 Suppl.), 535S–541S.

4. Fluoride in drinking water

a. *Actions/expected responses:* Chronic administration of aluminum fluoride and sodium fluoride in drinking water resulted in distinct morphological alterations in the brain, including effects on neurons and the cerbrovasculature.

b. *Routes/dosages/frequencies:* Chronic daily drinking of water with fluoride (either aluminum or sodium).

c. *Cautions:* Drinking water with fluoride in it may negatively affect blood vessels in the brain by altering the cerebral blood flow.

d. *Assessments:* Assess type of drinking water used.

e. *Tips on use:* Drink either distilled water or water that has passed through a reverse-osmosis filter.

f. *Other considerations:* Animals who were given fluoridated water had more infections and mortality than those who weren't given that treatment.

g. *References/other sources:*

Varner, J. A., Jensen, K. F., Horvath, W., & Isaacson, R. L. (1998). Chronic administration of aluminum-fluoride or sodium-fluoride to rats in drinking water: Alterations in neuronal and cerebrovascular integrity. *Brain Research, 784,* 284–298.

5. Hormone therapy

a. *Actions/expected responses:* Increased cardiovascular disease risk from discontinuing hormone therapy can be minimized by lifestyle change intervention.

b. *Routes/dosages/frequencies:* Women who want to reduce their risk for cardiovascular disease must decrease their weight (if they're overweight), eat healthy fats, and increase leisure physical activity.

c. *Cautions:* Cardiovascular disease is more likely when women discontinue hormones and omit protective lifestyle changes.

d. *Assessments:* Assess use of hormones and plans to discontinue their use. Assess knowledge of potential risks of cardiovascular disease without lifestyle change.

e. *Tips on use:* See http://exercise.lifetips.com

f. *Other considerations:* See http://www.tipsforlosingweight.com and http://www.thedietchannel.com/weightloss.htm

g. *References/other sources:*

Elsevier Health Sciences. (2007, May 16). Reducing cardiovascular disease risk factors when discontinuing hormone replacement therapy. *ScienceDaily.* Retrieved March 2, 2008, from, http://www.sciencedaily.com/releases/2007/05/070515074741.htm

6. Mercury and other air pollutants

a. *Actions/expected responses:* Mercury has been linked to heart disease, as have other forms of air pollution.

b. *Routes/dosages/frequencies:* Mercury activates an enzyme, which triggers a process leading to plaque buildup in blood vessel walls. Air pollution increases C-reactive protein (an indicator of risk for a cardiovascular event), 9-OHdG (a marker of oxidative stress), PAI-1 (a marker of inflammation), and decreases heart rate variability (a predictor of increased cardiovascular risk).

c. *Cautions:* Mercury can be harmful as methylmercury, thimerosal (in vaccines), or mercuric chloride. Air pollutants are especially harmful as particulate matter, sulfate, nitrate, and ozone.

d. *Assessments:* Assess exposure to mercury via the atmosphere, vaccines, or the food source, including closeness to mining, smelting, precious metal extraction, instrument manufacture, gilding industry, manufacture of drugs and health products using mercury, felting of fur, fingerprinting with mercury-chalk mixture, dental work, pulp and paper industries, landfills, dental preparations and laboratories using mercury, coal-burning emissions, hazardous wastes, improper disposal of products or wastes containing mercury, fish and seafood, poorly ventilated indoor spaces when exposed to elemental mercury or products containing mercury, topical mercury-based skin creams, infant teething powders, contact solutions, nasal sprays, broken fluorescent lights or thermometers, and vaccines/vaccinations. Assess exposure to air pollution by checking air pollution rates in city of residence.

e. *Tips on use:* To protect the heart, avoid exposure to mercury and air pollution whenever possible.

f. *Other considerations:* Chelation therapy, a process that removes metals from the body, and antioxidants both show signs of suppressing the activity of mercury. Eating more fruits, vegetables, and beans, especially as 1/2 cup blueberries, kidney or pinto or black beans, cranberries, cooked artichoke hearts, blackberries, prunes, raspberries, strawberries, cherries, granny smith or red delicious or gala apples, black plums, or 1 ounce of pecans can provide helpful antioxidants.

g. *References/other sources:*

American Thoracic Society. (2007, August 16). Air pollution linked to cardiovascular risk indices in healthy young adults. *ScienceDaily.* Retrieved January 21, 2008, from http://www.sciencedaily.com/releases/2008/08/070815085429.htm

Ohio State University Medical Center. (2007, May 31). Mercury's link to heart disease begins in blood vessel walls. Retrieved March 2, 2008, from http://www.sciencedaily.com/releases/2007/05/070531085829.htm

University of California-Los Angeles. (2007, July 27). Air pollution linked to clogged arteries. *ScienceDaily.* Retrieved March 4, 2008, from http://www.sciencedaily.com/releases/2007/07/070726090009.htm

7. Power-frequency fields
   a. *Actions/expected responses:* Cardiovascular effects are associated with electromagnetic fields (EMFs).
   b. *Routes/dosages/frequencies:* Current levels of long-term exposure to some kinds of electromagnetic fields are not protective of public health.
   c. *Cautions:* Scientific evidence raises concerns about the health impacts of mobile or cell phone radiation, power lines, interior wiring and grounding of buildings, and appliances such as microwaves, wireless technologies, and electric blankets.
   d. *Assessments:* Assess exposure to EMFs listed in item c.
   e. *Tips on use:* Until new public safety limits and limits on further deployment of risky technologies are warranted, avoid exposure to EMFs.
   f. *Other considerations:* An international working group of renowned scientists, researchers and public health policy professionals (The Bioinitiative Working Group) has released its report on electromagnetic fields and health. It raises serious concerns about the safety of existing public limits that regulate how much EMF is allowable from power lines, cell phones, and many other EMF sources of exposure in daily life.
   g. *References/other sources:*
      Hardell, L., & Sage, C. (2007). Biological effects from electromagnetic field exposure and public exposure standards. *Biomedical Pharmacotherapy, 62*(2), 104–109.
8. Social support
   a. *Actions/expected responses:* Casting a wide net when it comes to friends and family appears to be associated with a dramatically lower risk of suffering a heart attack, landing in a hospital, or dying from heart disease.
   b. *Routes/dosages/frequencies:* Having one or two casual friends was associated with better health outcomes, and the larger the social circle, the healthier the women were.
   c. *Cautions:* Choose friends carefully and do not disclose too much immediately.
   d. *Assessments:* Assess social support network.
   e. *Tips on use:* Find people with similar interests, to enhance good feelings.
   f. *Other considerations:* To meet new friends, join a group or class focused on valued activities. Church, recreational, or work groups may also be helpful.
   g. *References/other sources:*
      Ross, M. F. (2005, February 16). *Size, strength of social networks influence heart disease risk.* Press release, University of Florida, Gainesville, Office of News and Communication.
9. Sunshine
   a. *Actions/expected responses:* Vitamin D from sun exposure will protect against cardiovascular disease.
   b. *Routes/dosages/frequencies:* Expose the face, arms, hands, or back to midday sunlight for 10–15 minutes twice a week if fair-skinned or 35–40 minutes if dark-skinned.
   c. *Cautions:* Only expose face and arms to sun for 10–15 minutes if fair-skinned or 40 minutes if dark-skinned. Taking vitamin D supplements may suppress the immune system.

    d. *Assessments:* Assess exposure to midday sun. Assess ingestion of vitamin D supplements.

    e. *Tips on use:* Get sun exposure twice weekly.

    f. *Other considerations:* Avoid vitamin D supplements.

    g. *References/other sources:*

        American Heart Association. (2008, January 8). Lack of vitamin D may increase heart disease risk. *ScienceDaily.* Retrieved January 15, 2008, from http://www.sciencedaily.com/releases/2008/01/080107181600.htm

        Autoimmunity Research Foundation. (2008, January 27). Vitamin D deficiency study raises new questions about disease and supplements. *ScienceDaily.* Retrieved February 13, 2008, from http://www.science daily.com/releases/2008/01/080125223302.htm

        Martins, D., Wolf, M., Pan, D., Zadshir, A., Tareen, N., Thadhani, R., et al. (2007). Prevalence of cardiovascular risk factors and the serum levels of 250 hydroxy vitamin D in the United States: Data from the Third National Health and Nutrition Examination Survey. *Archives of Internal Medicine, 167*(11), 1159–1165.

10. Thyrotropin

    a. *Actions/expected responses:* Women's risk of fatal coronary heart disease (CHD) rises with levels of thryotropin a hormone that stimulates thyroid function, according to a recent study of 25,313 women.

    b. *Routes/dosages/frequencies:* This fatal risk occurs even when the levels are within the normal range.

    c. *Cautions:* If on thyrotropin, discuss lowering the range of the hormone with prescribing health care practitioner.

    d. *Assessments:* Ask prescribing health care practitioner to assess thyrotropin range.

    e. *Tips on use:* To reduce fatal CHD risk, investigate other ways to help thyroid function that don't include thyrotropin.

    f. *Other considerations:* None.

    g. *References/other sources:*

        Thyrotropin linked to fatal CHD risks in women. (2008, July). *The Clinical Advisor,* 10. (For more information about the study, go to http://www. sciencedaily.com /releases/2008/04/080428162532.htm)

Exercise/Movement

1. Aerobic training

    a. *Actions/expected responses:* Aerobic exercise training consisting of a warm-up, exercise on a stationary bicycle, followed by walking and jogging can decrease cardiovascular risk.

    b. *Routes/dosages/frequencies:* 10 minutes of stretching, followed by exercise on a stationary bicycle followed by 35 minutes of walking and jogging at a target intensity of 70%–85% of heart reserve.

    c. *Cautions:* Women with stable ischemic heart disease should participate in intense exercise.

    d. *Assessments:* Assess stability of ischemic heart disease. Assess interest in participating in an aerobic program. Assess cardiovascular risk prior to and after engaging in aerobic exercise.

e. *Tips on use:* Sitting has negative effects on fat and cholesterol metabolism. Computer-generated phone calls may be an effective low-cost way to encourage sedentary adults to exercise as well as stand instead of sitting while performing household chores, shopping, typing and more. For information on warm ups and cool downs prior to and after exercising, go to http://www.wellness.ma/adult-fitness/stretching-warmup.htm.

f. *Other considerations:* Exercise duration per session is the most important element of an exercise prescription for increasing HDL ("good") cholesterol. Exercise is more effective for women with initially high total cholesterol levels or low body mass index. Even moderate exercise can reduce the incidence of and rehabilitation from cardiovascular diseases by 49%.

g. *References/other sources:*

Blumenthal, J. A., Sherwood, A., Babyak, M. A., Watkins, L. L., Waugh, R., Georgiades, A., et al. (2005). Effects of exercise and stress management training on markers of cardiovascular risk in patients with ischemic heart disease. *Journal of the American Medical Association, 293,* 1626–1634.

Kodama, S., Tanaka, S., Saito, K., Shu, M., Sone, Y., Onitake, F., et al. (2007). Effect of aerobic exercise training on serum levels of high-density lipoprotein cholesterol: A meta-analysis. *Archives of Internal Medicine, 167*(10), 999–1008.

Kruk, J. (2007). Physical activity in the prevention of the most frequent chronic diseases: An analysis of the recent evidence. *Asian Pacific Journal of Cancer Prevention, 8*(3), 325–338.

Stanford University Medical Center. (2007, December 5). Computer calls can talk couch potatoes into walking, study finds. *ScienceDaily.* Retrieved December 10, 2007 from http://www.sciencedaily.com/releases/2007/12/071204122000.htm

University of Missouri-Columbia. (2007, November 20). Sitting may increase risk of disease. *ScienceDaily.* Retrieved March 3, 2008, from http://www.sciencedaily.com/releases/2007/11/071119130734.htm

2. Resistance training

a. *Actions/expected responses:* Women with chronic congestive heart failure (CHF), must maintain and/or increase muscle mass and strength.

b. *Routes/dosages/frequencies:* Dynamic resistance exercise is well tolerated in chronic stable CHF when (a) initial contraction intensity is low, (b) small muscle groups are involved, (c) work phases are kept short, (d) a small number of repetitions per set is performed, and (e) work-to-rest ratio is greater than or equal to 1:2. With resistance training programs lasting 12 weeks, maximal strength could be improved by 15%–50%.

c. *Cautions:* No differences were found between combined resistance/aerobic training and resistance training alone. Thus, resistance exercise can be assumed to be as safe as aerobic exercise in clinically stable CHF.

d. *Assessments:* Assess stability.

e. *Tips on use:* For information on strength training, go to http://www2.gsu.edu/~wwwfit/strength.html and http://www.internetfitness.com/articles/strength_benefits.htm

f. *Other considerations:* By following a 12-week resistance program, improvements in maximum exercise time and the total amount of oxygen needed and taken in were between 10%–18%.

    g. *References/other sources:*

       Meyer, K. (2006). Resistance exercise in chronic heart failure—Landmark studies and implications for practice. *Clinical Investigations in Medicine, 29*(3), 166–169.

3. Sports participation

    a. *Actions/expected responses:* Participating in sports reduces the risk of developing a blood clot in a lung artery by 46% and a blood clot in a leg vein by 24%.

    b. *Routes/dosages/frequencies:* Participation in sports at least once per week, regardless of the type of sport or its intensity, reduced the risk of developing a blood clot.

    c. *Cautions:* Go to http://www.lasting-weight-loss.com/dangers.html

    d. *Assessments:* Assess participation in sports.

    e. *Tips on use:* None.

    f. *Other considerations:* Women who did not participate in sports were more than four times as likely to develop a blood clot when obese (with a body mass index of 30 or greater) than when lean (with a body mass index of less than 25).

    g. *References/other sources:*

       Blackwell Publishing Ltd. (2007, November 21). Regular exercise reduces risk of blood clots, study suggests *Science Daily.* Retrieved November 29, 2007, from http://www.sciencedaily.com/releases/2007/11/071120124245.htm.

4. Tai chi

    a. *Actions/expected responses:* Tai chi improves quality of life in women with heart failure, increases results on a 6-minute walk test, and improves B-type natriuretic peptide levels in women with heart failure, compared to a control group.

    b. *Routes/dosages/frequencies:* 1-hour classes twice weekly participation in tai chi for 12 weeks.

    c. *Cautions:* None.

    d. *Assessments:* Assess attraction to tai chi. This exercise is appealing for women with congestive heart failure because it is low impact, not particularly strenuous, and easy to perform even for nonfit individuals.

    e. *Tips on use:* For directions on tai chi, go to http://www.everyday-taichi.com/tai-chi-instruction.html, http://www.everyday-taichi.com/, and http://www.activevideos.com/taichi.htm

    f. *Other considerations:* Meditative, mind-body techniques can modulate the neurohormonal axis and decrease sympathetic tone. The meditative aspects of breath control and relaxation have their own benefits.

    g. *References/other sources:*

       Kirn, T. (2004, February). Tai chi improves quality of life in heart failure. *Clinical Psychiatry,* 90.

5. Yoga

    a. *Actions/expected responses:* Practice of hatha yoga can improve strength and flexibility and may help control such physiological variables as blood pressure, respiration and heart rate, and metabolic rate to improve overall exercise capacity for women with cardiopulmonary disease.

    b. *Routes/dosages/frequencies:* Participate in a 30- to 60-minute yoga class or use a yoga tape (do a Google search for yoga tapes) at home.

c. *Cautions:* Go to http://yoga.lifetips.com/cat/56770/yoga-cautions/

d. *Assessments:* Assess for heavy menstrual flow, pregnancy, knee problems, and conditions that may affect yoga practice.

e. *Tips on use:* Because yoga exerts pressure on internal organs, wait at least 2 hours after a meal and 30 minutes to 1 hour after a snack to practice. For more information about yoga, go to www.mothernature.com/Library/Bookshelf/Books/21/54.cfm and http://www.santosha.com/asanas/asana.html

f. *Other considerations:* To avoid knee injury when doing yoga, keep the knees straight (especially in standing poses). The knees should be forward in line with the ankle and foot and should not twist inward or outward.

g. *References/other sources:*

Raub, J. A. (2002). Psychophysiologic effects of hatha yoga on musculo-skeletal and cardiopulmonary function: A literature review. *Journal of Alternative and Complementary Medicine, 8*(6), 797–812.

Herbs/Essential Oils

1. Chamomile tea

a. *Actions/expected responses:* Chamomile shows significant antiplatelet activity in vitro. Animal model studies indicate potent anti-inflammatory action and cholesterol-lowering activities, as well as antispasmotic and anxiolytic effects.

b. *Routes/dosages/frequencies:* Drink as a tea using either 2–4 ounces as needed or one to two tea bags per day.

c. *Cautions:* Avoid if sensitive to flowers. Avoid concurrent use of chamomile with anticoagulants and central nervous system depressants. Avoid during pregnancy; it is a known abortifacient.

d. *Assessments:* Assess for sensitivity to flower, pregnancy, or use of anticoagulants or central nervous system depressants.

e. *Tips on use:* Store chamomile in a tightly closed jar in a cool, dark place.

f. *Other considerations:* Chamomile can also be used to enhance sleep and topically to increase wound healing.

g. *References/other sources:*

McKay, D. L., & Blumberg, J. B. (2006). A review of the bioactivity and potential health benefits of chamomile tea (Matricaria recutita L.). *Phytotherapy Research, 20*(7), 519–530.

2. Fenugreek

a. *Actions/expected responses:* Fenugreek can lower blood lipid levels, reduce cholesterol, and improve hemorheological properties.

b. *Routes/dosages/frequencies:* One cup of tea made from a teabag per day for up to 6 weeks.

c. *Cautions:* This herb rapidly coats the intestinal system and may reduce absorption of medications used concurrently. Pregnant women should not use fenugreek; it may cause premature labor.

d. *Assessments:* Assess sensitivity to fenugreek and medications used.

e. *Tips on use:* Keep fenugreek teabags in a tightly closed container, away from heat and moisture.

f. *Other considerations:* Fenugreek can also lower blood glucose.

    g. *References/other sources:*

Xue, W. L., Li, S. X., Zhang, J., Liu, Y. H., Wang, Z. L., & Zhang, R. J. (2007). Effect of trigonella foenum-graecum (fenugreek) extract on blood glucose, blood lipid and hemorheological properties in streptozotocin-induced diabetic rats. *Asia Pacific Journal of Clinical Nutrition, 16,* (1 Suppl.), 422–426.

3. Green tea
    a. *Actions/expected responses:* Green tea consumption is associated with improved myocardial function and reduced mortality due to cardiovascular diseases.
    b. *Routes/dosages/frequencies:* Two to three cups of green tea a day.
    c. *Cautions:* Caffeine may increase restlessness and talkativeness; decaffeinated green tea is preferable.
    d. *Assessments:* Assess for allergies or sensitivity to the tea.
    e. *Tips for use:* Steep teabags in boiling water for 10 minutes; let cool and drink.
    f. *Other considerations:* The protective effect of green tea is strongest for women.
    g. *References/other sources:*

Hirai, M., Hotta, Y., Ishikawa, N., Wakida, Y., Fukuzawa, Y., Isobe, F., et al. (2007). Protective effects of EGCg or GCg, a green tea catechin epimer, against postischemic myocardial dysfunction in guinea-pig hearts. *Life Science, 80*(11), 1020–1032.

Kuriyama, S., Shimazu, T., Ohmori, K., Kikuchi, N., Nakaya, N., Nichino, Y., et al. (2006). Green tea consumption and mortality due to cardiovascular disease, cancer and all causes in Japan. *Journal of the American Medical Association, 296*(10), 1255–1265.

4. Hawthorn
    a. *Actions/expected responses:* Hawthorn produces a significant benefit in symptom control and physiologic outcomes as a treatment for chronic heart failure.
    b. *Routes/dosages/frequencies:* Take daily 1/4–1/2 tsp three times a day or 100–250 mg three times a day.
    c. *Cautions:* Avoid hawthorn if sensitive to it or if pregnant or lactating. Adverse effects to watch for include low blood pressure, arrhythmias, fatigue, nausea, vomiting, loss of appetite. Hawthorn may increase effects of antihypertensives, cardiac glycosides, and central nervous system depressants; avoid using concurrently. This herb may increase the absorption of iron salts; separate by 2 hours.
    d. *Assessments:* Assess hypersensitivity reactions. Assess symptoms prior to and after taking hawthorn.
    e. *Tips of use:* Store hawthorn in a cool, dry place.
    f. *Other considerations:* Hawthorn increases blood supply to the heart, increases the force of contractions and indirectly inhibits angiotensin-converting enzyme (ACE). The herb also stabilizes collagen, reduces atherosclerosis, and decreases cholesterol.
    g. *References/other sources:*

Pittler, M., Guo, R., & Ernst, E. (2008). Hawthorn extract for treating chronic heart failure. *Cochrane Database System Review, 1,* CD005312.

Skidmore-Roth, L. (2006). Hawthorn. In *Mosby's handbook of herbs and natural supplements* (pp. 555–559). St. Louis, MO: ElsevierMosby.

5. Mate tea

   a. *Actions/expected responses:* Mate (yerba mate) tea lowers cholesterol when compared to drinking milk or coffee. Blood levels of the cardio-protective enzyme paraoxonase-1 increased an averaged of 10% for mate tea drinkers only. Yerba mate tea has a natural sweetness.

   b. *Routes/dosages/frequencies:* Steep four to five bags in a quart of boiling water for up to 15 minutes and drink when cooled.

   c. *Cautions:* Go to http://www.mundomatero.com/yerba/Health-Benefits.html

   d. *Assessments:* Assess cholesterol prior to and after drinking mate tea.

   e. *Tips on use:* Go to http://www.mundomatero.com/yerba/How-Use.html

   f. *Other considerations:* For another way to prepare the tea, go to http://www.mundomatero.com/yerba/How-prepare.html

   g. *References/other sources:*

University of Illinois at Urbana-Champaign. (2007, October 26). Mate tea lowers cholesterol. *ScienceDaily.* Retrieved November 12, 2007, from http://www.sciencedaily.com/releases/2007/10/071023163949.htm

Mindset

1. Affirmations

   a. *Actions/expected responses:* Self-affirmation of personal values and beliefs buffers neuroendocrine and psychological stress.

   b. *Routes/dosages/frequencies:* Repeat aloud or write positive affirmations up to 20 times a day such as, "I accept and love my life" and "I move through life easily."

   c. *Cautions:* Ensure affirmations are positive and acceptable.

   d. *Assessments:* Assess anxiety prior to and after completing affirmations for a week.

   e. *Tips on use:* Write favorite affirmations on 3 by 5 cards and place them where they will be read frequently.

   f. *Other considerations:* Find more affirmations information at www.success consciousness.com/index_00000a.htm

   g. *References/other sources:*

Hay, L. (2000). *Heal your body.* Carlsbad, CA: Hay House.

Schwarzer, R., Babler, J., Kwiatek, P., Schroder, K., & Zang, J. W. (1997). The assessment of optimistic self-beliefs: Assessment of general perceived self-efficacy in thirteen cultures. *World Psychology, 3*(1–2), 177–190.

2. Cognitive-behavioral therapy (CBT)

   a. *Actions/expected responses:* CBT improves depression in women following coronary artery bypass graft surgery.

   b. *Routes/dosages/frequencies:* 8-week program of individual CBT.

   c. *Cautions:* None.

   d. *Assessments:* Assess signs of depression (poor sleep, increased or decreased appetite, worry, sense of guilt) prior to and after taking part in CBT.

  e. *Tips on use:* It may be helpful to keep a diary of depression symptoms during the 8 weeks.

  f. *Other considerations:* Between-session assignments are often given to help apply concepts learned during sessions.

  g. *References/other sources:*

DeRubeis, R. J., Hollon, S. D., & Amsterdam, J. D. (2005). Cognitive therapy vs. medications in the treatment of moderate to severe depression. *Archives of General Psychiatry, 62,* 409–416.

Jancin, B. (2005, July). CBT improves post-CABG depression in women. *Clinical Psychiatry News,* 57.

National Association of Cognitive-Behavioral Therapists. Retrieved August 1, 2008 from, www.nacbt.org/whatiscbt.htm

Nutrition

1. Alpha-linolenic acid

  a. *Actions/expected responses:* A new study has shown that consuming vegetable oils rich in alpha-linolenic acid (ALA) is associated with significant reductions in the risk of nonfatal myocardial infarction (heart attack/MI).

  b. *Routes/dosages/frequencies:* Eating soybean, canola and/or flaxseed oil every day.

  c. *Cautions:* None.

  d. *Assessments:* Assess intake of ALA.

  e. *Tips on use:* Just half a teaspoon a day of flaxseed oil or one to two teaspoons of soybean oil is sufficient to increase ALA intake.

  f. *Other considerations:* Using salad dressings using canola or soybean oil would be enough to increase intake to cardioprotective levels.

  g. *References/other sources*

Barclay, L. (2008, July 11). Alpha-linolenic acid reduces risk of nonfatal MI. *Medscape CME.* Retrieved August 7, 2008, from http://www.medscape.com/viewarticle/577420?sssdmh=dm1.367895&src=nldne

2. Animal protein versus antioxidant foods

  a. *Actions/expected responses:* Antioxidants prevent cardiovascular disease naturally, and cholesterol changes can be made through dietary changes alone. Heme iron from red meat, fish, and poultry is associated with heart disease, as are ham, salami, and butter, but not eggs. Foods containing high amounts of heart-protective antioxidants include beans (small red, kidney, pinto, and black), fruits (apples with peels, berries, avocados, cherries, green and red pears, fresh or dried plums, pineapple, oranges, and kiwi), vegetables (artichokes, spinach, red cabbage, red and white potatoes with peels, sweet potatoes, and broccoli), green tea, nuts (especially walnuts, pistachios, pecans, hazelnuts, and almonds), oats, ground cloves, cinnamon or ginger, dried oregano leaf, and turmeric powder.

  b. *Routes/dosages/frequencies:* By mouth, 5–10 servings of fruits and vegetables a day. A handful of nuts daily. Oatmeal with ground cloves, cinnamon, or ginger daily. Use oregano leaf and turmeric spice on vegetables or in soups or salads.

  c. *Cautions:* Some women may be sensitive to certain fruits or vegetables.

d. *Assessments:* Assess for sensitivity to and affinity for various fruits and/or vegetables, nuts, and oats.

e. *Tips on use:* Go to http://www.cooks.com/rec/ch/vegetables.html, http://www.ahealthyme.com/topic/fruitvegkids (useful for adults, too).

f. *Other considerations:* Fruits and vegetables contain a plethora of helpful substances including carotenoids, vitamins C and E, selenium, dietary fiber, flavonoids, polyphenols, and many other health-producing compounds. A low-fat diet rich in vegetables, fruits, whole grains, and beans had twice the cholesterol-lowering power as a conventional low-fat diet. Apples, berries, and onion are especially associated with reduced risk of coronary heart disease because they contain quercetin. The American Heart Association adds soy protein and nuts to round out an eating regimen found to be as effective as taking statin medication, and with none of the side effects. The more soy isoflavones women eat, the lower their risk for cerebral and myocardial infarctions. Eating soy as tempeh allows for higher protein digestibility.

g. *References/other sources:*

Djousse, L., & Gaziano, J. M. (2008). Egg consumption in relation to cardiovascular disease and mortality: The Physicians' Health Study. *American Journal of Clinical Nutrition, 87*(4), 964–969.

Gardner, C. D., Coulston, A., Chatterjee, L., Rigby, A., Spiller, G., & Farquhar, J. W. (2005). The effect of a plant-based diet on plasma lipids in hypercholesterolemic adults: A randomized trial. *Annals of Internal Medicine, 142*(9), 725–733.

Jenkins, D. J., Kendall, C. W., Marchie, A., Faulkner, D. A., Wong, J. M., de Souze, R., et al. (2003). Effects of a dietary portfolio of cholesterol-lowering foods vs. Lovastatin on serum lipids and C-reactive protein. *Journal of American Medical Association, 290*(4), 502–510.

Kokubo, Y., Iso, H., Ishihara, J., Okada, K., Inoue, M., & Tsugane, S. (2007). Association of dietary intake of soy, beans and isoflavones with risk of cerebral and myocardial infarctions in Japanese populations: The Japan Public Health Center-based (JHPC) study cohort. *Circulation, 116*(22), 2553–2562.

Kris-Etherton, P. M., Hecker, K. D., Bonanome, A., Coval, S. M., Binkoski, A. E., Hilpert, K. F., et al. (2002). Bioactive compounds in foods: Their role in the prevention of cardiovascular disease and cancer. *American Journal of Medicine, 113*(9B Suppl.), 71S–88S.

Lee, J. O., Park, M. H., Choi, Y. H., Ha, Y. L., & Ryu, C. H. (2007). New fermentation technique for complete digestion of soybean protein. *Journal of Microbiology and Biotechnology, 17*(11), 1904–1907.

Mayo Clinic. (2007, September 13). Antioxidants prevent diseases naturally. *ScienceDaily*. Retrieved September 13, 2007, from http://www.sciencedaily.com/releases/2007/09/070908001613.htm

Qi, L., van Dam, R. M., Rexrode, K., & Hu, F. B. (2007). Heme iron from diet as a risk factor for coronary heart disease in women with type 2 diabetes. *Diabetes Care 30* (1), 101–106.

University of Michigan Health System. (2008, March 6). Many patients can reach LDL cholesterol goal through dietary changes alone, study shows. *ScienceDaily*. Retrieved March 9, 2008, from http://www.sciencedaily.com/releases/2008/03/080304105817.htm

3. Calcium
   a. *Actions/expected responses:* Foods high in calcium increase the so-called good (HDL) cholesterol.
   b. *Routes/dosages/frequencies:* Eat high-calcium foods daily.
   c. *Cautions:* None unless sensitive to a particular food, then avoid.
   d. *Assessments:* Assess intake of calcium-rich foods.
   e. *Tips on use:* Eat at least 1/2 cup daily of the following foods whenever possible to enhance calcium intake: soy drinks, tofu, soybeans, sardines, collards, spinach, turnip greens, oatmeal, ocean perch, and low-fat yogurt. Take several tablespoons of blackstrap molasses a day (can be placed in drinks, used instead of sugar in cooking or baking, or eaten off the spoon.
   f. *Other considerations:* For more information on calcium-rich foods, go to http://www.health.gov/dietaryguidelines/dga2005/document/html/appendixB.htm
   g. *References/other sources:*
      Drouillet, P., Balkau, B., Charles, M. A., Vol, S., Bedouet, M., Ducimetiere, P. (2007). Calcium consumption and insulin resistance syndrome parameters. *Nutrition and Metabolism in Cardiovascular Disease, 17*(7), 486–492.
      Olatunji, L. A., Soladoye, A. O., & Oyeyipo, P. I. (2008). Effect of increased dietary calcium on hemorheological, lipid and lipid peroxidation in oral contraceptive-treated female rats. *Clinical Hemorheological Microcirculation, 38*(2), 135–142.
4. Cherries
   a. *Actions/expected responses:* Tart cherries may reduce heart inflammation, lower cholesterol and triglycerides, and help lose weight.
   b. *Routes/dosages/frequencies:* 1.5 cups a day of tart cherries or dried and mixed into a food.
   c. *Cautions:* These findings are based on animal studies, but a human trial is underway.
   d. *Assessments:* Assess amount of tart cherries consumed.
   e. *Tips on use:* For a tasty breakfast, mix 1.5 cups of dried cherries with 1–2 cups lowfat or nonfat plain yogurt, 1 packet of stevia, and 1 banana. Place in blender and blend to preferred consistency.
   f. *Other considerations:* None.
   g. *References/other sources:*
      University of Michigan Health System. (2008, April 10). Tart cherries may reduce factors associated with heart disease and diabetes. *ScienceDaily.* Retrieved April 20, 2008, from http://www.sciencedaily.com/releases/2008/04/080407114647.htm
5. Cinnamon
   a. *Actions/expected responses:* Cinnamon lowers total cholesterol and triacylglycerol.
   b. *Routes/dosages/frequencies:* 2 1/2 tsp of cinnamon used as a spice in a bowl of oatmeal or rice.
   c. *Cautions:* Until more research is conducted, avoid during pregnancy and lactation in large doses. Can be used safely as a spice.
   d. *Assessments:* Assess use of cinnamon and hypersensitivity, including wheezing or rash.

e. *Tips on use:* Store cinnamon in a cool, dry place.

f. *Other considerations:* Sprinkle cinnamon on oatmeal, rice, or pears and try it on other foods such as stews, prunes, cereals, yogurt, and soups.

g. *References/other sources:*

Hlebowicz, J., Darwiche, G., Bjorgell, O., & Almer, L. O. (2007). Effect of cinnamon on postprandial blood glucose, gastric emptying, and satiety in healthy subjects. *American Journal of Clinical Nutrition, 85*(6), 1552–1556.

Skidmore-Roth, L. (2006). Cinnamon. In *Mosby's handbook of herbs and natural supplements* (pp. 302–305). St. Louis, MO: ElsevierMosby.

6. Coffee, tea, and soft drinks

a. *Actions/expected responses:* Green tea is associated with a lowered heart disease risk (even for smokers), lowers the so-called bad cholesterol, increases the heart-protective HDL cholesterol, and can reduce the risk of cardiovascular disease in diabetes with a significant improvement in lipid metabolism. Coffee (black or decaffeinated) elevates cholesterol. Habitual coffee consumption is associated with heightened acute inflammatory response in the blood vessels to mental stress. Use of soft drinks is linked to increase in risk factors for heart disease, including obesity.

b. *Routes/dosages/frequency* By mouth, daily. Green tea is available in capsules, extract, or bags. Drink two to five cups per day.

c. *Cautions:* Caffeinated green tea should not be used by women with hypersensitivity to green tea or by those with kidney inflammation, gastrointestinal ulcers, insomnia, cardiovascular disease, or increased intraocular pressure. High doses of caffeinated green tea can result in palpitations and irregular heart beat, anxiety, nervousness, insomnia, nausea, heartburn, and increased stomach acid. The decaffeinated form may be a better choice for these reasons.

d. *Assessments:* Assess women for hypersensitivity to forms and brands of tea and counsel women to use the one they are not sensitive to.

e. *Tips on use:* Store green tea in a cool, dry place. To brew tea, put one bag in a large cup, fill with boiling water, and let steep for 5 minutes before drinking. Add lemon juice (helps decrease degradation of catechins in digestive tract) and/or stevia (helps repair DNA).

f. *Other considerations:* Antacids may decrease the therapeutic effects of green tea, and green tea may interact with anticoagulants/antiplatelets, increasing risk of bleeding. Avoid drinking green tea while taking MAOIs or bronchodilators.

g. *References/other sources:*

American Heart Association. (2007, July 25). Diet and regular soft drinks linked to increase in risk factors for heart disease. *ScienceDaily.* Retrieved March 8, 2008, from http://www.sciencedaily.com/releases/2007/07/070723163526.htm

Anandh Babu, P. V., Sabitha, K. E., & Shyamaladevi, C. S. (2006). Green tea extract impedes dyslipidaemia and development of cardiac dysfunction in streptozotocin-diabetic rats. *Clinical Experimental Pharmacology and Physiology, 33*(12), 1184–1189.

Baylor College of Medicine. (2007, June 15). How coffee raises cholesterol. *ScienceDaily*. Retrieved March 8, 2008, from http://www.sciencedaily. com/releases/2007/06/070614162223.htm

Ghanta, S., Banerjee, A., Poddar, A., & Chattopadhyay, S. (2007), Oxidative DNA damage preventive activity and antioxidant potential of Stevia rebaudiana Bertoni, a natural sweetener. *Journal of Agricultural and Food Chemistry, 55*(26), 10962–10967.

Hamer, M., Eilliams, E. D., Vuononvirta, R., Gibson, E. L., & Steptoe, A. (2006). Association between coffee consumption and markers of inflammation and cardiovascular function during mental stress. *Journal of Hypertension, 24*(11), 2191–2197.

Maron, D. J., Lu, G. P., Caik, N. S., Wu, G., Li, Y. H., Chen, H., et al. (2003). Cholesterol-lowering effect of a theaflavin-enriched green tea extract. *Archives of Internal Medicine, 163,* 1448–1453.

MLA Purdue University. (2007, November 14). Citrus juice, vitamin C give staying power to green tea antioxidants. *ScienceDaily*. Retrieved August 2, 2008, from http://www.sciencedaily.com/releases/2007/11/071113163016.htm

Sego, S. (2007, July). Green tea. *The Clinical Advisor,* 139–140.

Skidmore-Roth, L. (2006). Green tea. In *Mosby's handbook of herbs and natural supplements* (3rd ed., pp. 535–539). St. Louis, MO: ElsevierMosby.

7. Curcumin (turmeric)
   a. *Actions/expected responses:* Curcumin can prevent heart failure, relax blood vessels, and reduce the atherogenic properties of cholesterol.
   b. *Routes/dosages/frequencies:* Curcumin, from the curry spice turmeric, possesses the ability to inhibit hypertrophy of cardiomyocytes.
   c. *Cautions:* The herb is safe in food doses and up to 12 grams a day. In larger quantities it can have strong activity in the common bile duct that might aggravate the passage of gallstones in women currently suffering from the condition.
   d. *Assessments:* Assess sensitivity to curcumin.
   e. *Tips on use:* Counsel caregivers to serve curry or food seasoned with curcumin at least once a week; doing so more often may produce better results.
   f. *Other considerations:* None.
   g. *References/other sources:*
   Anand, P., Kunnumakkara, A. B., Newman, R. A., & Aggarwal, B. B. (2007). Bioavailability of curcumin: Problems and promises. *Molecular Pharmacology, 4*(6), 807–818.

   Morimoto, T., Sunagawa, Y., Kawamaura, T., Takaya, T., Wada, H., et al. (2008). The dietary compound curcumin inhibits p300 histone acetyltransferase activity and prevent heart failure in rats. *Journal of Clinical Investigation, 118*(3), 868–878.

8. Garlic
   a. *Actions/expected responses:* The raw form of garlic and some of its preparations are widely recognized as antiplatelet agents that may contribute to the prevention of cardiovascular disease.
   b. *Routes/dosages/frequencies:* Eat 1–2 crushed cloves of garlic and juice; cook using moderate heat for no more than 5 minutes.
   c. *Cautions:* Garlic can stimulate labor and cause colic in infants and should not be used medicinally, but dietary amounts are safe. Avoid using prior

to surgery as clotting times may be increased. Avoid use if sensitive or if the use of garlic results in stomach inflammation or gastritis. In the latter case, powdered garlic or garlic capsules may be used. Avoid concurrent use with insulin and antidiabetic agents: garlic has a hypoglycemic effect, and dosages may need to be readjusted. Garlic may decrease the action of oral contraceptives and anticoagulants. Separate intake of garlic by three hours from fish oil capsules (may increase the risk of bleeding) or acidophilus (which may decrease the absorption of garlic).

d. *Assessments:* Assess pregnancy, upcoming surgery, and sensitivity to garlic.

e. *Tips on use:* Oven-heating garlic or immersing it in boiling water for 3 minutes or less did not affect the ability of garlic to inhibit platelet aggregation, as compared to raw garlic. Heating for 6 minutes completely suppressed the antiaggregatory activity in uncrushed garlic, but not in previously crushed samples.

f. *Other considerations:* The addition of raw garlic juice to microwaved, uncrushed garlic restored a full complement of antiplatelet activity that was completely lost without the juice addition. Aged garlic extract may be safe for women on warfarin therapy.

g. *References/other sources:*

Cavagnaro, P. F., Camargo, A., Galmarini, C. R., & Simon, P. W. (2007). Effect of cooking on garlic (Allium sativum L.) antiplatelet activity and thiosulfinates content. *Journal of Agriculture and Food Chemistry, 55*(4), 1280–1288.

Macan, H., Uykimpang, R., Alconcel, M., Takasu, J., Razon, R. Amagase, H., et al. (2006). Aged garlic extract may be safe for patients on warfarin therapy. *Journal of Nutrition, 136*(3 Suppl.), 793S–795S.

9. Magnesium

a. *Actions/expected responses:* Magnesium has been shown to significantly decrease plasma lipids such as cholesterol, triglycerides and phospholipids.

b. *Routes/dosages/frequencies:* Increased intake of dietary magnesium can decrease plasma lipids.

c. *Cautions:* Organic forms of foods are less likely to include genetically modified forms and pesticides.

d. *Assessments:* Assess intake of magnesium-rich foods, including 1 ounce of roasted pumpkin and squash seeds, almonds, Brazil nuts, pine nuts, or bran cereal; 3 ounces of halibut or tuna; 1/2 cup cooked spinach, soybeans, black or white beans, artichoke hearts, lima beans, and beet greens.

e. *Tips on use:* For more information, go to http://www.health.gov/dietary guidelines/dga2005/document/html/appendixB.htm

f. *Other considerations:* None.

g. *References/other sources:*

Takeda, R., & Nakamura, T. (2008). Effects of high magnesium intake on bone mineral status and lipid metabolism in rats. *Journal of Nutritional Science and Vitaminology, 54*(1), 66–75.

10. Pomegranate juice

a. *Actions/expected responses:* Pomegranate juice may improve stress-induced myocardial ischemia in women who have coronary heart disease.

b. *Routes/dosages/frequencies:* 1 ounce a day of pomegranate juice.

    c. *Cautions:* Pomegranate is an abortifacient; do not to use during the first trimester of pregnancy. Do not use if hypersensitive to pomegranate.

    d. *Assessments:* Assess pregnancy status.

    e. *Tips on use:* Keep pomegranate in a sealed container, away from heat and moisture.

    f. *Other considerations:* Pomegranate has been used to reduce blood glucose level and diarrhea, as an antiviral, a gargle for sore throat, and to treat hemorrhoids and intestinal worms.

    g. *References/other sources:*

        Sumner, M. D., Elliott-Eller, M., Weidner, G., Daubenmier, J. J., Chew, M. H., Marlin, R., et al. (2005). Effects of pomegranate juice consumption on myocardial perfusion in patients with coronary heart disease. *American Journal of Cardiology, 96*(6), 810–814.

11. Sucrose

    a. *Actions/expected responses:* Sucrose (table sugar) may increase serum triglycerides and decrease high density lipoprotein (the so-called good cholesterol).

    b. *Routes/dosages/frequencies:* Eating sugary foods often.

    c. *Cautions:* Avoid sucrose to protect their hearts.

    d. *Assessments:* Assess whether sucrose is eaten (table sugar, many desserts, sodas, and other sweet products).

    e. *Tips on use:* Ingesting additional fiber via fresh fruits and vegetables or whole grains may protect somewhat against carbohydrate-induced lipemia but has no effect on cholesterol during very high carbohydrate diets.

    f. *Other considerations:* Lowering dietary sucrose intake may be beneficial for women who may have low levels of the so-called good cholesterol (HDL-C). For a sweetener, use stevia, which also repairs DNA, has no calories and no side effects.

    g. *References/other sources:*

        Archer, S. L., Liu, K., Dyer, A. R., Ruth, K. J., Jacobs, D. R., Jr., Van Horn, L., et al. (1998). Relationship between changes in dietary sucrose and high density lipoprotein cholesterol: The CARDIA study. Coronary Artery Risk Development in Young Adults. *Annals of Epidemiology, 8*(7), 433–438.

        Ghanta, S., Banerjee, A., Poddar, A., & Chattopadhyay, S. (2007). Oxidative DNA damage preventive activity and antioxidant potential of Stevia rebaudiana Bertoni, a natural sweetener. *Journal of Agricultural and Food Chemistry, 55*(26), 10962–10967.

12. Trans fat versus low fat versus low carbohydrate diets

    a. *Actions/expected responses:* High trans fat consumption is a significant risk factor for coronary heart disease. Low-fat diets are more effective in preserving and promoting a healthy cardiovascular system then are low-carbohydrate, Atkins-like diets, which are high in saturated fats and dietary cholesterol.

    b. *Routes/dosages/frequencies:* The more trans fat consumed, the higher the level of trans isomers in erthrocytes. The higher the fat content, the more detrimental to heart health, putting the dieter at risk of atherosclerosis (hardening of the arteries) because low carbohydrate diets don't contain enough folic acid to lower homocysteine.

c. *Cautions:* Eating foods containing trans fat and following an Atkins-like diet is linked to coronary heart disease.

d. *Assessments:* Assess intake of trans fats (partially hydrogenated vegetable oils, produced by the food industry to create solid fats from liquid oils to increase the shelf life of products; examples include margarines, high-fat baked goods, especially doughnuts, cookies, and cakes, and any product with a label that says, "partially hydrogenated vegetables oils"). Assess intake of an Atkins-like diet.

e. *Tips on use:* Read all food labels carefully before buying products containing partially hydrogenated vegetable oils, and avoid Atkins-like diets.

f. *Other considerations:* French fries and potato chips may also contain partially hydrogenated vegetables oils.

g. *References/other sources:*

Medical College of Wisconsin. (2008, March 3). Low-fat diets more likely to reduce risk of heart disease than low-carb diets. *Science-Daily.* Retrieved March 9, 2008, from http://www.sciencedaily.com/releases/2008/02/080229141756.htm

Sun, Q., Jing, M., Campos, H., Hankinson, S. E., Manson, J. E., Stampfer, M. J., et al. (2008). A prospective study of trans fatty acids in erythrocytes and risk of coronary heart disease. *Circulation, 115,* 1858–1865.

13. Walnuts, pecans, and olive oil

a. *Actions/expected responses:* Both walnuts and olive oil lessen the sudden onset of inflammation and oxidation in the arteries after a meal of animal fat (salami and cheese sandwich and full-fat yogurt). Pecans may inhibit unwanted oxidation of blood lipids, helping reduce the risk of heart disease.

b. *Routes/dosages/frequencies:* After every high-fat animal meal, inflammation and oxidation in the arteries increases.

c. *Cautions:* High fat meals are only a problem with animal fat, not with vegetable fats or oils.

d. *Assessments:* Assess intake of animal fats.

e. *Tips on use:* Eat vegetable, not animal fats.

f. *Other considerations:* Walnuts preserve the elasticity and flexibility of the arteries, regardless of cholesterol level. Pecans are especially rich in one form of vitamin E—gamma tocopherol—which protects fats from oxidation, and lowers levels of LDL cholesterol by 16.5%.

g. *References/other sources:*

Cortex, B., Nunez, I., Cofan, M., Gilabert, R., Perez-Heras, A. Casals, E., et al. (2006). Acute effects of high-fat meals enriched with walnuts or olive oil on postprandial endothelial function. *Journal of the American College of Cardiology, 48*(8), 1666–1671.

Halton, T. L., Willett, W. C., Liu, S., Manson, J. E., Albert, C. M., Rexrode, K., et al. (2006). Low-carbohydrate-diet score and the risk of coronary heart disease in women. *New England Journal of Medicine, 355*(19), 1991–2002.

Loma Linda University. (2006, October 3). Antioxidant-rich pecans can protect against unhealthy oxidation. *ScienceDaily.* Retrieved March 2, 2008, from http://www.sciencedaily.com/releases/2006/09/06092909346.htm

Stress Management

1. Laughter
   a. *Actions/expected responses:* Laughter, along with an active sense of humor, can help protect against a heart attack, whereas mental stress is associated with impairment of the endothelium, the protective barrier lining the blood vessels. Stress sets up a series of inflammatory reactions that lead to fat and cholesterol build-up in the coronary arteries and ultimately to a heart attack.
   b. *Routes/dosages/frequencies:* Watch comedies, find humor in life situations, and make it a point to laugh at least 5 times a day.
   c. *Cautions:* None.
   d. *Assessments:* Assess laughter frequency.
   e. *Tips on use:* Discuss favorite comedies with at least one other person and what makes the show/movie funny for them.
   f. *Other considerations:* For more humor ideas, go to http://www.healthlit eracy.com/article.asp?PageID=3797, http://www.aath.org, and http://www. worldlaughtertour.com
   g. *References/other sources:*
      Miller, M. (2000). *Laughter is the best medicine for your heart.* Presented at the American Heart Association's 73rd Scientific Sessions, November 15, New Orleans, LA.
2. Stress management training
   a. *Actions/expected responses:* Participating in an education component (information about ischemic heart disease and myocardial ischemia, structure and function of the heart, traditional risk factors, and emotional stress), skill training (ways to reduce the affective, behavioral, cognitive, and physiological components of stress), and group interaction and social support resulted in improvements on several cardiovascular risk markers (improvements in flow-mediated dilation and baroreflex sensitivity, smaller reduction in left ventricular ejection fraction during mental stress and exercise testing, and reduced wall motion abnormalities).
   b. *Routes/dosages/frequencies:* 1 1/2 hours of stress management training a week for 16 weeks.
   c. *Cautions:* Improvements in psychosocial functioning are not necessarily associated with improved clinical (heart disease) outcomes.
   d. *Assessments:* Assess interest in participating in a similar group.
   e. *Tips on use:* For more information on developing stress management programs, go to http://www.imt.net/~randolfi/WorkStress.html
   f. *Other considerations:* http://www.mindtools.com/smpage.html
   g. *References/other sources:*
      Blumenthal, J. A., Sherwood, A., Babyak, M. A., Watkins, L. L., Waugh, R., Georgiades, A., et al. (2005). Effects of exercise and stress management training on markers of cardiovascular risk in patients with ischemic heart disease. *Journal of American Medical Association, 293,* 1626–1634.
3. Yoga lifestyle program
   a. *Actions/expected responses:* Yoga reduces risk factors for cardiovascular disease (serum total cholesterol, low-density lipoprotein [LDL] cholesterol,

the ratio of total cholesterol to high-density lipoprotein [HDL] cholesterol, and total triglycerides), and raises the so-called good HDL cholesterol.

b. *Routes/dosages/frequencies:* An 8-day program includes asanas (yoga postures), pranayamas (breathing exercises), relaxation techniques, group support, individualized advice, lectures and films on the philosophy of yoga and the place of yoga in daily life, meditation, stress management, nutrition, and knowledge about cardiovascular disease.

c. *Cautions:* Go to http://yoga.lifetips.com/cat/56770/yoga-cautions/

d. *Assessments:* Assess cardiovascular risk factors prior to and after completing yoga and lifestyle program.

e. *Tips on use:* Because yoga exerts pressure on internal organs, women should wait at least 2 hours after a meal and 30 minutes to 1 hour after a snack to practice. For more information about yoga, go to www.motherna ture.com/Library/Bookshelf/Books/21/54.cfm

f. *Other considerations:* To avoid knee injury when doing yoga, keep the knees straight (especially in standing poses). The knees should be forward in line with the ankle and foot and women should not allow their knees to twist inward or outward.

g. *References/other sources:*

Bijlani, R. L., Vempati, R. P., Yadav, R. K., Ray, R. B., Gupta, V., Sharma, R., et al. (2005). A brief but comprehensive lifestyle education program based on yoga reduces risk factors for cardiovascular disease and diabetes mellitus. *Journal of Alternative and Complementary Medicine, 11*(2), 267–274.

Jancin, B. (2003, June 3). Yoga improves endothelia dysfunction in heart patients. *Clinical Psychiatry News,* 70.

Supplements

1. Coenzyme Q10 (CoQ10)

a. *Actions/expected responses:* CoQ10 helps cells regenerate and improves the survival of heart cells during and after an infarct (heart attack). CoQ10 has also been shown to reduce heart size in congestive heart failure.

b. *Routes/dosages/frequencies:* Take orally daily as an oil-filled capsule. Dosages range from 50 to 120 mg.

c. *Cautions:* No significant side effects have been observed at lower doses. At higher doses, watch for mild reactions such as nausea, vomiting, GI upset, heartburn, diarrhea, loss of appetite, skin itching, rash, insomnia, headache, dizziness, irritability, increased light sensitivity, fatigue, or flu-like symptoms. These effects are mild and brief, resolving without treatment.

d. *Assessments:* Assess symptoms prior to and after taking CoQ10.

e. *Tips on use:* Start at a low dosage and gradually build if needed to obtain effect.

f. *Other considerations.* CoQ10 may reduce the toxic effects on the heart caused by the chemotherapy medications, daunorubicin, and doxorubicin, enhance the effect of blood pressure medications, and reduce the heart-related side effects of timolol drops, a beta blocker used to treat glaucoma.

    g. *References/other sources:*
        Kalenikova, E. I., Gorodetskaya, E. A., Kolokolchikova, E. G., Shashurin, D. A., & Medvedev, O. S. (2007). Chronic administration of coenzyme Q10 limits postinfarct myocardial remodeling in rats. *Biochemistry, 72*(3), 332–338.
        Sego, S. (2007, October). Coenzyme Q10. *The Clinical Advisor,* 126–128.

2. Psyllium
    a. *Actions/expected responses:* Psyllium lowers serum LDL cholesterol concentrations, without affecting HDL cholesterol, and is inversely associated with cardiovascular disease.
    b. *Routes/dosages/frequencies:* Stir in 1 tsp of psyllium husks into a glass of water and drink before it gels.
    c. *Cautions:* Drink sufficient water when increasing fiber, preferably 8–10 glasses a day. Observe for hypersensitivity reactions.
    d. *Assessments:* Assess cholesterol level prior to and after using psyllium.
    e. *Tips on use:* Separate use of psyllium from vitamins, minerals, herbs and drugs to ensure adequate absorption. Store psyllium in a cool, dry spot.
    f. *Other considerations:* It is most likely that water-soluble fibers lower the reabsorption of particular bile acids. As a result the liver converts more cholesterol into bile acids, which leads to increased LDL uptake by the liver.
    g. *References/other sources:*
        Theuwissen, E., & Mensink, R. P. (2008). Water-soluble dietary fibers and cardiovascular disease. *Physiology and Behavior.* Retrieved January 2008, from http://www.ncbi.nlm.nih.gov/pubmed/18302966?ordinalpos=2&itool=EntrezSystem2.PEntrez.Pubmed.Pubmed_ResultsPanel.Pubmed_RVDocSum

3. Pycnogenol
    a. *Actions/expected responses:* Pycnogenol was effective in decreasing the number of deep venous thrombosis and superficial vein thrombosis during long-haul flights. The supplement has also been shown superior to Daflon for treating chronic venous insufficiency and venous microangiopathy.
    b. *Routes/dosages/frequencies:* By mouth, 150 mg or 300 mg daily for 8 weeks.
    c. *Cautions:* Until more research is completed, pregnant and lactating women should not use this supplement.
    d. *Assessments:* Assess for venous insufficiency and deep venous thrombosis prior to and after taking pycnogenol.
    e. *Tips on use:* Store pycnogenol in a cool, dry place.
    f. *Other considerations:* A reduction in ankle edema (swelling) is a sign of reduction in venous insufficiency.
    g. *References/other sources:*
        Belcaro, G., Cesarone, M. R., Rohdewald, P., Ricci, A., Ippolito, E., Dugall, M., et al. (2004). Prevention of venous thrombosis and thrombophlebitis in long-haul flights with pycnogenol. *Clinical Application of Thrombosis and Hemostasis, 10*(4), 373–377.
        Cesarone, M. R., Belcaro, G., Rohdewald, P., Pellegrini, L., Ledda, A., Vinciguerra, G., et al. (2006). Comparison of pycnogenol and daflon in treating chronic venous insufficiency: A prospective, controlled study. *Clinical Application of Thrombosis and Hemostasis, 12*(2), 205–212.

4. Vitamins and minerals
   a. *Actions/expected responses:* In women, the intake of vitamins B, E, and selenium is associated with reducing the inflammatory process underlying atherosclerosis.
   b. *Routes/dosages/frequencies:* By mouth, B-complex, up to 100 mg twice a day, vitamin E up to 1,000 IU daily, selenium, 200–400 mcg daily.
   c. *Cautions:* Check with their primary care practitioner prior to taking vitamin E and not to exceed maximum doses.
   d. *Assessments:* Assess current intake of vitamins and minerals and sensitivity to them.
   e. *Tips on use:* Store vitamins and minerals in a cool, dry place.
   f. *Other considerations:* None.
   g. *References/other sources:*

   Scheurig, A. C., Thorand, B., Fischer, B., Heier, M., & Hoenig, W. (2008). Association between the intake of vitamins and trace elements from supplements and C-reactive protein: Results of the MONICA/KORA Augsburg study. *European Journal of Clinical Nutrition, 62*(1), 127–137.

Touch

1. Acupressure
   a. *Actions/expected responses:* Continuous wristband acupressure points experienced significantly lower incidence of nausea and/or vomiting following acute myocardial infarction compared with placebo. The severity of symptoms and the need for antiemetic drugs were also reduced in the acupressure group. Acupressure to the lower limbs for the treatment of peripheral arterial occlusive diseases caused a significant increase in lower limb blood flow.
   b. *Routes/dosages/frequencies:* Continuous pressure to PC6 for nausea and 3-minute pressure to acupoints GB34, ST36, SP9, and SP6 for lower limb blood flow.
   c. *Cautions:* Only gentle acupressure should be used in injured or sore areas.
   d. *Assessments:* Rate symptoms before and after treatment on a scale of 1 (none) to 10 (very bad).
   e. *Tips on use:* For more information on using acupressure, go to http://www.eclecticenergies.com/acupressure/howto.php
   f. *Other considerations:* Changes in mood may begin to occur immediately and continue for several days.
   g. *References/other sources:*

   Dent, H. E., Dewhurst, N. G., Mills, S. Y., & Willoughby, M. (2003). Continuous PC6 wristband acupressure for relief of nausea and vomiting associated with acute myocardial infarction: a partially randomized, placebo-controlled trial. *Complementary Therapy in Medicine, 11*(2), 72–77.

   Li, S., Hirokawa, M., Inoue, Y., Sugano, N., Qian, S., & Iwai, T. (2007). Effects of acupressure on lower limb blood flow for the treatment of peripheral arterial occlusive diseases. *Surgery Today, 37*(2), 103–108.

Incontinence

Medical treatments for incontinence include medications, surgery, and medical devices. Effective and safe complementary procedures are available for this condition.

Environment

1. Biofeedback
   a. *Actions/expected responses:* Biofeedback can reduce incontinence episodes by a mean of 80.7% and is significantly more effective than drug treatment.
   b. *Routes/dosages/frequencies:* Four sessions over 8 weeks.
   c. *Cautions:* Biofeedback therapy is not recommended for persons with severe psychosis, depression, or obsessional neurosis, nor for debilitated clients or those with psychopathic personalities. Women using insulin or other medications should consult with their primary care practitioner as biofeedback may affect the dosage of drugs.

    d. *Assessments:* Assess knowledge of biofeedback and provide information as needed.

    e. *Tips on use:* For more information, go to http://www.minddisorders.com/A-Br/Biofeedback.html

    f. *Other considerations:* None.

    g. *References/other sources:*

        Burgio, K. L., Locher, J. L., Goode, P. S., Hardin, J. M., McDowell, B. J., Dombrowski, M., et al. (1998). Behavioral vs drug treatment for urge urinary incontinence in older women. *Journal of the American Medical Association, 280,* 1995–2000.

2. Going outdoors

    a. *Actions/expected responses:* Going outside after age 70 is associated with fewer complaints of urinary incontinence.

    b. *Routes/dosages/frequencies:* Not going out daily at age 70 is predictive of subsequent urinary incontinence at age 77.

    c. *Cautions:* To protect against skin cancer, fair-skinned women should only expose their arms, faces or backs to sunlight for 15 minutes a day; dark-skinned women can be in the sunshine for up to 40 minutes. After that amount of daily exposure in the summer or in Southern states, women should wear a broad-brimmed hat, long sleeves, and pants.

    d. *Assessments:* Assess frequency of going outside.

    e. *Tips on use:* Teach women about the connection between going outside and the number of fewer new complaints of musculoskeletal pain, sleep problems, urinary incontinence, and decline in activities of daily living (ADLs).

    f. *Other considerations:* Women are less likely than men to go out daily.

    g. *References/other sources:*

        Jacobs, J. M., Cohen, A., Hammerman-Rozenberg, R., Azoulay, D., Maaravi, Y., & Stessman, J. (2008). Going outdoors daily predicts long-term functional and health benefits among ambulatory older people. *Journal of Aging and Health, 20*(3), 259–272.

3. Hysterectomy

    a. *Actions/expected responses:* Hysterectomy greatly increases the risk of urinary incontinence.

    b. *Routes/dosages/frequencies:* Hysterectomy is the most common gynecological abdominal operation in the world. It is normally performed as a cure for benign medical problems in order to improve quality of life.

    c. *Cautions:* Women who have had a hysterectomy are more than twice as likely to undergo surgery for urinary incontinence as women with intact uteri.

    d. *Assessments:* Assess if women are considering hysterectomy.

    e. *Tips on use:* The highest likelihood of incontinence was noted within 5 years of the removal of the uterus, but the higher risk remains throughout a woman's life.

    f. *Other considerations:* Be aware of the greater risks of hysterectomy. The risk for incontinence increased most for women who had a hysterectomy before menopause or who had several deliveries.

    g. *References/other sources:*

        Karolinski Institutet. (2007, October 30). Removal of uterus increases risk of urinary incontinence. *ScienceDaily.* Retrieved November 12, 2007, from http://www.sciencedaily.com/releases/2007/10/071026095008.htm

Exercise/Movement

1. Kegels and bladder training
   a. *Actions/expected responses:* Compared to regular care, Kegels (pelvic floor muscle training) and bladder training resolved urinary incontinence.
   b. *Routes/dosages/frequencies:* Teach women to empty their bladder and then hold the muscle that voluntarily stops the stream of urine for a count of 10 seconds, then relax for another count of 10 to a daily total of 35. The bladder can be trained by resisting a premature signal to void and holding urine 5 minutes longer, adding 5 minutes each week until 4 hours elapse between urinations. Vaginal weights can also be purchased to help identify and use the correct muscles.
   c. *Cautions:* Oral hormone administration increases rates of urinary incontinence compared with placebo in most randomized controlled trials. When the muscle tires, stop and go back to exercising later.
   d. *Assessments:* Assess urinary incontinence prior to and after completing Kegels and bladder training.
   e. *Tips on use:* Start a 2-day diary of urination history, including incontinence and what triggered each event, and voiding into a measured container to keep track of amounts passed. For information on instructing women about vaginal weights, see Johnson (2000). If Kegels are unsuccessful, go to http://www.massagetoday.com/mpacms/mt/article.php?id=13515
   f. *Other considerations:* None.
   g. *References/other sources:*
      Johnson, S. T. (2000). From incontinence to confidence. *American Journal of Nursing, 100*(2), 69–75.
      Shamliyan, T. A., Kane, R. L., Wyman, J., & Wilt, T. J. (2008). Systematic review: Randomized, controlled trials of nonsurgical treatments for urinary incontinence in women. *Annals of Internal Medicine, 148*(6), 459–473.
2. Physical activity
   a. *Actions/expected responses:* Old women who self-reported middle and high levels of physical activity were respectively 29% and 42% less likely to report incontinence.
   b. *Routes/dosages/frequencies:* Daily moderate to high levels of physical activity.
   c. *Cautions:* Wear appropriate clothes and shoes and only move or exercise on safe surfaces.
   d. *Assessments:* Assess incontinence prior to and after increasing activity.
   e. *Tips on use:* Choose more than one activity and vary them to reduce boredom.
   f. *Other considerations:* Share their level of activity with their primary health care practitioner.
   g. *References/other sources:*
      Kikuchia, A., Niua, K., Ikedab, Y., Hozawac, A., Nakagawab, H., Guoa, H., et al. (2007). Association between physical activity and urinary incontinence in a community-based elderly population aged 70 years and over. *European Urology, 52,* 868–875.

Mindset

1. Affirmations
   a. *Actions/expected responses:* Self-affirmation of personal values and beliefs buffers neuroendocrine and psychological stress.
   b. *Routes/dosages/frequencies:* Repeat aloud or write positive affirmations up to 20 times a day such as, "I experience my emotions without trying to control them" and "I feel safe expressing what I feel."
   c. *Cautions:* Ensure affirmations are positive and acceptable.
   d. *Assessments:* Assess anxiety prior to and after completing affirmations for a week.
   e. *Tips on use:* Write favorite affirmations on 3 by 5 cards and place them where they will be read frequently.
   f. *Other considerations:* Find more affirmations information at www.success consciousness.com/index_00000a.htm
   g. *References/other sources:*
      Hay, L. (2000). *Heal your body.* Carlsbad, CA: Hay House.
      Schwarzer, R., Babler, J., Kwiatek, P., Schroder, K., & Zang, J. W. (1997). The assessment of optimistic self-beliefs: Assessment of general perceived self-efficacy in thirteen cultures. *World Psychology, 3*(1–2), 177–190.

Nutrition

1. Irritating foods and fluids
   a. *Actions/expected responses:* Too little or too much fluid (more than 1,500 ml a day) or consumption of caffeinated and carbonated drinks, artificial sweeteners, honey, tomato products, nicotine, spicy foods, alcohol, and acidic juices can irritate the bladder and are correlated with urge urination.
   b. *Routes/dosages/frequencies:* At any time.
   c. *Cautions:* Even small amounts of irritating substances can set off urinary incontinence.
   d. *Assessments:* Assess use of irritating substances.
   e. *Tips on use:* Avoid substances that irritate the bladder.
   f. *Other considerations:* Keep a food/drink/urgency diary to identify specific triggers for incontinence.
   g. *References/other sources:*
      Bradley, C. S., Kennedy, C. M., & Nygaard, I. E. (2005). Pelvis floor symptoms and life style factors in older women. *Journal of Women's Health, 14*(2), 128–135.
2. Nutrients that may decrease overactive bladder
   a. *Actions/expected responses:* Nutrients significantly associated with decreased risk of overactive bladder include vitamin D, protein, and potassium. Niacin and vitamin B6 are also associated with decreased risk, but not significantly.
   b. *Routes/dosages/frequencies:* Vitamin D is metabolized by humans from the sun. Vitamin D3 is produced in light-skinned by 4–10 minutes of exposure of face, arms, or back to the noonday sun, and by 60–80 minutes of exposure for darker-skinned individuals. Individuals living at latitudes north of

35 degrees or who may not receive exposure to the sun or who are older than 49 years may need to take a tablespoon of cod liver oil daily. Foods rich in potassium include baked and sweet potatoes, white beans, and bananas. For more potassium-rich foods, go to www.health.gov/dietaryguidelines/dga2005/document/html/appendixB.htm. Dietary surveys indicate 15%–25% of older women don't consume enough niacin. Foods rich in niacin (vitamin B3) include peanuts, white meat chicken, tuna, corn grits, and peanut butter. For other niacin-rich foods, go to www.feinberg.northwestern.edu/nutrition/factsheets/vitamin-b3.html. Foods rich in pyridoxine (vitamin B6) include baked potatoes with skin, bananas, garbanzo beans, oatmeal, rainbow trout, and sunflower seeds. For more foods rich in vitamin B6, go to http://dietary-supplements.info.nih.gov/factsheets/vitaminb6.asp

c. *Cautions:* Vitamin D supplements can suppress the proper operation of the immune system.

d. *Assessments:* Assess level of incontinence before and after exposure to sun and/or ingesting cod liver oil, eating additional protein, eating potassium-rich foods, and eating foods rich in vitamin B6 and niacin.

e. *Tips on use:* Vitamin D2 that is added to so-called fortified foods and many multivitamins and is usually written in prescriptions is inefficiently metabolized in humans; only 20%–40% is metabolized into biologically active vitamin D3.

f. *Other considerations:* Women using corticosteroids may require additional vitamin D. Women taking diuretics or drinking alcohol may require additional vitamin B.

g. *References/other sources:*

Armstrong, D. J., Meenagh, G. K., Bickle, I., Lee, A. S., Curran, E. S., & Finch, M. B. (2007). Vitamin D deficiency is associated with anxiety and depression in fibromyalgia. *Clinical Rheumatology, 26*(4), 551–554.

Autoimmunity Research Foundation. (2008, January 27). Vitamin D deficiency study raises new questions about disease and supplements. *ScienceDaily.* Retrieved February 13, 2008, from http://www.sciencedaily.com/releases/2008/01/080125223302.htm

Dallosso, H. M., McGrother, C. W., Matthews, R. J., & Donaldson, M. M. K. (2003). The association of diet and other lifestyle factors with overactive bladder and stress incontinence: A longitudinal study in women. *British Journal of Urology International, 92*(1), 69.

Dallosso, H. M., McGrother, C. W., Matthews, R. J., Donaldson, M. M., & Leicestershire, M. R. C. (2004). Nutrient composition of the diet and the development of overactive bladder: A longitudinal study in women. *Neurourology Urodynamics, 23*(3), 204–210.

Jockers, B. S. (2007). Vitamin D sufficiency: An approach to disease prevention. *The American Journal for Nurse Practitioners, 11*(10), 43–50.

Stress Management

1. Cognitive-behavioral therapy (CBT)
   a. *Actions/expected responses:* Audio-taped cognitive strategies and a voiding diary, designed to augment the effects of an education program on

urinary frequency and incontinence, provided improved control over urination and enhanced comfort.

b. *Routes/dosages/frequencies:* Listening to audiotapes daily, attending a CBT educational class or therapy session daily.

c. *Cautions:* None.

d. *Assessments:* Assess incontinence prior to and after taking part in CBT.

e. *Tips on use:* For more information, go to http://www.mind.org.uk/Informa tion/Booklets/Making+sense/MakingSenseCBT.htm

f. *Other considerations:* Significant changes in bladder function may take up to 3 months to become apparent.

g. *References/other sources:*

Dowd, T., & Dowd, E. T. (2006). A cognitive therapy approach to promote continence. *Journal of Wound Ostomy Continence, 33*(1), 63–68.

Dowd, T., Kolcaba, K., & Steiner, R. (2000). Using cognitive strategies to enhance bladder control and comfort. *Holistic Nursing Practice, 14*(2), 91–103.

Garley, A., & Unwin, J. (2006). A case series to pilot cognitive behaviour therapy for women with urinary incontinence. *British Journal of Health Psychology, 11*(Pt. 3), 373–386.

Touch

1. Foot reflexology and massage

a. *Actions/expected responses:* Foot reflexology resulted in a significant change in the frequency of daytime urination, when compared to a foot massage group.

b. *Routes/dosages/frequencies:* Twice a week for 40 minutes. Self-administered foot reflexology treatments may also be of benefit.

c. *Cautions:* Pregnant women should avoid foot reflexology because certain manipulations can lead to premature labor. Those with foot problems, gout, arthritis, and vascular conditions such as varicose veins should be careful using this procedure.

d. *Assessments:* Evaluate urinary incontinence prior to and after foot reflexology sessions.

e. *Tips on use:* For foot charts, see http://groups.msn.com/AlternativesTo PainandDisease/reflexologyinstructionspg1.msnw

f. *Other considerations:* For a specific urinary incontinence technique, go to http://www.naturalhealthtechniques.com/HealingTechniques/urinary incontinence_technique.htm

g. *References/other sources:*

Mak, H. L., Wong, T., Liu, Y. S., & Tong, W. M. (2007). Randomized controlled trial of foot reflexology for patients with symptomatic idiopathic detrusor overactivity. *International Urogynecology Journal Pelvic Floor Dysfunction, 18*(6), 653–658.

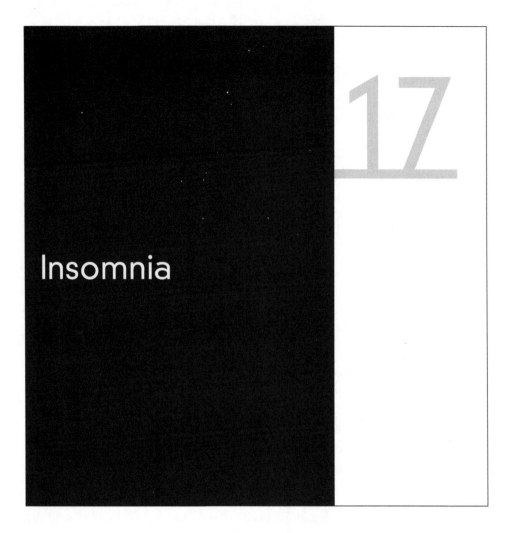

Insomnia

Medical treatments for insomnia include medications that may have a rebound effect. Recent research provides evidence that complementary approaches can be effective without negative results.

Environment

1. Environmental behavioral training
   a. *Actions/expected responses:* A master's level adult psychiatric and primary care nurse practitioner provided four individually tailored instructions to women suffering from insomnia: (a) reduce the time spent in bed to closely match their number of hours of sleep, (b) get up at the same time every day of the week, (c) not to go to bed unless they were sleepy, and (d) not to stay in bed unless they were asleep. Participating in this program significantly improved scores on the Pittsburgh Sleep Quality Index (PSQ), decreased the time it took to fall asleep, and decreased the amount of wake time after sleep onset.

b. *Routes/dosages/frequencies:* A 45-minute training session followed 2 weeks later by a 30-minute booster session.

c. *Cautions:* Avoid taking worries to bed and refrain from drinking alcohol, coffee, or other caffeinated drinks, foods, or drugs. If snoozing is necessary, limit the time to less than 1 hour by setting an alarm clock or timer. Avoid late night meals.

d. *Assessments:* Assess insomnia prior to and after using the four directives, including keeping a sleep diary.

e. *Tips on use:* At the booster session, sleep schedules can be modified if necessary. For example, if you fall asleep in less than 30 minutes, increase time in bed by 15 minutes, and maintain that new time in bed for 1 week. After a week if you are still falling asleep in less than 30 minutes and waking up during the night for less than 30 minutes, increase time in bed by another 15 minutes. In contrast, if it takes longer than 30 minutes to fall asleep and you are awake during the night for more than 30 minutes, decrease time in bed by 15 minutes.

f. *Other considerations:* Average time to fall asleep fell significantly from 38 minutes to 17 minutes in the treatment group, and from 30 minutes to 27 minutes in the control group.

g. *References/other sources:*

Finn, R. (2007, March). Brief behavioral training improves insomnia. *Clinical Psychiatry News,* 21.

Germain, A., Moul, D. E., Franzen, P. L., Miewald, J. M., Reynolds, C. F., 3rd, Monk, T. H., et al. (2006). Effects of a brief behavioral treatment for late-life insomnia: Preliminary findings. *Journal of Clinical Sleep Medicine, 2*(4), 403–406.

2. Music therapy paired with progressive relaxation

a. *Actions/expected responses:* A report of a study pairing music listening with progressive muscle relaxation (as compared to a control group) found the treatment produced a significant effect on sleep quality.

b. *Routes/dosages/frequencies:* Half an hour for at least 5 consecutive nights listening to self-selected music with a progressive muscle relaxation script.

c. *Cautions:* Go to http://www.intelihealth.com/IH/ihtIH/WSIHW000/8513/34968/358865.html?d=dmtContent#potentialdangers

d. *Assessments:* Assess insomnia prior to and after music therapy and progressive relaxation.

e. *Tips on use:* Find relaxation tapes with background music online.

f. *Other considerations:* None.

g. *References/other sources:*

Hernandez-Reuiz, E. (2005). Effect of music therapy on the anxiety levels and sleep patterns of abused women in shelters. *Journal of Music Therapy, 42*(2), 140–158.

Exercise/Movement

1. Exercise

a. *Actions/expected responses:* Exercise is an inexpensive, safe means of improving sleep.

    b. *Routes/dosages/frequencies:* Daily exercise, 50–60 minutes a day or as tolerated.

    c. *Cautions:* Wear appropriate clothes and shoes and exercise on safe surfaces.

    d. *Assessments:* Assess vital signs and balance, and consult with primary care giver prior to undertaking an exercise program. Assess insomnia prior to and after 2 weeks of exercise.

    e. *Tips on use:* Complete warm-up prior to exercising and cool-downs afterwards. For suggestions, go to http://www.aarp.org/health/fitness/walking/warm_up.html

    f. *Other considerations:* None.

    g. *References/other sources:*

        Youngstedt, S. D. (2005). Effects of exercise on sleep. *Clinical Sports Medicine, 24*(2), 355–365.

Herbs/Essential Oils

1. Aromatherapy

    a. *Actions/expected responses:* Women receiving either lavender or sweet almond essential oil via an Aromastream device showed an improvement and less insomnia.

    b. *Routes/dosages/frequencies:* Prior to bedtime; diffused through the air.

    c. *Cautions:* None known unless women are sensitive to aromatherapy oils.

    d. *Assessments:* Assess level of insomnia prior to and after being exposed to aromatherapy.

    e. *Tips on use:* Women and younger volunteers with a milder insomnia improved more than other participants.

    f. *Other considerations:* None.

    g. *References/other sources:*

        Lewith, G. T., Godfrey, A. D., & Prescott, P. (2005). A single-blinded, randomized pilot study evaluating the aroma of Lavandula augustifolia as a treatment for mild insomnia. *Journal of Alternative and Complementary Medicine, 11*(4), 631–637.

2. Black cohosh

    a. *Actions/expected responses:* Review of the published clinical data suggests that black cohosh may be useful for the treatment of insomnia, especially for menopausal women.

    b. *Routes/dosages/frequencies:* 40–80 mg per day.

    c. *Cautions:* Transient adverse events such as nausea, vomiting, headaches, dizziness, mastalgia, and weight gain have been observed in clinical trials.

    d. *Assessments:* Assess insomnia prior to and after taking black cohosh.

    e. *Tips on use:* Store black cohosh in a cool, dry place.

    f. *Other considerations:* The most recent data suggest black cohosh is not estrogenic.

    g. *References/other sources:*

        Mahady, G. B. (2005). Black cohosh (Actaea/Cimicifuga racemosa): Review of the clinical data for safety and efficacy in menopausal symptoms. *Treatment in Endocrinology, 4*(3), 177–184.

3. Chamomile
   a. *Actions/expected responses:* Classified as a mild sleep aid or sedative by the German Commission on Herbal Medicines.
   b. *Routes/dosages/frequencies:* A cup of tea prior to bedtime.
   c. *Cautions:* No known adverse reactions unless sensitive to dried chamomile.
   d. *Assessments:* Assess insomnia prior to and after drinking chamomile tea.
   e. *Tips on use:* Store chamomile tea or teabags in a cool, dry place.
   f. *Other considerations:* Chamomile is inexpensive and has no side effects unless hypersensitive to the flowers.
   g. *References/other sources:*
      Blumenthal, M., Hall, T., Rister, R., & Steinhoff, B. (Eds.). (1996). *The Complete German Commission E Monographs: Therapeutic guide to herbal medicines.* Austin, TX: American Botanical Council.

Mindset

1. Affirmations
   a. *Actions/expected responses:* Self-affirmation of personal values and beliefs buffers neuroendocrine and psychological stress.
   b. *Routes/dosages/frequencies:* Repeat aloud or write positive affirmations up to 20 times a day such as, "I release the day and slip into peaceful and relaxing sleep" and "Tomorrow is soon enough to take care of things."
   c. *Cautions:* Ensure affirmations are positive and acceptable.
   d. *Assessments:* Assess anxiety prior to and after completing affirmations for a week.
   e. *Tips on use:* Write favorite affirmations on 3 by 5 cards and place them where they will be read frequently.
   f. *Other considerations:* Find more affirmations information at www.success consciousness.com/index_00000a.htm
   g. *References/other sources:*
      Hay, L. (2000). *Heal your body.* Carlsbad, CA: Hay House.
      Schwarzer, R., Babler, J., Kwiatek, P., Schroder, K., & Zang, J. W. (1997). The assessment of optimistic self-beliefs: Assessment of general perceived self-efficacy in thirteen cultures. *World Psychology, 3*(1–2), 177–190.
2. Cognitive-behavioral therapy (CBT)
   a. *Actions/expected responses:* Cognitive-behavioral self-help treatment decreased total wake time by 52 minutes as compared to using hypnosis alone (increased total wake time by 17 minutes) to help taper off the chronic use of sleep hypnotics.
   b. *Routes/dosages/frequencies:* 8-week program.
   c. *Cautions:* None.
   d. *Assessments:* Assess insomnia prior to and after taking part in CBT.
   e. *Tips on use:* For more information, go to http://www.mind.org.uk/Informa tion/Booklets/Making+sense/MakingSenseCBT.htm
   f. *Other considerations:* The addition of a self-help treatment focusing on insomnia, a readily available and cost-effective alternative to individual psychotherapy, produced greater sleep improvement.

g. *References/other sources:*

Belleville, G., Guay, C., Guay, B., & Morin, C. M. (2007). Hypnotic taper with or without self-help treatment of insomnia: A randomized clinical trial. *Journal of Consulting and Clinical Psychology, 75*(2), 325–335.

Touch

1. Acupressure
   a. *Actions/expected responses:* Acupressure massage of key points improves the quality of sleep and does so in a noninvasive way. Sleep log data revealed the acupressure group significantly decreased wake time and improved quality of sleep.
   b. *Routes/dosages/frequencies:* 3-minute massage of the mid-helix of the ears and at the base of foot at the middle toe, three times a week for 4 weeks.
   c. *Cautions:* Avoid if there are ear or foot injuries in the area of the acupoints.
   d. *Assessments:* Assess insomnia prior to and after acupressure treatments.
   e. *Tips on use:* Go to http://www. mothernature.com/Library/Bookshelf/Books/21/3.cfm
   f. *Other considerations:* Keep a sleep log to identify patterns of sleep and the effect of acupoint massage.
   g. *References/other sources:*
Tsay, S. L., Rong, J. R., & Lin, P. F. (2003). Acupoints massage in improving the quality of sleep and quality of life in patients with end-stage renal disease. *Journal of Advanced Nursing, 42*(2), 134–142.
2. Back massage
   a. *Actions/expected responses:* A review of 16 studies indicate that back massage promotes relaxation and sleep.
   b. *Routes/dosages/frequencies:* Nightly for 5–15 minutes.
   c. *Cautions:* None unless back is injured.
   d. *Assessments:* Assess insomnia prior to and after back massage.
   e. *Tips on use:* Go to http://www.ehow.com/video_8066_give-back-massage.html
   f. *Other considerations:* http://www.videojug.com/film/how-to-give-a-deep-stress-relief-back-massage, http://searchwarp.com/swa7981.htm
   g. *References/other sources:*
Schiff, A. (2006). Literature review of back massage and similar techniques to promote sleep in elderly people. *Pflege, 19*(3), 163–173.

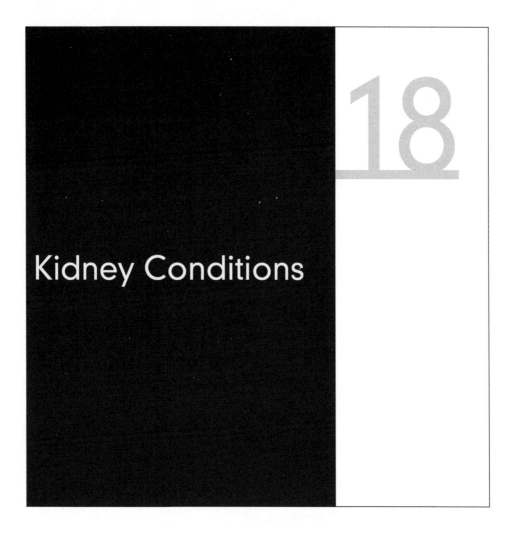

18

Kidney Conditions

Medical treatment for kidney conditions includes surgery and medications. Complementary approaches may engender fewer negative results, and research provides evidence they can be effective.

Environment

1. Sunlight
    a. *Actions/expected responses:* Researchers at the Moores Cancer Center at University of California, San Diego (UCSD) have shown a clear association between deficiency in exposure to sunlight, specifically ultraviolet B (UVB), and kidney cancer.
    b. *Routes/dosages/frequencies:* For light-skinned women, 10–15 minutes of direct midday sun at least twice a week on the face, arms, hands, or back is sufficient, according to the National Institutes of Health. Darker-skinned women may require three to six times as much exposure.
    c. *Cautions:* More frequent exposure could result in skin cancer. Insufficient exposure to the sun can result in improper absorption of calcium and

phosphorus, leading to imperfect skeletal formation as well as bone disorders. Vitamin D supplements can suppress the immune system.

d. *Assessments:* Assess the amount of time women spend in direct sunlight.

e. *Tips on use:* Help women to develop a plan for obtaining sufficient sunlight, depending on their lifestyle. Eating lunch outside when weather permits could be one solution. In colder climes, women can take a tablespoon of cod liver oil daily, eat fatty fish and fish oils, and egg yolks. Supplements of vitamin D3 (calciferol) may be necessary for certain women.

f. *Other considerations:* Vitamin D2, found in fortified foods, especially breads and cereals, is poorly metabolized by the body. Certain drugs can interfere with vitamin metabolism, including corticosteroids, phenytoin, heparin, cimetidine, isoniazid, rifampin, phenobarbital, and primidone. Counsel women to find alternate medications whenever possible so they can metabolize vitamin D3. Taking vitamin D supplements can actually block vitamin D nuclear receptor gene (VDR) activation, the opposite effect to that of sunshine.

g. *References/other sources:*

Autoimmunity Research Foundation. (2008, January 27). Vitamin D deficiency study raises new questions about disease and supplements. *ScienceDaily.* Retrieved February 13, 2008, from http://www.sciencedaily.com/releases/2008/01/080125223302.htm

Demgrow, M. (2007, June). High vitamin D: Treatment for cancer prevention? *The Clinical Advisor, 54,* 57.

Jockers, B. S. (2007). Vitamin D sufficiency: An approach to disease prevention. *The American Journal for Nurse Practitioners, 11*(10), 43–50.

University of California-San Diego. (2006, September 19). Global view shows strong link between kidney cancer, sunlight exposure. *ScienceDaily.* Retrieved March 21, 2008, from http://www.sciencedaily.com/releases/2006/09/060918164649.htm

Exercise/Movement

1. Exercise

a. *Actions/expected responses:* Regular exercise leads to better blood pressure control, lower levels of blood fats (cholesterol and triglycerides), better, deeper sleep, and better weight control. High blood pressure, high blood fats, kidney disease, and being overweight increase risk of developing heart disease, while exercise may lessen this risk. Exercise may also help to prevent a weakening of bones—a problem that women who undergo dialysis and transplant often have. Women who exercise are usually less depressed, worry less, are better able to do things for and feel better about themselves. Combined aerobic exercise and resistance training during dialysis improves muscle strength, work output, cardiac fitness, and possibly dialysis adequacy.

b. *Routes/dosages/frequencies:* At least 3 days a week, working up to 30–60 minutes each session.

c. *Cautions:* See http://www.medscape.com/viewarticle/561596_3

d. *Assessments:* Assess current exercise and exercise preferences.

e. *Tips on use:* See http://72.14.205.104/search?q=cache:CvrRF_nMD1EJ: www.kidney.org/atoz/pdf/stayfit.pdf+exercise+and+kidney+disease&hl= n&ct=clnk&cd=2&gl=us

f. *Other considerations:* Go to http://www.wellness.ma/adult-fitness/stretch ing-warmup.htm

g. *References/other sources:*

Moinuddin, I., & Leehey, D. J. (2008). A comparison of aerobic exercise and resistance training in patients with and without chronic kidney disease. *Advances in Chronic Kidney Disease, 15*(1), 83–96.

Herbs/Essential Oils

1. Aromatherapy
   a. *Actions/expected responses:* Laboratory studies and animal studies have shown that certain essential oils have antibacterial, calming, or energizing effects. Aromatherapy may work by sending chemical messages to the part of the brain that affects moods and emotions. Lavender and rosemary protect the body from oxidative stress by decreasing the stress hormone cortisol. Women with kidney cancer may use aromatherapy mainly to improve their quality of life.
   b. *Routes/dosages/frequencies:* Lavender and rosemary oils can calm. Sniff aroma of essential oils for 5 minutes.
   c. *Cautions:* Safety testing on essential oils has found very few bad side effects.
   d. *Assessments:* Assess negative emotions prior to and after using aromatherapy. Assess for hypersensitivity (skin reactions, nausea, or anorexia).
   e. *Tips on use:* Keep aromatherapy products away from heat and moisture in a sealed container.
   f. *Other considerations:* Can use one or the other essential oil or both to protect against oxidative stress.
   g. *References/other sources:*

   Atsumi, T., & Tonosaki, K. (2007). Smelling lavender and rosemary increases free radical scavenging activity and decreases cortisol level in saliva. *Psychiatry Research, 150*(1), 89–96.

2. Basil leaf extract
   a. *Actions/expected responses:* Basil leaf extract was highly effective in inhibiting carcinogen-induced tumors in the kidney.
   b. *Routes/dosages/frequencies:* 1–2 ml three to five times a day. The dried leaf can also be used in cooking.
   c. *Cautions:* Except when used in cooking, basil leaf extract in large amounts may increase the hypoglycemic effects of insulin and oral antidiabetes agents; avoid using concurrently. Not recommended for therapeutic use during pregnancy and lactation.
   d. *Assessments:* Assess use of oral antidiabetes agents and insulin.
   e. *Tips on use:* Avoid using basil leaf extract concurrently with oral antidiabetes agents or insulin.
   f. *Other considerations:* Basil has been used to increase immunity and metabolic function.

g. *References/other sources:*

Dasgupta, T., Rao, A. R., & Yadava, P. K. (2004). Chemmodulatory efficacy of basil leaf (Ocimum basilicum) on drug metabolizing and antioxidant enzymes, and on carcinogen-induced skin and forestomach papillo-magenesis. *Phytomedicine, 11*(2), 139–151.

Skidmore-Roth, L. (2006). Basil. In *Mosby's handbook of herbs and natural supplements* (pp. 84–88). St. Louis, MO: ElsevierMosby.

3. Milk thistle (Silybum marianum)
    a. *Actions/expected responses:* Silymarin, a mixture of flavanoid complexes, is the active component of milk thistle that protects the kidney cells from cancer and the toxic effects of chemotherapy.
    b. *Routes/dosages/frequencies:* 200–400 mg silymarin per day.
    c. *Cautions:* Adverse effects are rare but may include stomach pain, nausea, vomiting, diarrhea, headache, rash, joint pain, and anaphylaxis in allergic women. Pregnant and lactating women or those who are hypersensitive (have a known sensitivity to ragweed, marigolds, or chrysanthemums) should not use milk thistle.
    d. *Assessments:* Assess hypersensitivity to milk thistle.
    e. *Tips on use:* Store milk thistle in a cool, dry place, away from heat and moisture.
    f. *Other considerations:* Preliminary research suggests that silybin may enhance the tumor fighting effects of cisplatin and doxorubicin.
    g. *References/other sources:*

Bokemeyer, C., Fells, L. M., & Dunn, T. (1996). Silibinin protects against cisplatin-induced nephrotoxicity without compromising cisplatin on isosfamide anti-tumor activity. *British Journal of Cancer, 74,* 2036–2041.

Post-White, J., Ladas, E. J., & Kelly, K. M. (2007). Advances in the use of milk thistle (Silybum marianum). *Integrative Cancer Therapy, 2,* 104–109.

Zi, X., Mukhtar, H., & Agarwal, R. (1997). Novel cancer chemopreventive effects of a flavonoid antioxidant silymarin: Inhibition of RNA expression of an endogenous tumor promoter TNF-alpha. *Biochemical Biophysical Research Communication, 239,* 334–339.

Mindset

1. Affirmations
    a. *Actions/expected responses:* Self-affirmation of personal values and beliefs buffers neuroendocrine and psychological stress.
    b. *Routes/dosages/frequencies:* Repeat aloud or write positive affirmations up to 20 times a day such as, "I can safely grow and mature," "I find good everywhere," and "The right thing is happening at the right time."
    c. *Cautions:* Ensure affirmations are positive and acceptable to the woman.
    d. *Assessments:* Assess anxiety prior to and after completing affirmations for a week.
    e. *Tips on use:* Write favorite affirmations on 3 by 5 cards and place them where they will be read frequently.
    f. *Other considerations:* Find more affirmations information at www.success consciousness.com/index_00000a.htm

g. *References/other sources:*

Hay, L. (2000). *Heal your body*. Carlsbad, CA: Hay House.

Schwarzer, R., Babler, J., Kwiatek, P., Schroder, K., & Zang, J. W. (1997). The assessment of optimistic self-beliefs: Assessment of general perceived self-efficacy in thirteen cultures. *World Psychology, 3*(1–2), 177–190.

Nutrition

1. Healthy diet
   a. *Actions/expected responses:* Garlic protects the kidney against oxidative damage. The high protein Atkins diet is associated with reduced kidney function. Over time, individuals who consume very large amounts of protein, particularly animal protein, risk significant kidney damage. The American Academy of Family Physicians notes that high animal protein intake is largely responsible for the high prevalence of kidney stones in the United States and other developed countries, and it recommends protein restriction for the prevention of recurrent kidney stones. Carbonated beverages, especially cola consumption, may increase the risk of chronic kidney disease. Green tea may help strengthen metabolic defense against toxins capable of causing cancer. Homocysteine, a normal by-product of protein metabolism, derived primarily from meat and dairy products, is linked to kidney disease. The Mediterranean diet (vegetables, legumes, fruits, nuts, whole grains, fish) is associated with reduced deaths due to cancer.
   b. *Routes/dosages/frequencies:* Daily ingestion of helpful foods.
   c. *Cautions:* None.
   d. *Assessments:* Assess intake of anticancer foods.
   e. *Tips on use:* Using organic forms of produce can provide more healthy amounts of selenium, an essential mineral and anticarcinogenic agent.
   f. *Other considerations:* None.
   g. *References/other sources:*

Allon, N., & Friedman, M. D. (2004). High-protein diets: Potential effects on the kidney in renal health and disease. *American Journal of Kidney Diseases, 44*(6), 950–962.

American Association for Cancer Research. (2007, August 12). Green tea boosts production of detox enzymes, rending cancerous chemicals harmless. *ScienceDaily*. Retrieved December 20, 2007, from http://www.sciencedaily.com/releases/2007/08/070810194923.htm

Divisi, D., Di Tommaso, S., Salvemini, S., Garramone, M., & Crisci, R. (2006). Diet and cancer. *Acta Biomedica, 77*(2), 118–123.

Homocysteine level linked to kidney disease. (2004, December). *The Clinical Advisor*, 14.

Irion, C. W. (1999). Growing alliums and brassicas in selenium-enriched soils increases their anticarcinogenic potentials. *Medical Hypotheses, 53*(3), 232–235.

Kabasakal, L., Sehirli, O., Cetinel, S., Cikler, E., Gedik, N., & Sener, G. (2005). Protective effect of aqueous garlic extract against renal ischemia/reperfusion injury in rats. *Journal of Medicinal Food, 8*(3), 319–326.

Mitrou, P. N., Kipnis, V., Thiebaut, A. C., Reedy, J., Subar, A. F., Wirfalt, E., et al. (2007). Mediterranean dietary pattern and prediction of all-cause mortality in a US population: Results from the NIH-AARP diet and health study. *Archives of Internal Medicine, 167*(22), 2461–2468.

Parcell, S. (2002). Sulfur in human nutrition and applications in medicine. *Alternative Medical Review, 7*(1), 22–44.

Saldana, T. M., Basso, O., Darden, R., & Sandler, D. P. (2007). Carbonated beverages and chronic kidney disease. *Epidemiology, 18*(4), 501–506.

Stress Management

1. Stress management techniques
   a. *Actions/expected responses:* A weak immune system is one of the major factors that promotes cancer metastases after an operation, chemotherapy, or radiation therapy. Fear and stress weaken the immune system. Adequate stress management prior to and after medical treatment may help to prevent metastases.
   b. *Routes/dosages/frequencies:* Daily practice of stress management techniques.
   c. *Cautions:* Use only stress management techniques that feel comfortable and that work well.
   d. *Assessments:* Assess interest in various stress management techniques. Assess fear and stress after using stress management techniques.
   e. *Tips on use:* See http://www.webmd.com/balance/stress-management/features/blissing-out-10-relaxation-techniques-reduce-stress-spot
   f. *Other considerations:* None.
   g. *References/other sources:*
      Tel Aviv University. (2008, February 29). Stress and fear can affect cancer's recurrence. *ScienceDaily.* Retrieved March 9, 2008, from http://www.sciencedaily.com/releases/2008/02/080227142656.htm

Supplements

1. Pycnogenol and ginkgo biloba extract
   a. *Actions/expected responses:* Either pycnogenol or ginkgo biloba extract can protect against antimutagenic activity in animal studies.
   b. *Routes/dosages/frequencies:* 5–100 microgram/mL.
   c. *Cautions:* Until more research is completed, pregnant and lactating women should not use these supplements, nor should they be given to children. Avoid taking ginkgo concurrently with anticoagulants.
   d. *Assessments:* Assess reaction to pycnogenol and ginkgo.
   e. *Tips on use:* Store supplements in a cool, dry place.
   f. *Other considerations:* Pycnogenol has also been found useful in preventing venous thrombosis, thrombophlebitis, gingival bleeding and plaque, inflammatory bowel disease, venous insufficiency, digestive conditions, and menopause symptoms.

g. *References/other sources:*

Krizkova, L., Chovanova, Z., Durackova, Z., & Krajcovic, J. (2008). Antimu-tagenic in vitro activity of plan polyphenols: Pycnogenol and Ginkgo biloba extract. *Phytotherapy Research, 22*(3), 384–388.

2. Quercetin

a. *Actions/expected responses:* Quercetin shows antihypertensive, protective and antioxidant effects in renovascular hypertension. In combination with vitamin E, it may even ameliorate the chronic toxic effects of the immuno-suppressive drug CsA for renal transplants.

b. *Routes/dosages/frequencies:* 400 mg quercetin twice a day between meals, 400 IU vitamin E daily.

c. *Cautions:* Avoid taking quercetin in the first trimester of pregnancy. If taking blood thinners, discuss the use of vitamin E with primary care practitioner.

d. *Assessments:* Assess transplant status.

e. *Tips on use:* Go to http://www.drweil.com/drw/u/id/QAA158469.

f. *Other considerations:* None.

g. *References/other sources:*

Behling, E. B., Sendao, M. C., Fancescato, H. D., Antunes, L. M., Costa, R. S., & Bianchi, M. L. (2006). Comparative study of multiple dosage of quer-cetin against cisplatin-induced nephrotoxicity and oxidative stress in rat kidneys. *Pharmacology Reports, 58*(4), 526–532.

Garcia-Saura, M. F., Galisteo, M., Villar, I. C., Bermejo, A., Zarzuelo, A., Vargas, F., et al. (2005). Effects of chronic quercetin treatment in ex-perimental renovascular hypertension. *Molecular Cell Biochemistry, 270*(1–2), 147–155.

Zal, F., Mostafavi-Pour, Z., & Vessal, M. (2007). Comparison of the effects of vitamin E and/or quercetin in attenuating chronic cyclosporine A-induced nephrotoxicity in male rats. *Clinical Experimental Pharmacology Physiology, 34*(8), 720–724.

Touch

1. Acupressure

a. *Actions/expected responses:* Women in end-stage renal disease who re-ceived acupressure showed significantly greater improvement in fatigue and depression than women in a control group.

b. *Routes/dosages/frequencies:* Acupressure massage for 12 minutes per day, 3 days per week, for 4 weeks.

c. *Cautions:* None unless there are wounds or injuries in acupressure point areas.

d. *Assessments:* Assess acquaintance with acupressure and interest in try-ing the procedure. Assess fatigue and depression prior to and after using acupressure.

e. *Tips on use:* Go to http://www.eclecticenergies.com/acupressure/index emotional.php

f. *Other considerations:* The Revised Piper Fatigue Scale (http://www.pdx in-ternational.com/docs/piper/Piper_Fatigue_Scale.PDF) and Beck's Depression Inventory (available at http://www.ibogaine.desk.nl/graphics/3639b1c_23.pdf) can be used to evaluate the effect of acupressure.

     g. *References/other sources:*
>   Cho, Y. C., & Tsay, S. L. (2004). The effect of acupressure with massage on fatigue and depression in patients with end-stage renal disease. *Journal of Nursing Research, 12*(1), 51–59.

2. Foot reflexology
    a. *Actions/expected responses:* Life satisfaction was significantly improved in the experimental group after foot reflexology. Combined with aromatherapy and foot soak, reflexology also relieves fatigue in women with cancer. Foot reflexology or self-administered foot reflexology also significantly enhances and strengthens the immune system so that it can catch and eliminate cancer cells and prevent tumors from developing.
    b. *Routes/dosages/frequencies:* Twice a week for 4 weeks. Three-minute foot soak contains warm water and lavender essential oil, and is followed by reflexology treatment with jojoba oil containing lavender for 10 minutes. Four 40-minute self-administered foot reflexology treatments can also be of benefit. See http://www.handbag.com/healthfit/complementary/acupressure
    c. *Cautions:* Avoid foot reflexology when pregnant because certain manipulations can lead to premature labor. Those with foot problems, gout, arthritis, and vascular conditions such as varicose veins should be careful using this procedure. Perform a patch test with lavender essential oil prior to foot soak.
    d. *Assessments:* Evaluate life satisfaction and fatigue prior to and after foot reflexology sessions. See http://employees.oneonta.edu/vomsaaw/w/handouts%20-%20happiness/life%20satisfaction%20WvS%20questionnaire.pdf. Evaluate fatigue with the Cancer Fatigue Scale before, 1 hour after, and 4 hours after treatment.
    e. *Tips on use:* For foot charts, see http://groups.msn.com/AlternativesToPainandDisease/reflexologyinstructionspg1.msnw
    f. *Other considerations:* Quality of life is the most important predictor of survival for advanced cancer clients. See http://groups.msn.com/AlternativesToPainandDisease/reflexologyinstructionspg2.msnw
    g. *References/other sources:*
>   Fox Chase Cancer Center. (2007, November 1). Quality of life is the most important predictor of survival for advanced cancer patients. *ScienceDaily.* Retrieved November 12, 2007, from http://www.sciencedaily.com/releases/2007/10/071030170208.htm
>   Kesselring, A. (1994). Foot reflex zone massage. *Schweizerische Medizinische Wochenschrift, 62,* 88–93.
>   National Cancer Institute. (2006). *Immunity and cancer.* Retrieved February 6, 2008, from http://www.nci.nih.gov/cancertopics/understanding cancer/immunesystem/Slide32

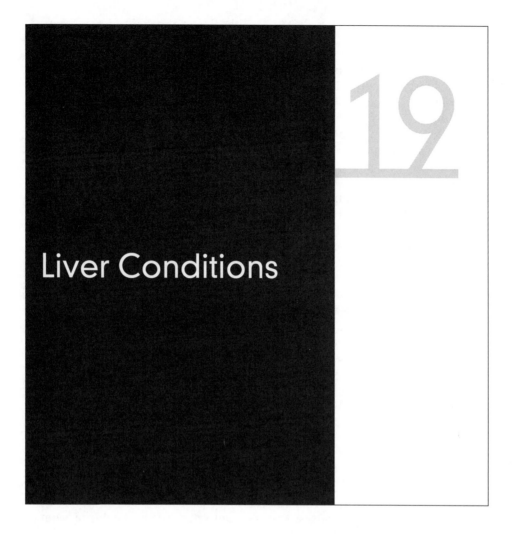

Liver Conditions

19

All drugs, whether prescribed or over-the-counter, stress the liver. Complementary approaches tend to cleanse and support the liver.

Environment

1. Sunlight
    a. *Actions/expected responses:* Studies show a strong correlation between adequate exposure to sunlight and a lower risk of cancer.
    b. *Routes/dosages/frequencies:* For light-skinned women, 10–15 minutes of direct midday sun at least twice a week on the face, arms, hands, or back is sufficient, according to the National Institutes of Health. Darker-skinned women may require three to six times as much exposure.
    c. *Cautions:* More frequent exposure could result in skin cancer. Insufficient exposure to the sun can result in improper absorption of calcium and phosphorus, leading to imperfect skeletal formation as well as bone disorders. Vitamin D supplements can suppress the immune system.
    d. *Assessments:* Assess the amount of time spent in direct sunlight.

e. *Tips on use:* Develop a plan for obtaining sufficient sunlight, depending on lifestyle. Eating lunch outside when weather permits could be one solution. In colder climes, women can take a tablespoon of cod liver oil daily, eat fatty fish and fish oils, and egg yolks. Supplements of vitamin D3 (calciferol) may be necessary for certain women.

f. *Other considerations:* Vitamin D2, found in fortified foods, especially breads and cereals, is poorly metabolized by the body. Certain drugs can interfere with vitamin D metabolism, including corticosteroids, phenytoin, heparin, cimetidine, isoniazid, rifampin, phenobarbital, and primidone. Find alternate medications whenever possible that do not interfere with the metabolism of vitamin D3. Taking vitamin D supplements can actually block vitamin D nuclear receptor (VDR) activation, the heart of immunity, having the opposite effect to that of sunshine. Quite nominal amounts of ingested vitamin D can suppress the proper operation of the immune system.

g. *References/other sources:*

Autoimmunity Research Foundation. (2008, January 27). Vitamin D deficiency study raises new questions about disease and supplements. *ScienceDaily.* Retrieved February 13, 2008, from http://www.science daily.com/releases/2008/01/080125223302.htm

Demgrow, M. (2007, June). High vitamin D: Treatment for cancer prevention? *The Clinical Advisor,* 54, 57.

Jockers, B. S. (2007). Vitamin D sufficiency: An approach to disease prevention. *The American Journal for Nurse Practitioners, 11*(10), 43–50.

Exercise/Movement

1. Exercise
   a. *Actions/expected responses:* Exercise can enhance the health of women with liver disease.
   b. *Routes/dosages/frequencies:* A good beginning regimen might include 10–20 minutes of aerobic exercise, followed by a few weight-bearing exercises, three times a week. Even standing instead of sitting while using the computer, watching TV, reading or talking on the phone can improve health. Physical inactivity throughout the day stimulates disease-promoting processes, while moving and standing stimulates enzymes that optimize metabolism throughout the day.
   c. *Cautions:* When in an acute phase of hepatitis or experiencing a severe exacerbation or relapse of disease, any form of intense exertion should be avoided.
   d. *Assessments:* Assess strength, current activities, and frequency of exercise.
   e. *Tips on use:* When feeling up to physical activity, be active. Be aware of personal limitations and know when it's time to rest, but do not be entirely inactive, which can be dangerous. Being inactive is associated with accumulations of dangerous abdominal fat, developing elevated blood lipids, a sign of prediabetes and cardiovascular disease. The liver has only so much energy to distribute to the rest of the body, so it's never wise to overdo it. Prior to commencing any exercise program discuss the prospect with the primary health care practitioner.

f. *Other considerations:* Women diagnosed with liver disease should drink at least six to eight 8-ounce glasses of water per day. It is especially important for women with chronic hepatitis B or C who are on interferon therapy to stay well-hydrated. These women should probably increase their water intake to at least 12 8-ounce glasses of water per day. Women with liver disease often find that drinking abundant amounts of water helps give them an improved sense of well-being. Women on interferon often find that liberal water consumption helps them with some of the side effects of the medication. On the other hand, individuals with ascites (the accumulation of fluid in the peritoneal cavity) are prone to excessive water retention. These individuals are advised to restrict their water intake to approximately three to four 8-ounce glasses of water per day, depending on the degree of fluid accumulation present. When drinking bottled mineral water, it is important to take note of the water's sodium content. In some instances, the sodium content may present a problem for individuals on sodium-restricted diets. Warm up prior to exercise and cool down afterward. For more information, go to http://www.wellness.ma/adult-fitness/stretching-warmup.htm

g. *References/other sources:*

Palmer, M. (2007). *The importance of exercise for liver disease.* Penguin Putnam. Retrieved April 24, 2008, from http://www.liverdisease.com/exercise_hepatitis.html

University of Missouri-Columbia. (2007, November 20). Sitting may increase risk of disease. *ScienceDaily.* Retrieved March 22, 2008, from http://www.sciencedaily.com/releases/2007/11/071119130734.htm

University of Missouri-Columbia. (2008, March 23). Killer stairs? Taking the elevator could be worse for your body. *ScienceDaily.* Retrieved March 23, 2008, from http://www.sciencedaily.com/releases/2008/03/080318182741.htm

Herbs/Essential Oils

1. Aromatherapy

a. *Actions/expected responses:* Laboratory studies and animal studies have shown that certain essential oils have antibacterial, calming, or energizing effects. Aromatherapy may work by sending chemical messages to the part of the brain that affects moods and emotions. Lavender and rosemary protect the body from oxidative stress by decreasing the stress hormone cortisol. Women with liver cancer may use aromatherapy mainly to improve their quality of life.

b. *Routes/dosages/frequencies:* Lavender and rosemary oils can calm. Sniff aroma of essential oils for 5 minutes.

c. *Cautions:* Safety testing on essential oils has found very few bad side effects.

d. *Assessments:* Assess negative emotions prior to and after using aromatherapy. Assess for hypersensitivity (skin reactions, nausea, or anorexia).

e. *Tips on use:* Keep aromatherapy products away from heat and moisture in a sealed container.

f. *Other considerations:* Can use one or the other essential oil or both to protect against oxidative stress.

g. *References/other sources:*
   Atsumi, T., & Tonosaki, K. (2007). Smelling lavender and rosemary increases free radical scavenging activity and decreases cortisol level in saliva. *Psychiatry Research, 150*(1), 89–96.

2. Milk thistle
   a. *Actions/expected responses:* Silymarin, the active substance in milk thistle, stimulates detoxification pathways, inhibits the growth of certain cancer cell lines, exerts direct cytotoxic activity toward certain cancer cell lines, and may increase the efficacy of certain chemotherapy agents. Milk thistle also protects the liver from drug or alcohol-related injury. Silibinin, a compound of milk thistle, may even prevent the development of liver cancer.
   b. *Routes/dosages/frequencies:* 200–400 mg silymarin per day.
   c. *Cautions:* Milk thistle is considered safe and well-tolerated with gastrointestinal upset, a mild laxative effect, and rare allergic reaction being the only adverse events reported when taken within the recommended dose range. Counsel pregnant and lactating women or those who are hypersensitive (have a known sensitivity to ragweed, marigolds, or chrysanthemums) not to use milk thistle. Avoid taking milk thistle concurrently with antipsychotics, phenytoin, and halothane.
   d. *Assessments:* Assess hypersensitivity to milk thistle.
   e. *Tips on use:* Milk thistle may protect against liver damage from antipsychotics, acetaminophen, phenytoin, and halothane.
   f. *Other considerations:* Preliminary research suggests that silybin may enhance the tumor fighting effects of cisplatin and doxorubicin.
   g. *References/other sources:*
      Bokemeyer, C., Fells, L. M., & Dunn, T. (1996). Silibinin protects against cisplatin-induced nephrotoxicity without compromising cisplatin on isosfamide anti-tumor activity. *British Journal of Cancer, 74,* 2036–2041.
      Post-White, J., Ladas, E. J., & Kelly, K. M. (2007). Advances in the use of milk thistle (Silybum marianum). *Integrative Cancer Therapy, 6*(2), 104–109.

3. Spearmint
   a. *Actions/expected responses:* Methanol extracts of spearmint possess antimutagenic qualities that inhibit carcinogen activation.
   b. *Routes/dosages/frequencies:* Brew spearmint leaves in hot water for 5 minute and drink as a tea.
   c. *Cautions:* Pregnant women should avoid spearmint, as should those with hiatal hernia or a gallstone attack.
   d. *Assessments:* Assess pregnancy, hiatal hernia, and gallstone status.
   e. *Tips on use:* See http://www.answers.com/topic/spearmint?cat=technology
   f. *Other considerations:* None.
   g. *References/other sources:*
      Yu, T. W., Xu, M., & Dashwood, R. H. (2004). Antimutagenic activity of spearmint. *Environmental Molecular Mutagens, 44*(5), 387–393.

Mindset

1. Affirmations
   a. *Actions/expected responses:* Self-affirmation of personal values and beliefs buffers neuroendocrine and psychological stress.

b. *Routes/dosages/frequencies:* Repeat aloud or write positive affirmations up to 20 times a day such as, "My heart is filled with love" and "I release whatever I no longer need."

c. *Cautions:* Ensure affirmations are positive and acceptable.

d. *Assessments:* Assess anxiety prior to and after completing affirmations for a week.

e. *Tips on use*: Write favorite affirmations on 3 by 5 cards and place them where they will be read frequently.

f. *Other considerations:* Find more affirmations information at www.successc onsciousness.com/index_00000a.htm

g. *References/other sources:*

Hay, L. (2000). *Heal your body.* Carlsbad, CA: Hay House.

Schwarzer, R., Babler, J., Kwiatek, P., Schroder, K., & Zang, J. W. (1997). The assessment of optimistic self-beliefs: Assessment of general perceived self-efficacy in thirteen cultures. *World Psychology, 3*(1–2), 177–190.

Nutrition

1. Antioxidant and antiproliferative activites of common vegetables

   a. *Actions/expected responses:* In rank order, consumption of spinach, cabbage, red pepper, onion, and broccoli show the high antiproliferative activity for preventing cancer.

   b. *Routes/dosages/frequencies:* Eat the above vegetables daily.

   c. *Cautions:* Avoid vegetables for which a sensitivity exists.

   d. *Assessments:* Assess intake of antiproliferative vegetables.

   e. *Tips on use:* Add antiproliferative vegetables to salads, stews, sauces, soups, sandwiches, fish, tofu, and other foods.

   f. *Other considerations:* Epidemiological studies have shown that consumption of fruits and vegetables is associated with reduced risk of chronic disease, including cancer.

   g. *References/other sources:*

   Chu, Y. F., Sun, J., Wu, X., & Liu, R. H. (2002). Antioxidant and antiproliferative activities of common vegetables. *Journal of Agriculture and Food Chemistry, 50*(23), 6910–6916.

   Gonzalez, C. A., & Riboli, E. (2006). Diet and cancer prevention: Where we are, where we are going. *Nutrition in Cancer, 56*(2), 225–231.

2. Curcumin (turmeric)

   a. *Actions/expected responses:* Curcumin exerts an antiproliferative effect on various tumor cell lines but leaves normal human tissue alone. Because of its qualities, curcumin may prevent the spread of liver cancer.

   b. *Routes/dosages/frequencies:* Sprinkle this spice in soups and stews, add to fish or chicken marinades, use in egg salads to ad a rich yellow color, make a tasty yellow rice pilaf using curcumin.

   c. *Cautions:* Pregnant women must check with their primary health care practitioner about using curcumin because in large doses it can be a uterine stimulant. Women with gallstones or biliary obstructions should avoid curcumin. In more than dietary use, this spice may interact with anticoagulants, NSAIDs, and immunosuppressants.

    d. *Assessments:* Assess for hypersensitivity, and use of anticoagulants, NSAIDs, and immunosuppressants.

    e. *Tips on use:* Store curcumin in a cool, dry place.

    f. *Other considerations:* Curcumin may also slow the progression of Alzheimer's by removing amyloid plaque buildup in the brain, it may be used as an antibacterial agent, and it prevents blood clots that could cause heart attack or stroke.

    g. *References/other sources:*

        Novak, K. R., Grbesa, I., Ivkic, M., Katdare, M., & Gall-Troselj, K. (2008). Curcumin downregulates H19 gene transcription in tumor cells. *Journal of Cell Biochemistry, 104*(5), 1781–1789.

3. Fast-food (avoid)

    a. *Actions/expected responses:* Diets high in fast food can be highly toxic to the liver and other internal organs.

    b. *Routes/dosages/frequencies:* Eating too many calories and too much fat and sugar.

    c. *Cautions:* It takes as little as a week to gain 4 pounds and see a sharp rise in liver enzymes after eating fast food and remaining sedentary.

    d. *Assessments:* Assess number of fast-food meals/week.

    e. *Tips for use:* Limit fast-food meals to no more than one a week. Consider a visit to a fast food restaurant as a treat.

    f. *Other considerations*: Liver damage can be prevented or reversed. When at a fast-food restaurant, try the burger without cheese and mayo and avoid fries and sugary soft drinks. Order a grilled chicken sandwich, a salad with low-fat dressing and bottled water. Start to exercise at least three times a week to help your body metabolize and process your food.

    g. *References/other sources:*

        Saint Louis University Medical Center. (2008, May 2). Fast-food liver damage can be reversed, experts say. *ScienceDaily.* Retrieved May 14, 2008, from http://www.sciencedaily.com/releases/2008/04/080430204519.htm

4. Folates

    a. *Actions/expected responses:* Dietary folates are protective against cancer, but folic acid fortification is associated with cancer. Because national surveys revealed most women did not consume adequate folate, a grain fortification program is in place.

    b. *Routes/dosages/frequencies:* Leafy green vegetables (like spinach and turnip greens), broccoli, fruits (citrus fruits and juices), and dried beans and peas are all natural sources of folate that can help meet the suggested amount of 1,000 micrograms (mcg) a day. Women on diets who do not eat breads, cereals or pasta, who abuse alcohol, or take medications that interfere with folate absorption may not receive sufficient amounts of the nutrient and may need additional amounts.

    c. *Cautions:* Medications and medical conditions that increase the need for folate or result in an increased excretion of folate include: anticonvulsant medications, metformin, sulfasalazine, triamterene, methotrexate, barbiturates, pregnancy and lactation, alcohol abuse, malabsorption, kidney dialysis, liver disease, and certain anemias. Because folate is a water-soluble B-vitamin, unneeded amounts will be eliminated in the urine.

    d. *Assessments:* Assess for signs of folate deficiency: anemia, diarrhea, loss of appetite, weight loss, weakness, sore tongue, headaches, heart palpitations, irritability, forgetfulness, behavioral disorders, and an elevated level of homocysteine.

 e. *Tips on use:* Avoid flour-fortified foods as a source of folic acid; new research has shown the introduction of flour fortified with folic acid into common foods has been linked to cancer.

 f. *Other considerations:* Exceeding 1,000 mcg per day of folate may trigger vitamin B12 deficiency. To compensate, take a multivitamin that contains B12 or eat at least one food daily that contains B12: nutritional yeast (unless susceptible to candida), clams, eggs, herring, kidney, liver, mackerel, seafood, milk, or dairy products.

 g. *References/other sources:*

  Blackwell Publishing Ltd. (2007, November 5). Folic acid linked to increased cancer rate, historical review suggests. *ScienceDaily.* Retrieved November 29, 2007, from http://www.sciencedaily.com/releases/2007/11/07/071102111956.htm

  Office of Dietary Supplements. (2005). *Dietary supplement fact sheet: Folate.* Bethesda, MD: NIH Clinical Center, National Institutes of Health. Retrieved November 25, 2007, from http://ods.od.nih.gov

5. Fruits, vegetables, and whole grains

 a. *Actions/expected responses:* The consumption of fruits, vegetables, and whole grains is linked to a decreased risk for cancers. Tomatoes are especially helpful. Tomatoes show a consistent pattern of protection when eaten raw and often. Consuming one serving of raw tomatoes per week reduced the risk of all cancers by 50% for older women. Watercress is linked to a reduced risk of cancer via decreased damage to DNA and possible modulation of antioxidant status by increasing carotenoid concentration.

 b. *Routes/dosages/frequencies:* Encourage women to eat 5–10 servings (1/2 cup) of fruits and vegetables daily, and 5 servings of whole grains (barley, buckwheat, bulgur/cracked wheat, millet, oatmeal, popcorn, whole-wheat bread and pasta, and/or wild rice).

 c. *Cautions:* Some women may be sensitive to certain fruits, vegetables, or grains (especially wheat).

 d. *Assessments:* Assess for sensitivity to and affinity for various fruits, vegetables, and grains.

 e. *Tips on use:* Go to http://www.cooks.com/rec/ch/vegetables.html and http://www.ahealthyme.com/topic/fruitvegkids (useful for adults, too).

 f. *Other considerations:* Fruits and vegetables contain a plethora of anticarcinogenic substances including carotenoids, vitamins C and E, selenium, dietary fiber, flavonoids, polphenols, and many other health-producing compounds. Grains to avoid: corn flakes, enriched macaroni or spaghetti, couscous, grits, pretzels, white bread, rye bread, white rice.

 g. *References/other sources:*

  Gill, C. I., Haldar, S., Boyd, L. A., Bennett, R., Whiteford, J., Butler, M., et al. (2007). Watercress supplementation in diet reduces lymphocyte DNA damage and alters blood antioxidant status in healthy adults. *American Journal of Clinical Nutrition, 85*(2), 504–510.

  Hord, N. G. (2005). The role of dietary factors in cancer prevention: Beyond fruits and vegetables. *Nutrition in Clinical Practice, 20*(4), 451–459.

6. Green tea
    a. *Actions/expected responses:* Green tea is protective against cancer before disease occurs and after onset, possibly by creating a detoxifying effect.
    b. *Routes/dosages/frequencies:* Two to five cups of decaffeinated tea daily (1 tsp tea leaves in 8 ounces of hot water).
    c. *Cautions:* May decrease iron absorption, so separate iron-rich foods or iron pills by at least 2 hours from green tea ingestion.
    d. *Assessments:* Assess for hypersensitivity reactions. Also assess for cardio-vascular (increased blood pressure, palpitations and irregular heartbeat), central nervous system (anxiety, nervousness, insomnia), and gastrointestinal (nausea, heartburn, increased stomach acid) effects.
    e. *Tips on use:* Caffeinated green tea can interact with MAOIs and lead to a hypertensive crisis. Counsel women not to take green tea with anticoagulants/antiplatelets (may increase risk of bleeding), beta-adrenergic blockers (can lead to increased inotropic effects), or benzodiazepines (may increase sedation). Teach women to store green tea in a cool, dry place.
    f. *Other considerations:* Dairy products may decrease the therapeutic effects of green tea, so separate their intake by several hours. Digestive process affects anticancer activity of tea in gastrointestinal cells; add citrus (such as lemon juice) or take ascorbic acid (vitamin C) to protect the catechins in green tea from digestive degradation.
    g. *References/other sources:*
        American Association for Cancer Research. (2007, August 12). Green tea boosts production of detox enzymes, rendering cancerous chemicals harmless. *ScienceDaily.* Retrieved December 20, 2007, from http://www.sciencedaily.com/releases/2007/08/070810194923.htm
        Federation of American Societies for Experimental Biology. (2008, April 10). Digestive process affects anti-cancer activity of tea in gastrointestinal cells. *ScienceDaily.* Retrieved April 20, 2008, from http://www.sciencedaily.com/releases/2008/04/080407172713.htm
        Pettit, J. L. (2001). Green tea. *Clinician Reviews, 11*(1), 71–72.
        Skidmore-Roth, L. (2006). Green tea. In *Mosby's handbook of herbs and natural supplements* (pp. 535–539). St. Louis, MO: ElsevierMosby.
7. Maitake mushrooms
    a. *Actions/Expected responses:* Animal and human studies have supported the use of maitake extraction for cancer. This mushroom is an immune modulator that helps to normalize the immune system. It exerts an anti-cancer action by activating interleukin-1 and increasing T-cells.
    b. *Routes/dosages/frequencies:* Eat as a part of a healthy diet to enhance the immune system.
    c. *Cautions:* Avoid if sensitive to this food. May interact with immunosuppressants and antidiabetes agents.
    d. *Assessments:* Assess sensitivity to maitake and use of immunosuppressants and antidiabetes agents.
    e. *Tips on use.* Store maitake in a clean, dry place. For recipes and ways to use maitake, go to http://theforagerpress.com/fieldguide/maitake/maitake-recipes.htm

f. *Other considerations:* Maitake and other mushrooms have been used for thousands of years in Asia for many purposes. Maitake is also available in capsules or as an extract.

g. *References/other sources:*

Kodama, N., Komuta, K., & Nanba, H. (2002). Can maitake MD-fraction aid cancer patients? *Alternative Medicine Review, 7*(3), 236–239.

8. Pomegranate juice

a. *Actions/expected responses:* Pomegranate juice can reduce liver stress.

b. *Routes/dosages/frequencies:* Drinking pomegranate juice daily.

c. *Cautions:* Avoid during the first trimester of pregnancy.

d. *Assessments:* Assess pregnancy status and sensitivity to pomegranate juice.

e. *Tips on use:* Keep pomegranate juice in a cool dry place.

f. *Other considerations:* Go to http://64.233.169.104/search?q=cache:Sx60Rjd NpCgJ:www.rimonest.com/doc/faq1.doc+dosage+of+pomegranate+seed+ oil&hl=en&ct=clnk&cd=12&gl=us

g. *References/other sources:*

Faria, A., Monteiro, R., Mateus, N., Azevedo, I., & Calhau, C. (2007). Effect of pomegranate (Punica granatum) juice intake on hepatic oxidative stress. *European Journal of Nutrition, 46*(5), 271–278.

Stress Management

1. Stress management techniques

a. *Actions/expected responses:* A weak immune system is one of the major factors that promotes cancer metastases after an operation, chemotherapy, or radiation therapy. Fear and stress weaken the immune system. Adequate stress management prior to and after medical treatment may help to prevent metastases.

b. *Routes/dosages/frequencies:* Daily stress management practice.

c. *Cautions:* Go to http://www.mindtools.com/pages/main/newMN_TCS.htm

d. *Assessments:* Assess stress level.

e. *Tips on use:* Go to http://www.mindtools.com/pages/main/newMN_TCS.htm

f. *Other considerations:* None.

g. *References/other sources:*

Tel Aviv University. (2008, February 29). Stress and fear can affect cancer's recurrence. *ScienceDaily*. Retrieved March 9, 2008, from http://www.sciencedaily.com/releases/2008/02/080227142656.htm

Supplements

1. Aged garlic extract

a. *Actions/expected responses:* Aged garlic extract attenuated histological liver damage and oxidative stress.

b. *Routes/dosages/frequencies:* 4 ml daily

c. *Cautions:* Should not be used medicinally during pregnancy because this extract can stimulate labor. Dietary amounts of garlic are acceptable.

Do not use garlic extract if suffering from hypothyroidism, right before surgery, if their stomach is inflamed, or if they're hypersensitive to garlic.

   d. *Assessments:* Assess for hypothyroidism, upcoming surgery, pregnancy or hypersensitivity to garlic.

   e. *Tips on use:* Keep aged garlic extract in a cool, dry place away from pets.

   f. *Other considerations:* Discontinue use of garlic prior to undergoing any invasive procedure. During pregnancy, monitor complete blood count (CBC) and coagulation time (when using extract at a high level). Seek supervision by a qualified herbalist if taking garlic extract long term.

   g. *References/other sources:*

      Kodai, S., Takemura, S., Minimiyama, Y., Hai, S., Yamamoto, S., Kubo, S., et al. (2007). S-allyl cysteine prevent CCl(4)-induced acute liver injury in rats. *Free Radical Research, 41*(4), 489–497.

2. Pycnogenol and ginkgo biloba extract

   a. *Actions/expected responses:* Either pycnogenol or ginkgo biloba extract can protect against antimutagenic activity in animal studies and may be helpful in cancers. Pycnogenol is also useful in protecting against and preventing liver toxicity.

   b. *Routes/dosages/frequencies:* 5–100 microgram/mL.

   c. *Cautions:* Until more research is completed, pregnant and lactating women should not use these supplements, nor should they be given to children. Avoid taking ginkgo concurrently with anticoagulants.

   d. *Assessments:* Assess reaction to pycnogenol and ginkgo.

   e. *Tips on use:* Store supplements in a cool, dry place.

   f. *Other considerations:* Pycnogenol has also been found useful in preventing venous thrombosis, thrombophlebitis, gingival bleeding and plaque, inflammatory bowel disease, venous insufficiency, digestive conditions, and menopause symptoms.

   g. *References/other sources:*

      Krizkova, L., Chovanova, Z., Durackova, Z., & Krajcovic, J. (2008). Antimutagenic in vitro activity of plan polyphenols: Pycnogenol and ginkgo biloba extract. *Phytotherapy Research, 22*(3), 384–388.

      Yang, Y. S., Ahn, T. H., Lee, J. C., Moon, C. J., Kim, S. H., Jun, W., et al. (2008). Protective effects of pycnogenol on carbon tetrachloride-induced hepatotoxicity in Sprague-Dawley rats. *Food Chemistry and Toxicology, 46*(1), 380–387.

Touch

1. Acupressure

   a. *Actions/expected responses:* Acupressure can reduce nausea and vomiting induced by chemotherapy.

   b. *Routes/dosages/frequencies:* Stimulate the PC6 point for at least 6 hours per day at the onset of chemotherapy. The PC6 point is situated in the middle of the front of the forearm above the wrist crease. Wristbands are available to stimulate this point. The point can be stimulated every 2–3 hours or as needed. See http://www.handbag.com/healthfit/complementary/acupressure

c. *Cautions:* Only gentle acupressure should be used in injured or sore areas.

d. *Assessments:* Rate symptoms before and after treatment.

e. *Tips on use:* For more information on using acupressure, go to http://www. eclecticenergies.com/acupressure/howto.php

f. *Other considerations:* Changes in mood may begin to occur immediately and continue for several days.

g. *References/other sources:*

Gardani, G., Cerrone, R., Biella, C., Mancini, L., Proserpio, E., Casiraghi, M., et al. (2006). Effect of acupressure on nausea and vomiting induced by chemotherapy in cancer patients. *Minerva Medicine, 97*(5), 391–394.

2. Foot reflexology

a. *Actions/expected responses:* Life satisfaction was significantly improved in the experimental group after foot reflexology. Combined with aromatherapy and foot soak, reflexology also relieves fatigue in clients with cancer. Foot reflexology or self-administered foot reflexology also significantly enhances and strengthens the immune system so it can catch and eliminate cancer cells and prevent tumors from developing.

b. *Routes/dosages/frequencies:* Twice a week for 4 weeks. Three-minute foot soak contains warm water and lavender essential oil, and is followed by reflexology treatment with jojoba oil containing lavender for 10 minutes. Four 40-minute self-administered foot reflexology treatments can also be of benefit. See http://www.handbag.com/healthfit/complementary/acupressure

c. *Cautions:* Pregnant women should avoid foot reflexology because certain manipulations can lead to premature labor. Those with foot problems, gout, arthritis, and vascular conditions such as varicose veins should be careful using this procedure. Perform a patch test with lavender essential oil prior to foot soak.

d. *Assessments:* Evaluate life satisfaction and fatigue prior to and after foot reflexology sessions. See http://employees.oneonta.edu/vomsaaw/w/handouts%20-%20happiness/life%20satisfaction%20WvS%20questionnaire.pdf. Evaluate fatigue with the Cancer Fatigue Scale before, 1 hour after, and 4 hours after treatment.

e. *Tips on use:* For foot charts, see http://groups.msn.com/AlternativesTo PainandDisease/reflexologyinstructionspg1.msnw

f. *Other considerations:* Quality of life is the most important predictor of survival for advanced cancer clients. See http://groups.msn.com/Alterna tivesToPainandDisease/reflexologyinstructionspg2.msnw

g. *References/other sources:*

Fox Chase Cancer Center. (2007, November 1). Quality of life is the most important predictor of survival for advanced cancer patients. *Science-Daily.* Retrieved November 12, 2007, from http://www.sciencedaily. com/releases/2007/10/071030170208.htm

Kesselring, A. (1994). Foot reflex zone massage. *Schweizerische Medizinische Wochenschrift, 62,* 88–93.

Kohara, H., Miyauchi, T., Suehiro, Y., Ueoka, H., Takeyama, H., & Morita, T. (2004). Combined modality treatment of aromatherapy, footsoak, and reflexology relieves fatigue in patients with cancer. *Journal of Palliative Medicine, 7*(6), 791–796.

Lee, Y. M. (2006). Effect of self-foot reflexology massage on depression, stress responses and immune functions of middle aged women. *Taehan Kanho Hakkoe Chi, 36*(1), 179–188.

3. Therapeutic touch (TT)

a. *Actions/expected responses:* Therapeutic touch treatments increase a sensation of well-being in women with terminal cancer.

b. *Routes/dosages/frequencies:* Three sessions of 15–20 minutes each.

c. *Cautions:* The aged, extremely ill, or dying should be given a 5-minute (or less) treatment by an experienced practitioner.

d. *Assessments:* Take a baseline measure for well-being prior to administering therapeutic touch and then take a measure after treatment.

e. *Tips on use:* Center and calm yourself by closing your eyes and focusing on breathing in your abdomen. When relaxed, rub your hands together and feel the tingling sensation as you slowly pull your hands apart. When able to feel the energies balancing between the hands, hold the intent to balance the other person's energy in your mind. Start above the head and keep an inch or so away from the body, bring your hands slowly down, sweeping down the body slowly, ending a few inches past the feet. For more information, go to http://www.healgrief.com/Site/Heal_Grief_in_Your_Body.html

f. *Other considerations:* Regular TT treatments may enhance the effect achieved.

g. *References/other sources:*

Giasson, M. (1998). Effect of therapeutic touch on the well-being of persons with terminal cancer. *Journal of Holistic Nursing, 16*(3), 383–398.

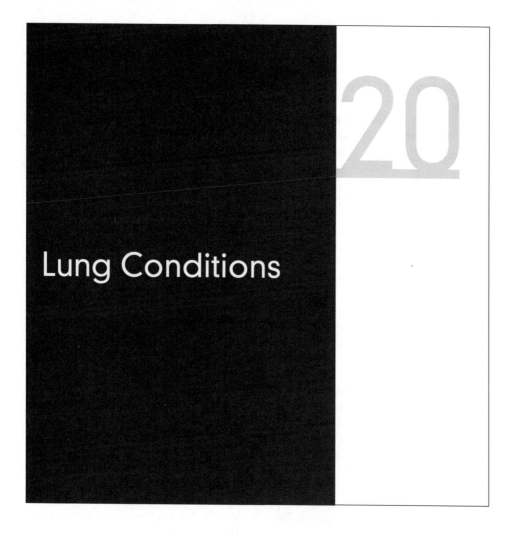

Lung Conditions

Many lung conditions are environmentally and nutritionally related. Recent research has demonstrated complementary approaches can reduce symptoms and heal underlying processes.

Environment

1. Computer game
   a. *Actions/expected responses:* Women with chronic obstructive pulmonary disease (COPD) may gain better control over their breathing and breathe more efficiently by using their breath to play a computer game that teaches them to inhalf more slowly and exhale more completely. A new randomized, controlled trial resulted in finding that a computer program could decrease the extent of air trapping during exercise and thus improve the results of rehabilitation in women with COPD.
   b. *Routes/dosages/frequencies:* Daily until breathing improves.
   c. *Cautions:* None known.
   d. *Assessments:* Assess breathing prior to and after playing the computer game.

   e. *Tips on use:* The game used in this study is not yet available commercially but investigate breathing games on the internet to find one that may be suitable.
   f. *Other considerations:* None.
   g. *References/other sources:*
      American Thoracic Society. (2008, April 17). Computer game helps COPD patients breath better, study shows. *ScienceDaily.* Retrieved April 24, 2008, from http://www.sciencedaily.com/releases/2008/04/080415075711.htm
2. Room mold
   a. *Actions/expected responses:* Almost one in five rooms studied with no visible mold was in fact "highly contaminated" by fungus that could aggravate conditions such as asthma.
   b. *Routes/dosages/frequencies:* By breathing in rooms with nonvisible mold in them.
   c. *Cautions:* Lack of ventilation or a ground floor apartment or accidental damage, such as water damage, are the significant factors in level of contamination.
   d. *Assessments:* Assess for lack of ventilation, accidental damage, or living on the ground floor apartment.
   e. *Tips on use:* If lung conditions plague one or more family members, consider moving to an apartment above ground level, enhancing in-home ventilation, and fixing any water damage.
   f. *Other considerations:* Age of building, presence of pets, and even outdoor or indoor temperature had little bearing on fungus concentration.
   g. *References/other sources:*
      Royal Society of Chemistry. (2008, May 1). One in five rooms is "highly contaminated" with hidden mold. *ScienceDaily.* Retrieved May 14, 2008, from http://www.sciencedaily.com/releases/2008/08/080430123552.htm
3. Sunlight
   a. *Actions/expected responses:* Researchers at the Moores Cancer Center at University of California, San Diego (UCSD) have shown a clear association between deficiency in exposure to sunlight, specifically ultraviolet B (UVB), and cancer.
   b. *Routes/dosages/frequencies:* For light-skinned women, 10–15 minutes of direct midday sun at least twice a week on the face, arms, hands, or back is sufficient, according to the National Institutes of Health. Darker-skinned women may require three to six times as much exposure.
   c. *Cautions:* More frequent exposure could result in skin cancer. Insufficient exposure to the sun can result in improper absorption of calcium and phosphorus, leading to imperfect skeletal formation as well as bone disorders. Vitamin D supplements can suppress the immune system.
   d. *Assessments:* Assess the amount of time spent in direct sunlight.
   e. *Tips on use:* Develop a plan for obtaining sufficient sunlight, depending on lifestyle. Eating lunch outside when weather permits could be one solution. In colder climes, take a tablespoon of cod liver oil daily; eat fatty fish and fish oils, and egg yolks. Supplements of vitamin D3 (calciferol) may be necessary for certain women.
   f. *Other considerations:* Vitamin D2, found in fortified foods, especially breads and cereals, is poorly metabolized by the body. Certain drugs can interfere

with vitamin D metabolism, including corticosteroids, phenytoin, heparin, cimetidine, isoniazid, rifampin, phenobarbital, and primidone. Find alternate medications whenever possible that do not interfere with metabolism of vitamin D3. Taking vitamin D supplements can actually block the immune system, the opposite effect to that of sunshine. Quite nominal amounts of ingested vitamin D can suppress the proper operation of the immune system.

g. *References/other sources:*

Autoimmunity Research Foundation. (2008, January 27). Vitamin D deficiency study raises new questions about disease and supplements. *ScienceDaily.* Retrieved February 13, 2008, from http://www.science-daily.com/releases/2008/01/080125223302.htm

Demgrow, M. (2007, June). High vitamin D: Treatment for cancer prevention? *The Clinical Advisor, 54,* 57.

Jockers, B. S. (2007). Vitamin D sufficiency: An approach to disease prevention. *The American Journal for Nurse Practitioners, 11*(10), 43–50.

Exercise/Movement

1. Exercise
   a. *Actions/expected responses:* It is dangerous to be inactive for just a couple of weeks and may even be the cause of many chronic diseases, including cancer. There is evidence that regular physical activity or exercise can decrease emotional stress and pain and can increase quality of life, maximal oxygen uptake, sleep patterns, and cognition.
   b. *Routes/dosages/frequencies:* Daily activity is important. Taking the stairs instead of the elevator, walking 10,000 steps a day, or standing when watching TV or talking on the phone can help. Low intensity aerobics walking, tai chi, or cycling can also decrease fatigue levels. Even women who are bedridden or in a wheelchair can benefit from exercise such as circling and bending the arms and legs.
   c. *Cautions:* Choose a level of activity that suits the level of disease.
   d. *Assessments:* Assess daily level of physical activity.
   e. *Tips on use:* Evaluate the effect of exercise on health status.
   f. *Other considerations:* For more information, go to http://exercise.lifetips.com
   g. *References/other sources:*

University of Missouri-Columbia. (2008, March 21). Killer stairs? Taking the elevator could be worse for your body. *ScienceDaily.* Retrieved March 23, 2008, from http://www.sciencedaily.com/releases/2008/03/080318182741.htm

Visovsky, C., & Dvorak, C. (2005). Exercise and cancer recovery. *Online Journal of Issues in Nursing, 26*(10), 7.

Herbs/Essential Oils

1. Milk thistle (silymarin)
   a. *Actions/expected responses:* Silymarin, the active substance in milk thistle, stimulates detoxification pathways, inhibits the growth of certain cancer

cell lines, exerts direct cytotoxic activity toward certain cancer cell lines, and may increase the efficacy of certain chemotherapy agents.

b. *Routes/dosages/frequencies:* 200 to 400 mg silymarin per day.

c. *Cautions:* Milk thistle is considered safe and well-tolerated with gastrointestinal upset, a mild laxative effect, and rare allergic reaction being the only adverse events reported when taken within the recommended dose range. Pregnant and lactating women or those who are hypersensitive (have a known sensitivity to ragweed, marigolds, or chrysanthemums) should not use milk thistle. Avoid taking milk thistle concurrently with antipsychotics, phenytoin, and halothane.

d. *Assessments:* Assess hypersensitivity to milk thistle.

e. *Tips on use:* Milk thistle may protect against liver damage from antipsychotics, acetaminophen, phenytoin, and halothane.

f. *Other considerations:* Preliminary research suggests that silybin may enhance the tumor-fighting effects of cisplatin and doxorubicin.

g. *References/other sources:*

Bokemeyer, C., Fells, L. M., & Dunn, T. (1996). Silibinin protects against cisplatin-induced nephrotoxicity without compromising cisplatin on isosfamide anti-tumor activity. *British Journal of Cancer, 74,* 2036–2041.

Post-White, J., Ladas, E. J., & Kelly, K. M. (2007). Advances in the use of milk thistle (Silybum marianum). *Integrative Cancer Therapy, 6*(2), 104–109.

Mindset

1. Affirmations

a. *Actions/expected responses:* Self-affirmation of personal values and beliefs buffers neuroendocrine and psychological stress.

b. *Routes/dosages/frequencies:* Repeat aloud or write positive affirmations up to 20 times a day such as, "I breathe in life easily and let it flow through me" and "I love life and live it to the fullest."

c. *Cautions:* Ensure affirmations are positive and acceptable.

d. *Assessments:* Assess anxiety prior to and after completing affirmations for a week.

e. *Tips on use:* Write favorite affirmations on 3 by 5 cards and place them where they will be read frequently.

f. *Other considerations:* Find more affirmations information at www.success consciousness.com/index_00000a.htm

g. *References/other sources:*

Hay, L. (2000). *Heal your body.* Carlsbad, CA: Hay House.

Schwarzer, R., Babler, J., Kwiatek, P., Schroder, K., & Zang, J. W. (1997). The assessment of optimistic self-beliefs: Assessment of general perceived self-efficacy in thirteen cultures. *World Psychology, 3*(1–2), 177–190.

Nutrition

1. Butter-flavored popcorn (avoid)

a. *Actions/expected responses:* Diacetyl, the chemical responsible for the odor and flavor of "butter" in popcorn has been shown to injure the lungs.

b. *Routes/dosages/frequencies:* Just the inhalation of this chemical can damage the lungs.

c. *Cautions:* Avoid areas in theaters or homes where butter-flavored popcorn is being produced. Diacetyl is easily vaporized at temperatures used in microwave popcorn production.

d. *Assessments:* Assess for exposure to diacetyl.

e. *Tips for use:* Avoid using butter-flavored microwavable popcorn at home or purchasing it at theaters.

f. *Other considerations:* Use a hot air popcorn matchine and kernels which have not been exposed to diacetyl.

g. *References: other sources:*

Butter-flavored popcorn ingredient suspected cause of lung disease. (2008, May 1). *ScienceDaily.* Retrieved May 14, 2008, from http://www.sciencedaily.com/releases/2008/04/080430090123.htm

2. Curcumin (turmeric)

a. *Actions/expected responses:* Curcumin exerts an antiproliferative effect on various tumor cell lines but leaves normal human tissue alone. Because of its qualities, curcumin may prevent the spread of lung cancer.

b. *Routes/dosages/frequencies:* Sprinkle this spice in soups and stews, add to fish or chicken marinades, use in egg salads to add a rich yellow color, or make a tasty yellow rice pilaf using curcumin.

c. *Cautions:* Pregnant women should check with their primary health care practitioner about using curcumin in large doses because it can be a uterine stimulant. Women with gallstones or biliary obstructions should avoid curcumin. In more than dietary use, this spice may interact with anticoagulants, NSAIDs and immunosuppressants.

d. *Assessments:* Assess for hypersensitivity, and use of anticoagulants, NSAIDs, and immunosuppressants.

e. *Tips on use:* Store curcumin in a cool, dry place.

f. *Other considerations:* Curcumin may also slow the progression of Alzheimer's by removing amyloid plaque buildup in the brain, be used as an antibacterial agent, and prevent blood clots that could cause heart attack or stroke.

g. *References/other* sources:

Novak, K. R., Grbesa, I., Ivkic, M., Katdare, M., & Gall-Troselj, K. (2008). Curcumin downregulates H19 gene transcription in tumor cells. *Journal of Cell Biochemistry, 104*(5), 1781–1789.

3. Folate

a. *Actions/expected responses:* Dietary folates are protective against cancer, but folic acid fortification is associated with cancer. Because national surveys revealed most women did not consume adequate folate, a grain fortification program is in place.

b. *Routes/dosages/frequencies:* Leafy green vegetables (like spinach and turnip greens), broccoli, fruits (citrus fruits and juices), and dried beans and peas are all natural sources of folate that can help meet the suggested amount of 1,000 micrograms (mcg) a day. Women on diets who do not eat breads, cereals, or pasta, who abuse alcohol, or who take medications that interfere with folate absorption may not receive sufficient amounts of the nutrient and may need additional amounts.

   c. *Cautions:* Medications and medical conditions that increase the need for folate or result in an increased excretion of folate include: anticonvulsant medications, metformin, sulfasalazine, triamterene, methotrexate, barbiturates, pregnancy and lactation, alcohol abuse, malabsorption, kidney dialysis, liver disease, and certain anemias. Because folate is a water-soluble B-vitamin, unneeded amounts will be eliminated in the urine.

   d. *Assessments:* Assess for signs of folate deficiency: anemia, diarrhea, loss of appetite, weight loss, weakness, sore tongue, headaches, heart palpitations, irritability, forgetfulness, behavioral disorders, and an elevated level of homocysteine.

   e. *Tips on use:* Avoid flour-fortified foods as a source of folic acid; new research has shown the introduction of flour fortified with folic acid into common foods has been linked to cancer.

   f. *Other considerations:* Exceeding 1,000 mcg per day of folate may trigger vitamin B12 deficiency. To compensate, take a multivitamin that contains B12 or eat at least one food daily that contains B12: nutritional yeast (unless susceptible to candida), clams, eggs, herring, kidney, liver, mackerel, seafood, milk, or dairy products.

   g. *References/other sources:*

     Blackwell Publishing Ltd. (2007, November 5). Folic acid linked to increased cancer rate, historical review suggests. *ScienceDaily.* Retrieved November 29, 2007, from http://www.sciencedaily.com-/releases/2007/11/07/071102111956.htm

4. Fruits, vegetables, and whole grains

   a. *Actions/expected responses:* The consumption of fruits and vegetables and whole grains are linked to a decreased risk for cancers. Tomatoes are especially helpful. Tomatoes show a consistent pattern of protection when eaten raw and often. Consuming one serving of raw tomatoes per week reduced the risk of all cancers by 50% for older women.

   b. *Routes/dosages/frequencies:* Encourage women to eat 5–10 servings (1/2 cup) of fruits and vegetables daily, and 5 servings of whole grains (barley, buckwheat, bulgur/cracked wheat, millet, oatmeal, popcorn, whole-wheat bread and pasta, and/or wild rice).

   c. *Cautions:* Some women may be sensitive to certain fruits, vegetables, or grains (especially wheat).

   d. *Assessments:* Assess for sensitivity to and affinity for various fruits, vegetables, and grains.

   e. *Tips on use:* Go to http://www.cooks.com/rec/ch/vegetables.html and http://www.ahealthyme.com/topic/fruitvegkids (useful for adults, too)

   f. *Other considerations:* Fruits and vegetables contain a plethora of anticarcinogenic substances including carotenoids, vitamins C and E, selenium, dietary fiber, flavonoids, polyphenols, and many other health-producing compounds. Grains to avoid: corn flakes, enriched macaroni or spaghetti, couscous, grits, pretzels, white bread, rye bread, and white rice.

   g. *References/other sources:*

     Hord, N. G. (2005). The role of dietary factors in cancer prevention: Beyond fruits and vegetables. *Nutrition in Clinical Practice, 20*(4), 451–459.

5. Green tea

   a. *Actions/expected responses:* Green tea is protective against cancer before disease occurs and after onset, possibly by creating a detoxifying effect.

b. *Routes/dosages/frequencies:* Two to five cups of decaffeinated tea daily (1 tsp tea leaves in 8 ounces of hot water).

c. *Cautions:* May decrease iron absorption, so separate iron-rich foods or iron pills by at least 2 hours from green tea ingestion.

d. *Assessments:* Assess for hypersensitivity reactions. Also assess for cardiovascular (increased blood pressure, palpitations, and irregular heartbeat), central nervous system (anxiety, nervousness, insomnia), and gastrointestinal (nausea, heartburn, increased stomach acid) effects.

e. *Tips on use:* Caffeinated green tea can interact with MAOIs and lead to a hypertensive crisis. Avoid taking green tea with anticoagulants/antiplatelets (may increase risk of bleeding), beta-adrenergic blockers (can lead to increased inotropic effects), or benzodiazepines (may increase sedation). Store green tea in a cool, dry place.

f. *Other considerations:* Dairy products may decrease the therapeutic effects of green tea, so separate their intake by several hours. Digestive process affects anticancer activity of tea in gastrointestinal cells; add citrus (such as lemon juice) or take ascorbic acid (vitamin C) to protect the catechins in green tea from digestive degradation.

g. *References/other sources:*

American Association for Cancer Research. (2007, August 12). Green tea boosts production of detox enzymes, rendering cancerous chemicals harmless. *ScienceDaily.* Retrieved December 20, 2007, from http://www.sciencedaily.com/releases/2007/08/070810194923.htm

Federation of American Societies for Experimental Biology. (2008, April 10). Digestive process affects anti-cancer activity of tea in gastrointestinal cells. *ScienceDaily.* Retrieved April 20, 2008, from http://www.sciencedaily.com/releases/2008/04/080407172713.htm

Pettit, J. L. (2001). Green tea. *Clinician Reviews, 11*(1), 71–72.

Skidmore-Roth, L. (2006). Green tea. In *Mosby's handbook of herbs and natural supplements* (pp. 535–539). St. Louis, MO: ElsevierMosby.

6. Maitake mushrooms

a. *Actions/expected responses:* Animal and human studies have supported the use of maitake for cancer. This mushroom is an immune modulator that helps to normalize the immune system. It exerts an anticancer action by activating interleukin-1 and increasing T-cells.

b. *Routes/dosages/frequencies:* Eat as a part of a healthy diet to enhance the immune system.

c. *Cautions:* Avoid if sensitive to this food. May interact with immunosuppressants and antidiabetes agents.

d. *Assessments:* Assess sensitivity to maitake and use of immunosuppressants and antidiabetes agents.

e. *Tips on use.* Store maitake in a clean, dry place. For recipes and ways to use maitake, go to http://theforagerpress.com/fieldguide/maitake/maitake-recipes.htm

f. *Other considerations:* Maitake and other mushrooms have been used for thousands of years in Asia for many purposes. Maitake is also available in capsules or as an extract.

g. *References/other sources:*

Kodama, N., Komuta, K., & Nanba, H. (2002). Can maitake MD-fraction aid cancer patients? *Alternative Medicine Review, 7*(3), 236–239.

7. Red and processed meat, onions and garlic
   a. *Actions/Expected responses:* Consumption of red and processed meat is positively associated with lung cancer, while onions and garlic may reduce risk.
   b. *Routes/dosages/frequencies:* Eliminate red and processed meat from the diet. Eat onions and garlic daily.
   c. *Cautions:* Red and processed meat is linked with lung cancer.
   d. *Assessments:* Assess intake of red and processed meat, onions and garlic.
   e. *Tips on use:* Add powdered or fresh garlic and onions to salads, stews, sauces, soups, sandwiches, fish, tofu, and other foods.
   f. *Other considerations:* Garlic and onions are toxic for many animals. Keep garlic and onions away from their pets.
   g. *References/other sources:*
      Cross, A.J., Leitzann, M. E., Gail, M. H., Hollenbeck, A. R., Schatzkin, A., & Sinha, R. (2007). A prospective study of red and processed meat intake in relation to cancer risk. *PLoSMed, 4*(12), e325.
      Galeon, C. (2006). Onion and garlic use and human cancer. *American Journal of Clinical Nutrition, 84,* 1027–1032.
      Gonzalez, C. A., & Riboli, E. (2006). Diet and cancer prevention: Where we are, where we are going. *Nutrition in Cancer, 56*(2), 225–231.

Stress Management

1. Stress management techniques
   a. *Actions/expected responses:* A weak immune system is one of the major factors that promote cancer metastases after an operation, chemotherapy, or radiation therapy. Fear and stress weaken the immune system. Adequate stress management prior to and after medical treatment may help to prevent metastases.
   b. *Routes/dosages/frequencies:* Daily stress management practice.
   c. *Cautions:* Use stress management practices that are appealing and suit current lifestyle.
   d. *Assessments:* Assess levels of stress and fear. Assess stress management knowledge.
   e. *Tips on use:* For stress management information and techniques, go to http://www.mindtools.com/smpage-new-all.htm
   f. *Other considerations:* None.
   g. *References/other sources:*
      Tel Aviv University. (2008, February 29). Stress and fear can affect cancer's recurrence. *ScienceDaily.* Retrieved March 9, 2008, from http://www.sciencedaily.com/releases/2008/02/080227142656.htm

Supplements

1. Pomegranate fruit extract
   a. *Actions/expected responses:* Pomegranate fruit extract can significantly inhibit lung tumors.

b. *Routes/dosages/frequencies:* Ingesting one to two capsules of pomegranate fruit extract daily.

c. *Cautions:* Avoid during the first trimester of pregnancy.

d. *Assessments:* Assess pregnancy status and sensitivity to pomegranate juice.

e. *Tips on use:* Keep pomegranate juice in a cool dry place.

f. *Other considerations:* Go to http://64.233.169.104/search?q=cache:Sx60Rjd NpCgJ:www.rimonest.com/doc/faq1.doc+dosage+of+pomegranate+seed+ oil&hl=en&ct=clnk&cd=12&gl=us

g. *References/other sources:*

  Khan, N., Afaq, F., Kweon, M. H., Kim, K., & Mukhtar, H. (2007). Oral consumption of pomegranate fruit extract inhibits growth and progression of primary lung tumors in mice. *Cancer Research, 67*(7), 3475–3482.

2. Pycnogenol and ginkgo biloba extract

a. *Actions/expected responses:* Either pycnogenol or ginkgo biloba extract can protect against antimutagenic activity in animal studies. They have potential as antimutagenic agents for lung cancer.

b. *Routes/dosages/frequencies:* 5–100 microgram/mL.

c. *Cautions:* Until more research is completed, pregnant and lactating women should not use these supplements, nor should they be given to children. Ginkgo should not be taken concurrently with anticoagulants.

d. *Assessments:* Assess reaction to pycnogenol and ginkgo.

e. *Tips on use:* Store supplements in a cool, dry place.

f. *Other considerations:* Pycnogenol has also been found useful in preventing venous thrombosis, thrombophlebitis, gingival bleeding and plaque, inflammatory bowel disease, venous insufficiency, digestive conditions, and menopause symptoms.

g. *References/other sources:*

  Krizkova, L., Chovanova, Z., Durackova, Z., & Krajcovic, J. (2008). Antimutagenic in vitro activity of plan polyphenols: Pycnogenol and ginkgo biloba extract. *Phytotherapy Research, 22*(3), 384–388.

3. Vitamins A, B-complex, C, E, and selenium

a. *Actions/expected responses:* A study showed that micronutrient supplementation was associated with reduced rates of TB recurrence. Both HIV-infected and uninfected women with pulmonary TB receiving the supplements had a decreased risk of TB recurrence during the next few months after the TB culture had become negtative (45% overall and 63% in HIV-infected clients). Supplementation also reduced the incidence of peripheral neuopathy by 57%, irrespective of HIV status, and increased immune response in HIV-uninfected clients.

b. *Routes/dosages/frequencies:* Start with a multivitamin.

c. *Cautions:* Consult with an experienced nutritionist if higher dosages are necessary.

d. *Assessments:* Assess effect of multivitamins on peripheral neuropathy.

e. *Tips for use:* Follow directions on multivitamin/multimineral bottles.

f. *Other considerations:* None.

g. *References/other sources:*

  Common vitamin and other micronutrient supplements reduce risks of TB recurrence, study suggests. (2008). *ScienceDaily*. Retrieved May 14, 2008, from http://www.sciencedaily.com/releases/2008/04/080425112208.htm

Touch

1. Acupressure
   a. *Actions/expected responses:* Acupressure can reduce nausea and vomiting induced by chemotherapy.
   b. *Routes/dosages/frequencies:* Stimulate the PC6 point for at least 6 hours per day at the onset of chemotherapy. The PC6 point is situated in the middle of the front of the forearm above the wrist crease. Wristbands are available to stimulate this point. The point can be stimulated every 2–3 hours or as needed. See http://www.handbag.com/healthfit/complemen tary/acupressure.
   c. *Cautions:* Only gentle acupressure should be used in injured or sore areas.
   d. *Assessments:* Rate symptoms before and after treatment.
   e. *Tips on use:* For more information on using acupressure, go to http://www.eclecticenergies.com/acupressure/howto.php
   f. *Other considerations:* Changes in mood may begin to occur immediately and continue for several days.
   g. *References/other sources:*
      Gardani, G., Cerrone, R., Biella, C., Mancini, L., Proserpio, E., Casiraghi, M., et al. (2006). Effect of acupressure on nausea and vomiting induced by chemotherapy in cancer patients. *Minerva Medicine, 97*(5), 391–394.
2. Foot reflexology
   a. *Actions/expected responses:* Life satisfaction was significantly improved in the experimental group after foot reflexology. Combined with aromatherapy and foot soak, reflexology also relieves fatigue in clients with cancer. Foot reflexology or self-administered foot reflexology also significantly enhances and strengthens the immune system so it can catch and eliminate cancer cells and prevent tumors from developing.
   b. *Routes/dosages/frequencies:* Twice a week for 4 weeks. Three-minute foot soak contains warm water and lavender essential oil, and is followed by reflexology treatment with jojoba oil containing lavender for 10 minutes. Four 40-minute self-administered foot reflexology treatments can also be of benefit. For more information, see http://www.reflexology-research.com/whatis.htm
   c. *Cautions:* Pregnant women should avoid foot reflexology because certain manipulations can lead to premature labor. Those with foot problems, gout, arthritis, and vascular conditions such as varicose veins should be careful using this procedure. Perform a patch test with lavender essential oil prior to foot soak.
   d. *Assessments:* Evaluate life satisfaction and fatigue prior to and after foot reflexology sessions. See http://employees.oneonta.edu/vomsaaw/w/hand outs%20-%20happiness/life%20satisfaction%20WvS%20questionnaire.pdf. Evaluate fatigue with the Cancer Fatigue Scale before, 1 hour after, and 4 hours after treatment.
   e. *Tips on use:* For foot charts, see http://groups.msn.com/AlternativesTo PainandDisease/reflexologyinstructionspg1.msnw
   f. *Other considerations:* Quality of life is the most important predictor of survival for advanced cancer clients. See http://groups.msn.com/Alterna tivesToPainandDisease/reflexologyinstructionspg2.msnw

g. *References/other sources:*

Fox Chase Cancer Center. (2007, November 1). Quality of life is the most important predictor of survival for advanced cancer patients. *Science-Daily.* Retrieved November 12, 2007, from http://www.sciencedaily.com/releases/2007/10/071030170208.htm

Kesselring, A. (1994). Foot reflex zone massage. *Schweizerische Medizinische Wochenschrift, 62,* 88–93.

3. Therapeutic touch (TT)

a. *Actions/expected responses:* Therapeutic touch treatments increase a sensation of well-being in women with terminal cancer.

b. *Routes/dosages/frequencies:* Three sessions of 15–20 minutes each.

c. *Cautions:* The aged, extremely ill, or dying should be given a 5-minute (or less) treatment by an experienced practitioner.

d. *Assessments:* Take a baseline measure for well-being prior to administering therapeutic touch and then take a measure after treatment.

e. *Tips on use:* Center and calm yourself by closing your eyes and focusing on breathing in your abdomen. When relaxed, rub your hands together and feel the tingling sensation as you slowly pull your hands apart. When able to feel the energies balancing between the hands, hold the intent to balance the other person's energy. Start above the head and keep an inch or so away from the body, bring your hands slowly down, sweeping down the body slowly, ending a few inches past the feet. For more information, go to http://www.healgrief.com/Site/Heal_Grief_in_Your_Body.html

f. *Other considerations:* Regular TT treatments may enhance the effect achieved.

g. *References/other sources:*

Giasson, M., & Bouchard, L. (1998). Effect of therapeutic touch on the well-being of persons with terminal cancer. *Journal of Holistic Nursing, 16*(3), 383–398.

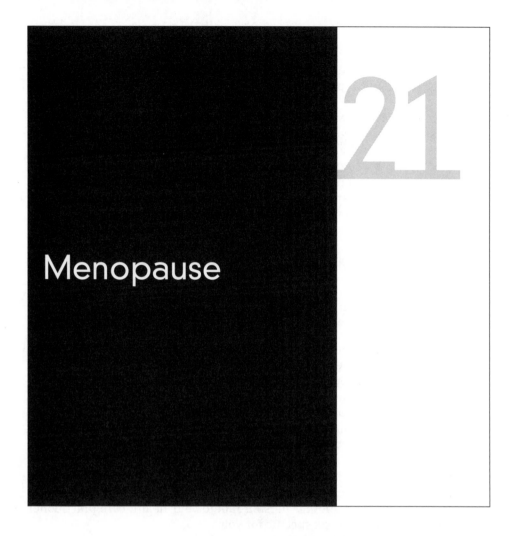

Menopause

21

Menopause is a normal part of the life cycle, not a medical condition. Many complementary approaches exist that can provide relief from the challenges of menopause.

Environment

1. Prempro
   a. *Actions/expected responses:* To prevent breakthrough bleeding in post-menopausal women age 50–69.
   b. *Routes/dosages/frequency:* 0.625 mg daily.
   c. *Cautions:* Compared with placebo, Prempro (or Premarin or Premique) increased the risk of cardiovascular events in older women, including a significantly increased risk of major cardiovascular disease (CVD): venous thromboembolism, unstable angina requiring hospitalization, heart attack, or sudden coronary death. Discontinuing hormones can also lead to an increased risk of breast cancer and heart disease.
   d. *Assessments:* Assess intake of postmenopausal hormones.

e. *Tips on use:* Lifestyle approaches are both safe and effective for CVD risk-factor reduction in postmenopausal women who have discontinued hormone use.

f. *Other considerations:* Decreasing weight (see chapter 25, "Overweight/Obesity"), improving nutrition, and increasing leisure physical activity can decrease risks to the heart.

g. *References/other sources:*

Alper, B. S. (2008, January). Evidence-based medicine: HRT increases risk of cardiovascular disease in older women. *The Clinical Advisor,* 97.

Elsevier Health Sciences. (2007, May 16). Reducing cardiovascular disease risk factors when discontinuing hormone replacement therapy. *ScienceDaily.* Retrieved March 2, 2008, from http://www.sciencedaily.com/releases/2007/05/070515074741.htm

Exercise/Movement

1. Brisk walking

a. *Actions/expected responses:* Women in premenopause and postmenopause who walked regularly every week reduced oxidative stress, thereby improving their sleep status and their perceived mood, including anxiety and depression.

b. *Routes/dosages/frequency:* The most beneficial reactions occurred in women who walked for an hour and a half at least five times a week. Women who walked five times a week for 40 minutes, also benefited, but not as much.

c. *Cautions:* Do warmup first (e.g., swinging arms, doing backstrokes, reaching for the ceiling), then start walking slowly. If walking outside, walk with at least one other person. Never walk faster than you can easily carry on a conversation with another person. Talk to your health care practitioner about any other cautions specific for you.

d. *Assessments:* Assess the level of exercise.

e. *Tips on use:* Wear clothing appropriate for the weather. Layers are preferable so you can take off a sweat shirt or jacket and tie it around your waist as you start to perspire. Wear walking shoes only. After walking, stretch your muscles by slowly reaching over the head, to the side and down toward the toes. Go inside and hold onto a chair if you need support. After perspiration, a shower and change to dry clothing is recommended. Avoid heavy exercise prior to sleep. Yoga and gentle stretches will help with relaxation and prepare for rest.

f. *Other considerations:* It is not necessary to go to the gym. Walking outside on city blocks or in shopping malls can be helpful as long as pollution is low. More frequent walking is associated with improved sleep.

g. *References/other sources:*

Temple University. (2008, January 4). Walk away menopausal anxiety, stress and depression. *ScienceDaily.* Retrieved January 5, 2008, from http://www.sciencedaily.com/releases/2008/01/080103090651.htm

Temple University. (2008, March 20). Reducing heart disease risk naturally post-menopause. *ScienceDaily.* Retrieved March 23, 2008, from http://www.sciencedaily.com/releases/2008/03/080318084333.htm

Wilbur, J., Miller, A. M., McDevitt, J., Wang, E., & Miller, J. (2005). Menopausal status, moderate-intensity walking, and symptoms in midlife women. *Research and Theory in Nursing Practice, 19*(2), 163–180.

2. Resistance training versus hormones for preventing bone loss.
    a. *Actions/expected responses:* Weight lifting (resistance training) alone was as effective as hormones for early postmenopausal women in preventing spinal bone loss.
    b. *Routes/dosages/frequencies:* Two free-weight exercises: hold weights in front of chest with elbows bent and slowly pull hands apart; feel the stretch in upper back and arms; do squats.
    c. *Cautions:* Continue to breathe while lifting weights to prevent increased blood pressure.
    d. *Assessments:* Assess bone mineral density (BMD) of the spine.
    e. *Tips on use:* Go to http://www.bodybuilding.com/fun/south30.htm
    f. *Other considerations:* Start with one-pound weights and build up gradually as strength increases.
    g. *References/other sources:*

Maddalozzo, G. F., Widrick, J. J., Cardinal, B. J., Winters-Stone, K. M., Hoffman, M. A., & Snow, C. M. (2006). The effects of hormone replacement therapy and resistance training on spine bone mineral density in early postmenopausal women. *Bone, 40*(5), 1244–1251.

Herbs/Essential Oils

1. Black cohosh
    a. *Actions/expected responses:* Black cohosh can reduce menopause symptoms as well as conjugated estrogens.
    b. *Routes/dosages/frequency:* Daily oral dose of 40 mg of black cohosh versus 0.6 mg/day of conjugated estrogens.
    c. *Cautions:* Tolerability was good in this study, but transient adverse effects such as slow heart rate, hypotension, uterine stimulation, miscarriage, nausea, vomiting, and anorexia have been noted. Black cohosh should not be used during pregnancy or lactation unless under the supervision of an expert herbalist.
    d. *Assessments:* Assess menopausal complaints prior to and after 4–6 weeks of ingesting black cohosh.
    e. *Tips on use:* Take only standardized products.
    f. *Other considerations:* Structurally, black cohosh more closely resembles estriol, which researchers believe offers protection against cancer of the endometrium, ovaries, and breast.
    g. *References/other sources:*

Geller, S. E., & Studee, I. (2006). Contemporary alternatives to plant estrogens for menopause. *Maturitas, 55*(Suppl 1), S3–S13.

Lupu, R., Mehmi, I., Atlas, E., Tsai, M. S., Pisha, E., Oketch-Rabah, H. A., et al. (2003). Black cohosh, a menopausal remedy, does not have estrogenic activity and does not promote breast cancer cell growth. *International Journal of Oncology, 23*(5), 1407–1412.

Mahady, G. B. (2005). Black cohosh (Actaea/Cimicifuga racemosa): Review of the clinical data for safety and efficacy in menopausal symptoms. *Treatments in Endocrinology, 4*(3), 177–184.

2. Spearmint
   a. *Actions/expected responses:* Spearmint can be an alternative to antiandrogenic treatment for excessive growth of hair.
   b. *Routes/dosages/frequency:* Brew spearmint leaves in hot water for 5 minutes and drink as a tea.
   c. *Cautions:* Women with hiatal hernia or a gallstone attack should avoid spearmint.
   d. *Assessments:* Assess hiatal hernia and gallstone status.
   e. *Tips on use:* Start with a weak tea and evaluate the results.
   f. *Other considerations:* For more information, go to http://www.answers.com/topic/spearmint?cat = technology
   g. *References/other sources:*
      Akdogan, M., Tamer, M. N., Cure, E., Cure, M. C., Koroglu, B. K., & Delibas, N. (2007). Effect of spearmint (Mentha spicata Labiatae) teas on androgen levels in women with hirsutism. *Phytotherapy Research, 21*(5), 444–447.

Mindset

1. Affirmations
   a. *Actions/expected responses:* Self-affirmation of personal values and beliefs buffers neuroendocrine and psychological stress.
   b. *Routes/dosages/frequency:* Repeat aloud or write positive affirmations up to 20 times a day such as, "All cycles and changes are in balance" and "I bless all parts of me with love and joy."
   c. *Cautions:* Insure affirmations are positive and acceptable.
   d. *Assessments:* Assess anxiety prior to and after completing affirmations for a week.
   e. *Tips on use:* Write favorite affirmations on 3 by 5 cards and place them in places where they will be read frequently.
   f. *Other considerations:* Find more affirmations information online at www.successconsciousness.com/index_00000a.htm
   g. *References/other sources:*
      Hay, L. (2000). *Heal your body*. Carlsbad, CA: Hay House.
      Schwarzer, R., Babler, J., Kwiatek, P., Schroder, K., & Zang, J. W. (1997). The assessment of optimistic self-beliefs: Assessment of general perceived self-efficacy in thirteen cultures. *World Psychology, 3*(1–2), 177–190.

Nutrition

1. Red meat
   a. *Actions/expected responses:* Consumption of heme iron from red meat may increase cardiovascular health risk among postmenopausal women compared to premenopausal women, especially for women with diabetes.
   b. *Routes/dosages/frequency:* The higher the consumption, the higher the risk.

c. *Cautions:* To eliminate this source of increased risk, substitute other forms of protein.

d. *Assessments:* Assess intake of red meat.

e. *Tips for use:* Go to http://www.armymedicine.army.mil/hc/healthtips/03/meatless.cfm

f. *Other considerations:* Good sources of protein include ocean salmon, mackerel, chunk light tuna, tofu, tempeh, chicken or turkey (without the skin), beans and rice, and vegetables and rice.

g. *References/other sources:*

Qi, L., van Dam, R. M., Rexrode, K., & Hu, F. B. (2007). Heme iron from diet as a risk factor for coronary heart disease in women with type 2 diabetes. *Diabetes Care, 30*(1), 101–106.

2. Soy

a. *Actions/expected responses:* High soy isoflavone intake reduces the risk of cerebral and myocardial infarctions, protects against hypertension, memory loss, hot flashes, and bone fracture, and improves quality of life and sexual scores in postmenopausal women.

b. *Routes/dosages/frequency:* 1/2 cup soy nuts divided into 3–4 portions spaced throughout the day, 1–2 glasses of soy milk, 1 cup cooked soybeans, 1 soy burger or soy cheese to a total of 100 mg isoflavones per day.

c. *Cautions:* Many nonorganic soy beans have been genetically modified (never researched for their long-term effects) and treated with dangerous chemicals so they should be avoided.

d. *Assessments:* Complete a food-frequency questionnaire about eating soy products (burgers, milk, cheese, tempeh, bars, nuts, or drinks) for a week.

e. *Tips on use:* The best sources of soy are organic fermented products like tempeh or miso because they are more easily digested.

f. *Other considerations:* More processed soy products (e.g., burgers) may cause flatulence or bloating. Experiment with forms that work best.

g. *References/other sources:*

File, S. E., Jarrett, N., Fluck, E., Duffy, R., Casey, K., & Wiseman, H. (2001). Eating soya improves human memory. *Psychopharmacology, 157*(4), 430–436.

Kokubo, Y., Iso, H., Ishihara, J., Okada, K., Inoue, M., & Tsugane, S. (2007). Association of dietary intake of soy, beans, and isoflavones with risk of cerebral and myocardial infarctions in Japanese populations: The Japan Public Health Center-based (JPHC) study cohort. *Circulation, 116*(22), 2553–2562.

Welty, F. K., Lee, K. S., Lew, N. S., Nasca, M., & Zhou, J.-R. (2007). The association between soy nut consumption and decreased menopausal symptoms. *Journal of Women's Health, 16*(3), 361–369.

Zhang, X., Shu, X.-O., Honglan, L., Yang, G., Qi, L., Yu-Tang, G., et al. (2005). Prospective cohort study of soy food consumption and risk of bone fracture among post-menopausal women. *Archives of Internal Medicine, 165,* 1890–1895.

3. Vitamin K

a. *Actions/expected responses:* An analysis of 13 clinical trials showed that vitamin K reduces postmenopausal fracture rates.

b. *Routes/dosages/frequency:* Eat daily servings of high vitamin K foods.

c. *Cautions:* Choose organic sources of food whenever possible to avoid pesticide residue and genetically engineered produce, the effects of which are unknown.

d. *Assessments:* Assess the intake of vitamin K-rich foods.

e. *Tips on use:* Good sources of vitamin K include asparagus, blackstrap molasses, broccoli, Brussels sprouts, cabbage, cauliflower, dark green leafy vegetables, egg yolks, liver, oatmeal, soybeans, and wheat.

f. *Other considerations:* None.

g. *References/other sources:*

Alper, B. S. (2007, January). Vitamin K appears to reduce post-menopausal fracture rates: Evidence-based medicine. *The Clinical Advisor,* 127.

Stress Management

1. Cognitive-behavioral group intervention

   a. *Actions/expected responses:* Cognitive-behavioral group interventions resulted in women showing significant improvements in anxiety, depression, partnership relations, sexuality, hot flashes, and cardiac complaints from pre- to postintervention.

   b. *Routes/dosages/frequency:* The women, all suffering from climacteric symptoms, participated in psychoeducation, group discussion, and coping skills training.

   c. *Cautions:* This pilot study points at possible effectiveness. Future studies are needed that use random assignment and a control group.

   d. *Assessments:* Assess level of anxiety, depression, partnership difficulties, sexuality, hot flashes, and cardiac complaints from pre- to postintervention.

   e. *Tips on use:* To turn irrational thinking into rational thought, write down specifics about: (a) a recent interchange between you and one other person that upset you; (b) rational observations of the other person, for example, she is new to the job and under a lot of pressure; (c) irrational ideas, for example, "I can't stand being humiliated in public" and "I'm falling apart"; (d) the main feelings evoked, for example, anger, rage, and humiliation; (e) refuting the irrational ideas, for example, "I'm not really falling apart— it's not pleasant, but I can handle it"; (f) the worst thing that could happen, for example, "I could retaliate and lose my job"; (g) good things that could occur as a result of the incident, for example, "I can learn to deal with difficult situations"; (h) alternate thoughts, for example, "I'm okay and it's okay to feel anger and know I can still function and learn to handle this kind of situation"; and (i) alternate emotions, for example, "I feel less angry now and calmer." For more information see http://www.mind.org.uk/Informa tion/Booklets/Making+sense/MakingSenseCBT.html

   f. *Other considerations:* Keep using the above model with emerging situations, make positive statements about their efforts, and identify ongoing irrational thoughts. Cognitive behavioral therapy has been shown to reduce blood pressure. If necessary, make an appointment to consult with a cognitive-behavioral therapist.

g. *References/other sources:*

Alder, J., Eymann, B. K., Armbruster, U., Decio, R., Gairing, A., Kang, A., & Bitzer, J. (2006). Cognitive-behavioural group intervention for climacteric syndrome. *Psychotherapy and Psychosomatics, 75*(5), 298–303.

Granath, J., Ingvarsson, S., von Thiele, U., & Lundberg, U. (2006). Stress management: A randomized study of cognitive behavioural therapy and yoga. *Cognitive Behavioural Therapy, 35*(1), 3–10.

Supplements

1. Flaxseed
   a. *Actions/expected responses:* Flaxseed can decrease hot flashes by 50% over 6 weeks in postmenopausal women who do not take estrogen.
   b. *Routes/dosages/frequency:* 40 g of crushed flaxseed daily in food or water.
   c. *Cautions:* Fourteen women experienced mild or moderate abdominal distention, eight women experienced mild diarrhea, and one women experienced flatulence.
   d. *Assessments:* Keep a daily hot flash and other symptom diary for 2 months while taking flaxseed.
   e. *Tips on use:* For better digestion, make flaxseed muffins or use the seeds in soups or stews.
   f. *Other considerations:* Flaxseed is as effective as oral estrogen-progesterone to improve mild menopausal symptoms and to lower glucose and insulin levels.
   g. *References/other sources:*

   Lemay, A., Dodin, S., Kadri, N., Jacques, H., & Forest, J. C. (2002). Flaxseed dietary supplement versus hormone replacement therapy in hypercholesterolemic menopausal women. *Obstetrics and Gynecology, 100*(3), 495–504.

   Patade, A., Devareddy, L., Lucas, E. A., Korlagunta, K., Daggy, B. P., & Arjmandi, B. H. (2008). Flaxseed reduces total and LDL cholesterol concentrations in Native American postmenopausal women. *Journal of Womens Health (Larchmt), 17*(3), 355–366.

   Pruthi, S., Thompson, S. L., Novotny, P. J., Barton, D. L., Kottschade, L. A., Tan, A. D., et al. (2007). Pilot evaluation of flaxseed for the management of hot flashes. *Journal of the Society for Integrative Oncology, 5*(3), 106–112.

2. Magnolia extract and magnesium
   a. *Actions/expected responses:* Magnolia bark extract and magnesium showed a significant effect on flushing, nocturnal sweating, palpitations, insomnia, asthenia, anxiety, mood depression, irritability, vaginal dryness and pain on intercourse, and loss of libido as opposed to taking soy isoflavones, lactobacilli, calcium, and vitamin D3.
   b. *Routes/dosages/frequency:* 60 mg of magnolia bark extract and 50 mg of magnesium.
   c. *Cautions:* This combination is safe at recommended dosages, but toxicity can occur at high doses and is contraindicated during pregnancy.

    d. *Assessments:* Assess level of flushing, nocturnal sweating, palpitations, insomnia, asthenia, anxiety, mood depression, irritability, vaginal dryness and pain on intercourse, and loss of libido prior to and after taking magnolia bark and magnesium.

    e. *Tips on use:* Store magnolia extract and magnesium in a cool, dry place away from heat and humidity.

    f. *Other considerations:* Magnolia bark is a popular herb from the Chinese pharmacopoeia. Called Hou Po, it is used for digestive upset and cough, but recent research has focused on anxiety and neurotransmitters.

    g. *References/other sources:*

        Mucci, M., Carraro, C., Mancino, P., Monti, M., Papadia, L. S., Volpini, G., et al. (2006). Soy isoflavones, lactobacilli, magnolia bark extract, vitamin D3 and calcium: Controlled clinical study in menopause. *Minerva Ginecology, 58*(4), 323–334.

        Xu, Q., Yi, L. T., Pan, Y., Wang, X., Li, Y. C., Li, J. M., et al. (2008). Antidepressant-like effects of the mixture of honokiol and magnolol from the barks of Magnolia officinalis in stressed rodents. *Progress in Neuropsychopharmacology and Biological Psychiatry, 32*(3), 715–725.

3. Pomegranate fruit extract

    a. *Actions/expected responses:* Pomegranate shows estrogenic activities and is clinically effective on a depressive state and bone loss in menopausal women.

    b. *Routes/dosages/frequency:* Ingesting 1–2 capsules of pomegranate fruit extract daily.

    c. *Cautions:* Should not be taken by women with hiatal hernia, gallstones, or sensitivity to pomegranate.

    d. *Assessments:* Assess hiatal hernia, gallstones, and sensitivity to pomegranate juice.

    e. *Tips on use:* Keep pomegranate fruit extract in a cool, dry place away from heat and humidity.

    f. *Other considerations:* Go to http://64.233.169.104/search?q=cache:Sx60R jdNpCgJ:www.rimonest.com/doc/faq1.doc+dosage+of+pomegranate+seed +oil&hl=en&ct=clnk&cd=12&gl=us

    g. *References/other sources:*

        Mori-Okamoto, J., Otawara-Homamoto, Y., Yamato, H., & Yoshimura, H. (2004). Pomegranate extract improves a depressive state and bone properties in menopausal syndrome model ovariectomized mice. *Journal of Ethnopharmacology, 92*(1), 93–101.

4. Pycnogenol

    a. *Actions/expected responses:* Pycnogenol improves all menopause symptoms.

    b. *Routes/dosages/frequency:* 200 mg daily.

    c. *Cautions:* No side effects were reported.

    d. *Assessments:* Assess menopause symptoms prior to and after taking pycnogenol.

    e. *Tips on use:* Keep pycnogenol in a cool, dry spot away from heat and humidity.

    f. *Other considerations:* Pycnogenol is French maritime pine bark extract and has also been found to alleviate menstrual pain and reduce hyperactivity.

g. *References/other sources:*

Yang, H. M., Liao, M. F., Zhu, S. Y., Liao, M. N., & Rohdewald, P. (2007). A randomized, double-blind, placebo-controlled trial on the effect of pycnogenol: On the climacteric syndrome in peri-menopausal women. *Acta obstetricia et Gynecologica Scandinavica, 86*(8), 978–985.

Touch

1. Massage with aromatherapy
   a. *Actions/expected responses:* Physical and mental health status of women with menopausal symptoms was significantly improved (using the Kupperman index, the self-rating depression scale, and consultation) after massage with aromatherapy.
   b. *Routes/dosages/frequencies:* Two 30-minute treatments one month apart.
   c. *Cautions:* Work with an experienced aromatherapist.
   d. *Assessment:* Assess menopausal symptoms.
   e. *Tips on use*: Aromatherapy oil kits can be bought and used in a massage. Some kits will even include a massage carrier oil, to which to add the essential oils. Start with a natural oil like jojoba oil or almond oil, or use olive oil as a carrier oil. Add the essential oil(s) and then massage it into the skin.
   f. *Other considerations:* For more directions, go to http://www.aromacures.com/aromacures-articles/aromatherapy-instructions.htm
   g. *References/other sources:*

Murakami, S., Shirota, T., Hayashi, S.,& Ishizuka, B. (2005). Aromatherapy for outpatients with menopausal symptoms in obstetrics and gynecology. *Journal of Alternative and Complementary Medicine, 11*(3), 491–494.

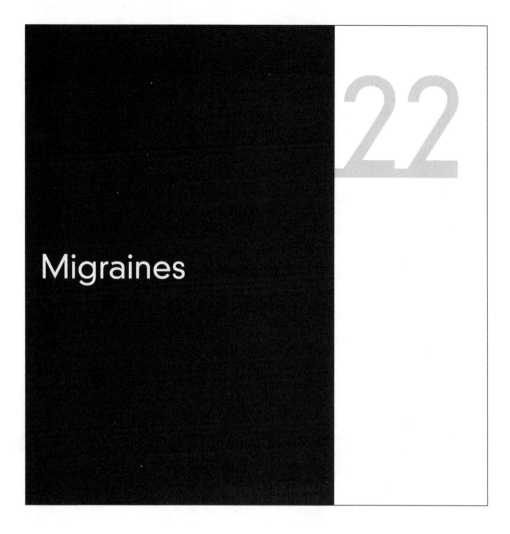

Migraines

22

The medical treatment for migraines includes medications that are usually taken early in the course of a migraine. Complementary treatment includes nutritional, environmental, and stress-related approaches.

Environment

1. Headache diary
   a. *Actions/expected responses:* By keeping a headache diary, women can identify triggers that bring on their migraines.
   b. *Routes/dosages/frequencies:* Write down exact symptoms (visual changes, a funny taste, yawning) that preceded a migraine, when the headache struck (in the morning, after work, after exercise, after a meal, after an argument, on the weekend, etc.), and why they thought it happened (stresses, travel, weather changes.)
   c. *Cautions:* Certain substances (or their lack) may be universal triggers, including alcohol, dehydration, preservatives (nitrates/nitrites, MSG), foods containing tyramine (aged cheese, pickled herring, sour cream, yogurt, yeast extracts, Chianti wine, dried smoked fish), beans, nuts, chocolate,

onions, dairy products, citrus fruits, caffeine (excess or withdrawal), fatty foods, aspartame, sleep deprivation, skipped meals, emotional stress, dental problems, and some medications (such as estrogen therapy, diuretics, asthma medications, nitroglycerin, antihypertensives, analgesic overuse, ergotamines), injury to head or neck, holding in anger, external locus of control (perceiving life events and circumstances as beyond their control), dependence on benzodiazepine anxiolytics to control pain-related anxiety, Lyme disease, thyroid disorders, exertion through sports or sexual activity, invasive diagnostic tests, bright or flickering or fluorescent lights, strong odors, industrial fumes, secondhand smoke, air pollution, perfumes, motion, complex visual patterns, travel, weather changes, fatigue, irregular eating or sleep habits, vitamin or mineral deficiencies, cigarette smoking, stress, and emotional letdown or disappointment.

   d. *Assessments:* Identify migraine triggers.

   e. *Tips on use:* Find lifestyle changes to avoid migraine triggers, including drinking nine cups of noncaffeinated beverages a day, preferably distilled water or water that has passed through a reverse-osmosis filter (http://www.mayoclinic.com/health/water/NU00283).

   f. *Other considerations:* None.

   g. *References/other sources:*

      Arrowsmith, F. M. (2007). Preventing the cycle of migraine: A review of patient issues for NPs. *The American Journal for Nurse Practitioners, 11*(8), 42–54.

      Behavior and psychology are important factors in headache management. (2005). *Neuropsychiatry Reviews, 6*(7), 12–13.

      Mahoney, D. (2004, April). Holding in anger exacerbates headache disability. *Clinical Psychiatry Review, 90.*

Exercise/Movement

1. Yoga

   a. *Actions/expected responses:* Women who participated in yoga experienced a significant reduction in migraine headache frequency and associated clinical features.

   b. *Routes/dosages/frequencies:* Perform 60-minute sessions over a period of 3 months.

   c. *Cautions:* Go to http://yoga.lifetips.com/cat/56770/yoga-cautions/

   d. *Assessments:* None.

   e. *Tips on use:* Because yoga exerts pressure on internal organs, women should wait at least 2 hours after a meal and 30 minutes to 1 hour after a snack to practice. For more information about yoga, go to www.mothernature.com/Library/Bookshelf/Books/21/54.cfm

   f. *Other considerations:* To avoid knee injury when doing yoga, keep the knees straight (especially in standing poses). The knees should be forward in line with the ankle and foot and should not twist inward or outward.

   g. *References/other sources:*

      John, P. J., Sharma, N., Sharma, C. M., & Kankane, A. (2007). Effectiveness of yoga therapy in the treatment of migraine without aura: A randomized controlled trial. *Headache, 47*(5), 654–661.

Herbs/Essential Oils

1. Butterbur
   a. *Actions/expected responses:* Butterbur significantly decreased migraine attack frequency per month by 48% as compared to placebo.
   b. *Routes/dosages/frequencies:* Orally, as an extract of 75 mg.
   c. *Cautions:* The most frequently reported adverse reactions were mild gastrointestinal events, predominantly burping.
   d. *Assessments:* Assess migraine frequency prior to and after taking butterbur.
   e. *Tips on use:* Store butterbur extract in a cool, dry place.
   f. *Other considerations:* Butterbur worked well for women aged 18 to 65 who had at least two to six attacks per month over the preceding 3 months.
   g. *References/other sources:*
   Lipton, R. B., Gobel, H., Einhaupl, K. M., Wilks, K., & Mauskop, A. (2004). Petasites ybridus root (butterbur) is an effective preventive treatment for migraine. *Neurology, 63*(12), 2240–2244.

Mindset

1. Affirmations
   a. *Actions/expected responses:* Self-affirmation of personal values and beliefs buffers neuroendocrine and psychological stress.
   b. *Routes/dosages/frequencies:* Repeat aloud or write positive affirmations up to 20 times a day such as, "Life flows through me with ease" and "Everything in my life is easy and free-flowing."
   c. *Cautions:* Ensure affirmations are positive and acceptable.
   d. *Assessments:* Assess anxiety prior to and after completing affirmations for a week.
   e. *Tips on use:* Write favorite affirmations on 3 by 5 cards and place them where they will be read frequently.
   f. *Other considerations:* Find more affirmations information at www.success consciousness.com/index_00000a.htm
   g. *References/other sources:*
   Hay, L. (2000). *Heal your body.* Carlsbad, CA: Hay House.
   Schwarzer, R., Babler, J., Kwiatek, P., Schroder, K., & Zang, J. W. (1997). The assessment of optimistic self-beliefs: Assessment of general perceived self-efficacy in thirteen cultures. *World Psychology, 3*(1–2), 177–190.

Stress Management

1. Autogenic training
   a. *Actions/expected responses:* Long-term autogenic training proved to be a significantly effective preventive intervention in migraine sufferers.
   b. *Routes/dosages/frequencies:* Every evening, preferably prior to going to sleep.
   c. *Cautions:* Go to http://www.autoaura.com/autogenic.html
   d. *Assessments:* Assess frequency and intensity of migraine headaches prior to and after practicing autogenic training for 6 months.

   e. *Tips on use:* Go to http://www.autoaura.com
   f. *Other considerations:* None.
   g. *References/other sources:*
      Juhasz, G., Zsombok, T., Gonda, X., Nagyne, N., Modosne, E., & Bagdy, G. (2007). Effects of autogenic training on nitroglycerin-induced headaches. *Headaches, 47*(3), 371–383.
2. Cognitive-behavioral therapy and relaxation training
   a. *Actions/expected responses:* Behavioral treatments enable women with recurrent headaches to handle related stress, modify reactions to their condition, and reduce migraine occurrence significantly (approximately 32%–49% as opposed to 5% reduction in a control group). The effects appear to be sustained over time with or without further contacts or booster sessions.
   b. *Routes/dosages/frequencies:* 3–12 or more sessions.
   c. *Cautions:* None.
   d. *Assessments:* Assess migraine frequency prior to and after treatment.
   e. *Tips on use:* For treatment details, go to http://www.migrainepage.com/top ics/relax. html and http://www.mind.org.uk/Information/Booklets/Making +sense/MakingSenseCBT.htm
   f. *Other considerations:* The U.S. Headache Consortium recommended that relaxation training and cognitive behavioral therapy be considered as treatment options for the prevention of migraine.
   g. *References/other sources:*
      Symvoulakis, E. K., Clark, L. V., Dowson, A. J., Jones, R., & Leone, R. (2007). Headache: A suitable case for behavioural treatment in primary care? *British Journal of General Practice, 57*(536), 231–237.

Supplements

1. Coenzyme Q10 (CoQ10)
   a. *Actions/expected responses:* Compared to placebo, CoQ10 was superior for attack-frequency, headache-days, and days-with-nausea.
   b. *Routes/dosages/frequencies:* 100 mg three times a day for 3 months.
   c. *Cautions:* Well-tolerated, but mild gastrointestinal reactions have been reported, including nausea, anorexia, diarrhea, and epigastric pain. CoQ10 may decrease the action of anticoagulants; avoid using concurrently. Drugs that can decrease the action of CoQ10 include beta-blockers, HMG-CoA reductase inhibitors, chlorpromazine, and tricyclic antidepressants.
   d. *Assessments:* Assess migraines prior to and after taking CoQ10 for 3 months.
   e. *Tips on use:* Store CoQ10 in a cool, dry place.
   f. *Other considerations:* CoQ10 may protect against chemotherapy, enhance the effectiveness of blood pressure medications, and reduce the heart-related side effects of a beta-blocker used to treat glaucoma.
   g. *References/other sources:*
      Sandor, E. S., Di Clemente, L., Coppola, G., Saenger, U., Fumal, A., Magis, D., et al. (2005). Efficacy of coenzyme Q10 in migraine prophylaxis: A randomized controlled trial. *Neurology, 64*(4), 713–715.
      Sego, S. (2007, October). Coenzyme Q10. *The Clinical Advisor, 126,* 128.

Touch

1. Massage therapy
   a. *Actions/expected responses:* Compared to control participants, massage participants exhibited greater improvements in migraine frequency and sleep quality during the intervention weeks and the 3 follow-up weeks. Massaging over the greater occipital nerve can reduce the intensity of migraine attacks.
   b. *Routes/dosages/frequencies:* Weekly massage sessions.
   c. *Cautions:* The aged, extremely ill, or dying individuals may require a gentle and brief massage. The head is also a sensitive area; only gentle sweeping motions are used, and energy is not concentrated in that area or in an area where cancer resides.
   d. *Assessments:* Assess migraine frequency and sleep quality prior to and after massage. Keep daily assessments for migraine experiences and sleep patterns.
   e. *Tips on use:* Go to http://www.wikihow.com/Do-a-Hard-Core-Advanced-Therapeutic-Massage
   f. *Other considerations:* None.
   g. *References/other sources:*
   Lawler, S. P., & Cameron, L. D. (2006). A randomized, controlled trial for massage therapy as a treatment for migraine. *Annals of Behavioral Medicine, 32*(1), 50–59.
   Piovesan, E. J., Di Stani, F., Kowacs, P. A., Mulinari, R. A., Radunz, V. H., Utiumi, M., et al. (2007). Massaging over the greater occipital nerve reduces the intensity of migraine attacks: Evidence for inhibitory trigemino-cervical convergence mechanisms. *Arquivos de neuro-psiquiatria, 65*(3A), 599–604.

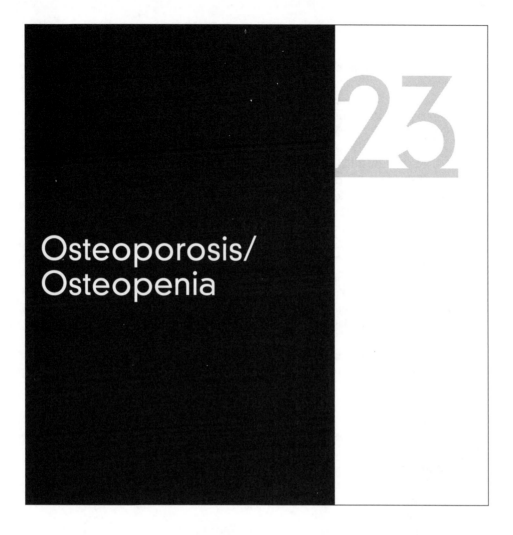

Osteoporosis/ Osteopenia

Medical treatment for osteoporosis/osteopenia includes hormone replacement therapy (which increases the risk of heart attack, cancer, stroke, breast cancer, blood clots, and vaginal bleeding). Biphosphonates, calcitonin, selected estrogen receptor modulators, and raloxifene may also be prescribed. Complementary approaches have been shown to be safe and effective.

Environment

1. Antidepressants
   a. *Actions/expected responses:* Antidepressant use is associated with increased risk of fractures at the spine and sites other than the hip or wrist, and women taking Prozac, Paxil, and Zoloft are more prone to bone loss.
   b. *Routes/dosages/frequencies:* Regular oral use.
   c. *Cautions:* Specific selective serotonin reuptake inhibitors (SSRIs) may increase bone loss in women.
   d. *Assessments:* Assess intake of SSRIs.

e. *Tips on use:* Women taking antidepressants may want to have bone mineral density and fracture assessments regularly.

f. *Other considerations:* None.

g. *References/other sources:*

Oregon Health and Science University. (2007, June 27). Antidepressants linked to bone loss, study suggests. *ScienceDaily.* Retrieved March 29, 2008, from http://www.sciencedaily.com/releases/2007/06/070626115436.htm

Spangler, L., Scholes, D., Brunner, R. L., Robbins, J., Reed, S. D., Newton, K. M., et al. (February 20, 2008). Depressive symptoms, bone loss, and fractures in postmenopausal women. *Journal of General Internal Medicine, 23(2),* 567–574.

2. Dieting

a. *Actions/expected responses:* Women whose diet does not supply enough energy to fuel their exercise level may harm their body's ability to form bone.

b. *Routes/dosages/frequencies:* Thousands of women severely restrict their diet and practice rigorous exercise programs (2 hours a day) for weight control.

c. *Cautions:* Because obvious signs of undernutrition may not be identified by women, they may think they're eating enough.

d. *Assessments:* Assess caloric intake by keeping a food diary for a week.

e. *Tips on use:* Appetite is not a good indicator of how much women should eat.

f. *Other considerations:* Eat enough food to protect the body from bone loss.

g. *References/other sources:*

Ohio University. (2007, June 5). Women up to age 30 at risk for bone loss, study finds. *ScienceDaily.* Retrieved March 29, 2008, from http://www.sciencedaily.com/releases/2007/06/070604123853.htm

3. Low vitamin D

a. *Actions/expected responses:* Women with low levels of vitamin D have a 77% increased risk of hip fracture.

b. *Routes/dosages/frequencies:* Vitamin D is manufactured in the skin after sun exposure and is not available in many foods other than fish liver oil. Vitamin D3 is produced in light-skinned women by 4–10 minutes of exposure of face, arms, or back to the noonday sun, and by 60–80 minutes of exposure for darker-skinned individuals. Women living at latitudes north of 35 degrees or who may not receive exposure to the sun or who are older than 49 years may need to take a tablespoon of cod liver oil daily.

c. *Cautions:* Taking amounts over 100,000 IU of vitamin D per day as a supplement may be toxic: signs of toxicity include anorexia, nausea/vomiting, polyuria, polydipsia, weakness, nervousness, and pruritus. Vitamin D supplements can suppress the proper operation of the immune system.

d. *Assessments:* Assess level of anxiety before and after exposure to sun and/or ingesting cod liver oil.

e. *Tips on use:* Vitamin D2 that is added to so-called fortified foods and many multivitamins and is usually written in prescriptions is inefficiently metabolized in humans; only 20%–40% is metabolized into biologically active vitamin D3.

f. *Other considerations:* Women using corticosteroids may require additional vitamin D.

g. *References/other sources:*

Armstrong, D. J., Meenagh, G. K., Bickle, I., Lee, A. S., Curran, E. S., & Finch, M. B. (2007). Vitamin D deficiency is associated with anxiety and depression in fibromyalgia. *Clinical Rheumatology, 26*(4), 551–554.

Autoimmunity Research Foundation. (2008, January 27). Vitamin D deficiency study raises new questions about disease and supplements. *ScienceDaily.* Retrieved February 13, 2008, from http://www. science daily.com/releases/2008/01/080125223302.htm

Jockers, B. S. (2007). Vitamin D sufficiency: An approach to disease prevention. *The American Journal for Nurse Practitioners, 11*(10), 43–50.

University of Pittsburgh Schools of the Health Sciences. (2007, September 21). Low vitamin D linked to higher risk of hip fracture. *ScienceDaily.* Retrieved March 29, 2008, from http://www.science daily.com/releases/2007/09/070920111402.htm

4. Smoking

a. *Actions/expected responses:* Smoking is linked with osteoporosis.

b. *Routes/dosages/frequencies:* The more women smoke, the more they increase the risk for osteoporosis.

c. *Cautions:* Reduce or eliminate smoking to help prevent osteoporosis.

d. *Assessments:* Assess smoking habits.

e. *Tips on use:* For smoking cessation ideas, go to http://www.helpguide. org/mental/quit_smoking_cessation.htm or http://www.cdc.gov/tobacco/ how2quit.htm

f. *Other considerations:* None.

g. *References/other sources:*

Aran-Arri, E., Gutierrez-Ibarluzea, I, Ecenarro, M. A., & Asua Batarrita, J. (2007). Prevalence of certain osteoporosis-determining habits among post menopausal women in the Basque country, Spain, in 2003. *Revista Espanola de salud publica, 81*(6), 647–656.

Exercise/Movement

1. Exercise

a. *Actions/expected responses:* Weighted exercises can help maintain bone mineral density (BMD) in postmenopausal women and increase BMD of the spine and hip in women with osteopenia and osteoporosis. Women in long-term care institutions are especially at risk for osteoporotic fractures owing to their lack of mobility, poor nutrition, and limited sun exposure. A comprehensive exercise program combined with vitamin D and calcium has been recommended by the Quebec symposium for the treatment of osteoporosis in long-term care institutions.

b. *Routes/dosages/frequencies:* 8–12 repetitions of two to three sets performed over 1 year duration.

   c. *Cautions:* See http://www.sportscoach.34sp.com/modules.php?op=modload &name=News&file=article&sid=469&mode=mode=thread&order =0&thold=0&POSTNUKESID=89638f8531c4c073f25c731ab26a70f7 and http://treadmarkz.wordpress.com/2008/02/16/wheelchair-weightlifting-tips-and-cautions/

   d. *Assessments:* Assess weight lifting knowledge and practice.

   e. *Tips on use:* See http://www.exrx.net/Exercise.html

   f. *Other considerations:* See http://www.exrx.net/WeightTraining/Instruc tions.html

   g. *References/other sources:*

      Duque, G., Mallet, L., Roberts, A., Gingrass, S., Kremer, R., Sainte-Marie, L. G. et al. (2007). To treat or not to treat, that is the question: Proceedings of the Quebec symposium for the treatment of osteoporosis in long-term care institutions. *Journal of Medical Directors Association, 8*(3 Suppl. 2), e67–e73.

      Zehnacker, C. H., & Bemis-Doughtery, A. (2007). Effect of weighted exercises on bone mineral density in post menopausal women: A systematic review. *Journal of Geriatric Physical Therapy, 30*(2), 79–88.

Mindset

  1. Affirmations

    a. *Actions/expected responses:* Self-affirmation of personal values and beliefs buffers neuroendocrine and psychological stress.

    b. *Routes/dosages/frequencies:* Repeat aloud or write positive affirmations up to 20 times a day such as, "Life supports me with love" and "I stand up tall and proud."

    c. *Cautions:* Ensure affirmations are positive and acceptable.

    d. *Assessments:* Assess anxiety prior to and after completing affirmations for a week.

    e. *Tips on use:* Write favorite affirmations on 3 by 5 cards and place them where they will be read frequently.

    f. *Other considerations:* Find more affirmations information at www.suc cessconsciousness.com/index_00000a.htm.

    g. *References/other sources:*

      Hay, L. (2000). *Heal your body.* Carlsbad, CA: Hay House.

      Schwarzer, R., Babler, J., Kwiatek, P., Schroder, K., & Zang, J. W. (1997). The assessment of optimistic self-beliefs: Assessment of general perceived self-efficacy in thirteen cultures. *World Psychology, 3*(1–2), 177–190.

  2. Hypnosis

    a. *Actions/expected responses:* Hypnosis may be capable of enhancing both anatomical and functional fracture healing.

    b. *Routes/dosages/frequencies:* Individual sessions and hypnotic audiotapes designed to augment fracture healing.

    c. *Cautions:* For information, go to http://hypnosisassociates.homestead. com/faq.html

d. *Assessments:* For information, go to http://www.hypnosisandsuggestion. org/measurement.html

e. *Tips on use:* Go to http://www.hypnotics.co.uk/index.htm

f. *Other considerations:* None.

g. *References/other sources:*

Ginandes, C. S., & Rosenthal, D. I. (1999). Using hypnosis to accelerate the healing of bone fractures; a randomized control pilot study. *Alternative Therapies in Health and Medicine, 5*(2), 67–75.

Nutrition

1. Acidic dietary patterns

   a. *Actions/expected responses:* Metabolic acidosis can have a negative effect on bone density. Those with the greatest potential renal acid load (PRAL) had higher intakes of meat, fish, eggs, and cereal and lower intakes of fruit and vegetables. PRAL was inversely associated with bone ultrasound measures in women. Fruits and vegetables provide magnesium, a mineral associated with an alkaline environment that reduces calcium excretion, thereby improving bone density.

   b. *Routes/dosages/frequently:* Daily intake of animal protein versus fruit and vegetables.

   c. *Cautions:* High intakes of meat, fish, eggs, and cereal can lead to reduced bone density.

   d. *Assessments:* Use a food-frequency questionnaire to access potential acid-base load.

   e. *Tips on use:* Eat 1/2 cups of 5–10 fruits and/or vegetables daily.

   f. *Other considerations:* A more acidic dietary intake (high PRAL) was significantly associated with lower calcaneal broadband ultrasound attenuation in women.

   g. *References/other sources:*

   Kitchin, B., & Morgan, S. L. (2007). Not just calcium and vitamin D: Other nutritional considerations in osteoporosis. *Current Rheumatology Reports, 9*(1), 85–92.

   New, S. A., Robins, S. P., Campbell, M. K., Martin, J. C., Garton, M. J., Bolton-Smith, C. et al. (2000). Dietary influences on bone mass and bone metabolism: Further evidence of a positive link between fruit and vegetable consumption and bone health? *American Journal of Clinical Nutrition, 71*(1), 142–151.

   Welch, A. A., Bingham, S. A., Reeve, J., & Khaw, K. T. (2007). More acidic dietary acid-base load is associated with reduced calcaneal broadband ultrasound attenuation in women but not in men: results from the EPIC-Norfolk cohort study. *American Journal of Clinical Nutrition, 85*(4), 1134–1141.

2. Calcium

   a. *Actions/expected responses:* Calcium has been found beneficial for bone health in young adult and menopausal women.

b. *Routes/dosages/frequencies:* Good sources of calcium include salmon with bones, sardines, seafood, cooked green leafy vegetables, broccoli, cabbage, figs, oatmeal, prunes, and low-fat yogurt.

c. *Cautions:* Oxalic acid (found in almonds, beet greens, cashews, chard, cocoa, kale, rhubarb, soybeans, and spinach) can interfere with calcium absorption when used in large amounts. Phytic acid, found in the bran of whole grains, nuts, and the skins of legumes, can bind to calcium to block intake of calcium. A diet high in protein, fat, and/or sugar affects calcium uptake. The average American diet of meats, refined grains, and soft drinks (high in phosphorus) leads to increased excretion of calcium. Consuming alcoholic beverages, coffee, junk foods, excess salt, and/or white flour products also leads to loss of calcium from the body.

d. *Assessments:* Assess intake of calcium-rich foods.

e. *Tips on use:* Eat more calcium-rich foods and decrease foods that lead to increased excretion of calcium, especially in the same meal.

f. *Other considerations:* None.

g. *References/other sources:*

Frasetto, L. A., Morris, R. C., Jr., Sellmety, D. E., & Sebastian, A. (2008). Adverse effects of sodium chloride on bone in the aging human population resulting from habitual consumption of typical American diets. *Journal of Nutrition, 138*(2), 419S–422S.

3. Chocolate

a. *Actions/expected responses:* Chocolate's oxalate content blocks calcium absorption and its sugar content boosts calcium excretion, making a negative impact on women's bone density and strength for total hip, femoral neck, tibia, and heel bones.

b. *Routes/dosages/frequencies:* Greatest risk to bone density and strength is when chocolate is eaten daily.

c. *Cautions:* The more frequently chocolate is eaten, the greater the risk.

d. *Assessments:* Assess chocolate intake.

e. *Tips on use:* Switch to carob; it has a natural sweetness and three times more calcium than milk. For more information on the advantages of carob, go to http://www.wholife.com/issues/10_5/02_article.html

f. *Other considerations:* None.

g. *References/other sources:*

Hodgson, J. M., Devine, A., Burke, V., Dick, I. M., & Prince, R. L. (2008). Chocolate consumption and bone density in older women. *American Journal of Clinical Nutrition, 87*(1), 175–180.

4. Coffee (avoid)

a. *Actions/expected responses:* A high coffee consumption significantly increased the risk of fracture, but tea didn't, probably because of its high level of flavonoids.

b. *Routes/dosages/frequencies:* Drinking four or more cups of coffee a day.

c. *Cautions:* Drinking coffee can increase osteoporotic fracture risk.

d. *Assessments:* Assess coffee intake.

e. *Tips on use:* Reduce or eliminate their coffee intake by drinking half caffeinated and half decaffeinated coffee. Switch to drinking black or green tea, but not the instant form.

f. *Other considerations:* Risk of osteoporotic fractures increased in women with a low intake of calcium. Increase intake of high calcium foods that don't include homocysteine: green leafy vegetables, asparagus, blackstrap molasses, broccoli, cabbage, carob, figs, filberts, oats, prunes, sesame seeds, and tempeh or miso.

g. *References/other sources:*

Hallstrom, H., Wolk, A., Glynne, A., & Michaelsson, K. (2006). Coffee, tea and caffeine consumption in relation to osteoporotic fracture risk in a cohort of Swedish women. *Osteoporosis International, 17*(7), 1055–1064.

Hegarty, V. M., May, H. J., & Khaw, K.-T. (2000). Tea drinking and bone mineral density in older women. *American Journal of Clinical Nutrition, 71*(4), 1003–1007.

Muraki, S., Yamamoto, S., Ishibashi, H., Okra, H., Yoshimura, N., Kawaguchi, H., et al. (2007). Diet and lifestyle associated with increased bone mineral density cross-sectional study of Japanese elderly women at an osteoporosis outpatient clinic. *Journal of Orthopedic Science, 12*(4), 317–320.

Washington University School of Medicine. (2005, January 25). Potentially harmful fluoride levels found in some instant teas. Retrieved March 30, 2008, at http://www.mednews.wustl.edu/news/page/normal/4607.html

5. Colas

a. *Actions/expected responses:* Intake of colas, but not other carbonated soft drinks, is associated with low bone mineral density at each hip site, but not the spine, in women.

b. *Routes/dosages/frequencies:* The mean bone mineral density of those with daily cola intake was 3.7% lower at the femoral neck and 5.4% lower at ward's area than of those who consumed less than one serving of cola a month. Similar results were seen for diet cola, although weaker, for decaffeinated cola.

c. *Cautions:* Drink no colas or noncaffeinated colas to protect their bones.

d. *Assessments:* Assess intake of colas.

e. *Tips on use:* No significant relations between noncola carbonated beverage consumption and bone mineral density were observed.

f. *Other considerations:* Drink water, fruit juices, or teas that don't compromise bone mineral density.

g. *References/other sources:*

Tucker, K. L., Morita, K. I., Qiao, N., Hannan, M. T., Cupples, L. A., & Kiel, D. P. (2006). Colas, but not other carbonated beverages, are associated with low bone mineral density in older women: The Framingham Osteoporosis Study. *The American Journal of Clinical Nutrition, 84*(4), 936–942.

6. Curcumin (turmeric)

a. *Actions/expected responses:* Curcumin elicits unique signaling pathways to orchestrate bioeffects in bone.

b. *Routes/dosages/frequencies:* Curcumin, from the curry spice turmeric, possesses potent antioxidant and anti-inflammatory properties and can be used daily to season salad dressing, baked potatoes, stews, soups, vegetables, meats, fish, and sauces.

c. *Cautions:* The herb is safe in food doses and up to 12 grams a day. In larger quantities it can have strong activity in the common bile duct that might aggravate the passage of gallstones in women currently suffering from the condition.

d. *Assessments:* Assess intake of curcumin.

e. *Tips on use:* Use curcumin as a food spice daily.

f. *Other considerations:* None.

g. *References/other sources:*

Anand, P., Kunnumakkara, A. B., Newman, R. A., & Aggarwal, B. B. (2007). Bioavailability of curcumin: Problems and promises. *Molecular Pharmacology, 4*(6), 807–818.

Jurutka, P. W., Bartik, L., Whitfield, G. K., Mathern, D. R., Barthel, T. K., Gurevich, M., et al. (2007). Vitamin D receptor: Key roles in bone mineral pathophysiology, molecular mechanism of action, and novel nutritional ligands. *Journal of Bone and Mineral Research. 22*(2 Suppl.), V2–10.

7. Homocysteine and vitamin B12

a. *Actions/expected responses:* Older women with high homocysteine (an amino acid produced by the body as a byproduct of consuming meat or drinking five or more cups of coffee) and low vitamin B12 levels have a 70% greater risk of hip fracture.

b. *Routes/dosages/frequencies:* Taking folic acid and vitamin B12 can reduce homocysteine blood levels; homocysteine compromises brain function by damaging the lining of blood vessels in the brain. Vegetarians and vegans (who avoid fish, dairy products, and eggs) are especially at risk for folate deficiency. Folic acid (the synthetic form of folate) is metabolized in the liver, while folate is metabolized in the gut, an easily saturated system. Fortification can lead to significant unmetabolized folic acid entering the blood stream, with the potential to cause a number of health problems. Undigested folic acid accelerates cognitive decline in older women with low vitamin B12 status. For sources of folate, counsel women to go to http://ohioline.osu.edu/hyg-fact/5000/5533.html

c. *Cautions:* Avoid foods fortified with folic acid and eat foods high in folate instead. Drinking five or more cups of coffee a day and eating meat raises homocysteine significantly and should be avoided by women at risk for osteoporosis.

d. *Assessments:* Take a baseline measure for osteoporosis and then take a measure after increasing vitamin B12 and folate.

e. *Tips on use:* Calcium supplementation can improve B12 absorption. Eat foods that provide good sources of vitamin B12 and folate, include them in daily menus, and reduce meat and coffee intake below five cups a day.

f. *Other considerations:* The following medications can lead to B12 deficiencies and a need for more foods high in folate: H2 blockers (such as ranitidine), proton pump inhibitors (e.g., omeprazole), colchicines, zicovudine, nitrous oxide anesthesia, metformin, phenformin, and potassium supplements.

g. *References/other sources:*

Dhonukshe-Rutten, R. A., Pluijm S. M., de Groot, L. C., Lips, P., Smit, J. H., & van Staveren, W. A. (2005). Homocysteine and vitamin B12 status relate to bone turnover markers, broadband ultrasound attenuation, and fractures in healthy elderly people. *Journal of Bone Mineral Research, 20*(6), 921–929.

Herrmann, W. (2006). Significance of hyperhomocysteinemia. *Clinical Laboratory, 52*(7–8), 367–374.

McClean, R. R., Jacques, P. F., Selhub, J., Fredman, L., Tucker, K. L., Samuelson, E. J., et al. (2008). Plasma B vitamins; homocysteine and their relation with bone loss and hip fracture in elderly men and women. *Journal of Clinical Endocrinology, 93*(6), 2206–2212.

Pettit, J. L. (2002). Vitamin B12. *Clinicians Review, 12*(7), 64, 66.

Wright, J., Dainty, J., & Fingles, P. (2007). Folic acid metabolism in human subjects: Potential implications for proposed mandatory folic acid fortification in the UK. *British Journal of Nutrition, 98,* 667–675.

8. Magnesium

a. *Actions/expected responses:* Eating high amounts of magnesium-rich foods can significantly improve bone density.

b. *Routes/dosages/frequencies:* A 10-fold daily increase in magnesium-rich foods.

c. *Cautions:* Choose organic foods whenever possible to avoid untested, genetically modified, and pesticide-laced items.

d. *Assessments:* Assess daily intake of magnesium-rich foods including dry-roasted pumpkin and squash seed kernels, Brazil nuts, halibut, spinach, dry-roasted cashews, cooked soybeans, and pine nuts.

e. *Tips on use:* Use the brands of nuts and seeds that do not contain added oils.

f. *Other considerations:* For more information on magnesium-rich foods, go to www.health.gov/dietaryguidelines/dga2005/document/html/appen dixB.htm

g. *References/other sources:*

Takeda, R., & Nakamura, T. (2008). Effects of high magnesium intake on bone mineral status and lipid metabolism in rats. *Journal of Nutritional Science and Vitaminology, 54*(1), 66–75.

9. Soy, omega-3 fatty acids, and fruit

a. *Actions/expected responses:* Omega-3 long chain fatty acids as in fish oil may be integral to preventing bone loss. When added to fish oil (salmon, sardines, tuna, mackerel, or other cold water fish), soy made vertebrae more resistant to fracture. High fruit intake is associated with higher bone mineral density.

b. *Routes/dosages/frequencies:* A daily diet containing soy, omega-3 fatty acids, and fruit.

c. *Cautions:* None unless women have a high risk of breast cancer, then a discussion with their primary care practitioner about soy use is suggested.

d. *Assessments:* Assess intake of omega-3 foods, fruit, and soy.

e. *Tips on use:* Suggest alternate sources of omega-3 foods and soy. Other sources of omega 3s include 1 cup winter squash, one handful of walnuts, 2 tbsp of olive oil, 1/4 cup beans, and 1–2 tsp of flaxseeds. Sources of soy include 1 cup soy milk, two slices soy cheese or soy meat, 1/4 cup soy nuts, one-third package of tempeh, or 1 cup miso soup.

f. *Other considerations:* None.

g. *References/other sources:*

Ho, S. C., Woo, J., Lam, S., Chen, Y., Sham, A., & Lau, J. (2003). Soy protein consumption and bone mass in early postmenopausal Chinese women. *Osteoporosis International, 14*(10), 835–842.

Ward, W. E., & Fonseca, D. (2007). Soy isoflavones and fatty acids: Effects on bone tissue postovariectomy in mice. *Molecular Nutrition and Food Research, 51*(7), 824–831.

Zalloua, P. A., Hsu, Y. H., Terwedow, H., Zang, T., Wu, D., Tang, G., et al. (2007). Impact of seafood and fruit consumption on bone mineral density. *Maturitas, 56*(11), 1–11.

10. Vitamin K

a. *Actions/expected responses:* Vitamin K reduced bone loss in 12 of 13 trials and was associated with reduced postmenopausal fracture rates in all 7 trials that evaluated this outcome.

b. *Routes/dosages/frequencies:* Daily ingestion of vitamin K-rich foods can strengthen bones. Foods to focus on include asparagus, blackstrap molasses (a tablespoon a day or use in cooking), broccoli, Brussels sprouts, cabbage, cauliflower, green leafy vegetables, egg yolks, liver, and oatmeal.

c. *Cautions:* Coumarin-based anticoagulants adversely affect vertebral bone mineral density and fracture risk.

d. *Assessments:* Assess intake of vitamin K-rich foods.

e. *Tips on use*: Eat more vitamin K-rich foods daily.

f. *Other considerations:* Clinicians should carefully assess women taking anticoagulants for osteoporosis risk, and should monitor bone mineral density.

g. *References/other sources:*

Pearson, D. A. (2007). Bone health and osteoporosis: The role of vitamin K and potential antagonism by anticoagulants. *Nutrition in Clinical Practice, 22*(5), 517–544.

Vitamin K appears to reduce post-menopausal fracture rates. (2007). *The Clinical Advisor,* 127.

Supplements

1. Calcium

a. *Actions/expected responses:* It may be difficult to attain the amount of daily calcium that postmenopausal women require. A supplement may be needed. Women over 50 who take calcium supplements suffer fewer fractures and enjoy a better quality of life. Women in long-term care institutions, where osteoporosis is underdiagnosed and undertreated, are especially at risk for osteoporotic fractures due to their immobility, poor nutrition, and limited sun exposure. These women should receive vitamin D (via sunshine or tablet), calcium, and a comprehensive exercise program.

b. *Routes/dosages/frequencies:* 1,500 mg a day for postmenopausal women, 1,200 mg for younger women.

c. *Cautions:* The results of a meta-analysis showed the importance of starting calcium supplements early in life, at about age 50, when bone mineral loss begins to accelerate.

d. *Assessments:* Assess intake of calcium.

e. *Tips on use:* For the types of calcium that are best to use, go to http://www.doctormurray.com/ask/bestcalcium.asp

f. *Other considerations:* The positive effects of daily calcium and vitamin D supplements have the potential to reduce the risk of fracture in older adults by almost a quarter.

g. *References/other sources:*

Duque, G., Mallet, L., Robers, A., Gingrass, S., Kremer, R., Sainte-Marie L. G., et al. (2007). To treat or not to treat, that is the question: Proceedings of the Quebec symposium for the treatment of osteoporosis in long-term care institutions. *Journal of American Medical Directors Association, 8*(3 Suppl. 2), e67–e73.

The Lancet. (2007, August 25). Calcium supplementation reduces risk of bone fracture and bone loss in older people. *ScienceDaily.* Retrieved May 23, 2008, from http://www.sciencedaily.com/releases/2007/08/070931204908.htm

University of Western Sydney. (2007, August 28). Case for daily calcium pill strengthened. *ScienceDaily.* Retrieved December 24, 2007, from http://www.sciencedaily.com/releases/2007/08/070

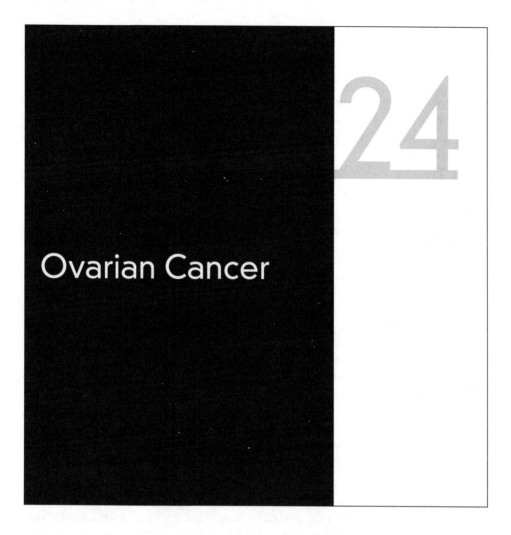

Ovarian Cancer

Treatment for ovarian cancer includes chemotherapy, surgery, radiation, and/or medications, all of which have side effects. Complementary approaches have been shown to be safe and effective with few, if any, side effects.

Environment

1. Computed Tomography (CT) scans
   a. *Actions/expected responses:* CT scans could be responsible for raising the risk of cancer.
   b. *Routes/dosages/frequencies:* A typical CT scan delivers 50 to 100 times more radiation than a conventional X-ray.
   c. *Cautions:* Brenner and Hall (2007) estimate that one-third of all CT scans might not be necessary.
   d. *Assessments:* Assess number of CT scans.
   e. *Tips on use:* Suggest using the safer options of ultrasound and magnetic resonance imaging, which do not expose women to radiation.

    f. *Other considerations:* An estimated 62 million CT scans were performed in 2006 compared to only 3 million in 1980.

    g. *References/other sources:*

        Brenner, D., & Hall, E. J. (2007). Computed tomography, an increasing source of radiation exposure. *New England Journal of Medicine, 357*(22), 2277–2284.

2. Hair dyes

    a. *Actions/expected responses:* Use of hair dyes increases relative risk for ovarian cancer.

    b. *Routes/dosages/frequencies:* Dyes applied to the hair one or more times.

    c. *Cautions:* Women who had ever used hair dye had a relative risk for ovarian cancer.

    d. *Assessments:* Assess women's use of hair dyes.

    e. *Tips on use:* Only one or two studies examined this risk. Further investigation is needed. In the meantime, women can use henna to color and thicken their hair. This herb has none of the possible dangerous effects of hair dye.

    f. *Other considerations:* None.

    g. *References/other sources:*

        Takkouche, B., Etmian, H., & Montes-Martinez, A. (2005). Personal use of hair dyes and risk of cancer. *Journal of the American Medical Association, 293*(20), 2516–2525.

3. Perineal talc

    a. *Actions/expected responses:* Women who dust their perineum with talc-containing powders may have a 50% increase in their risk for ovarian cancer.

    b. *Routes/dosages/frequencies:* Many years of usage of talc.

    c. *Cautions:* Counsel women not to use talc-containing powders.

    d. *Assessments:* Assess use of talc-containing powders.

    e. *Tips on use:* All available data indicate that associations between talc exposure and ovarian cancer have suggested a causal relationship; the application of perineal powder containing cornstarch is not a risk factor for ovarian cancer.

    f. *Other considerations:* None.

    g. *References/other sources:*

        Mills, P. K., Riordan, D. G., Cress, R. D., & Young, H. A. (2004). Perineal talc exposure and epithelial ovarian cancer risk in the Central Valley of California. *International Journal of Cancer, 112*(3), 458–464.

        Salehi, F., Dunfield, L., Phillips, K. P., Krewski, D., & Vanderhyden, B. C. (2008). Risk, factors for ovarian cancer: An overview with emphasis on hormonal factors. *Journal of Toxicology and Environmental Health, 11*(3–4), 301–321.

        Whysner, J., & Mohan, M. (2000). Perineal application of talc and cornstarch powders: Evaluation of ovarian cancer risk. *American Journal of Obstetrics and Gynecology, 182*(3), 720–724.

4. Sunlight

    a. *Actions/expected responses:* A deficiency of vitamin D is linked to increased incidence of ovarian cancer.

    b. *Routes/dosages/frequencies:* For White women, 10–15 minutes of direct midday sun at least twice a week on the face, arms, hands, or back is sufficient, according to the National Institutes of Health. Darker-skinned women may require three to six times as much exposure.

   c. *Cautions:* More frequent exposure could result in skin cancer. Insufficient exposure to the sun can result in improper absorption of calcium and phosphorus, leading to imperfect skeletal formation as well as bone disorders. Vitamin D supplements can suppress the immune system.

   d. *Assessments:* Assess the amount of time women spend in direct sunlight.

   e. *Tips on use:* Help women to develop a plan for obtaining sufficient sunlight, depending on their lifestyle. Eating lunch outside when weather permits could be one solution. In colder climes, women can take a tablespoon of cod liver oil daily, eat fatty fish and fish oils, and egg yolks. Supplements of vitamin D3 (calciferol) may be necessary for certain women.

   f. *Other considerations:* Vitamin D2, found in fortified foods, especially breads and cereals, is poorly metabolized by the body. Certain drugs can interfere with vitamin D metabolism, including corticosteroids, phenytoin, heparin, cimetidine, isoniazid, rifampin, phenobarbital, and primidone. Counsel women to find alternate medications whenever possible so they can metabolize vitamin D3.

   g. *References/other sources:*

     Demgrow, M. (2007, June). High vitamin D: Treatment for cancer prevention? *The Clinical Advisor, 54,* 57.

     Jockers, B. S. (2007). Vitamin D sufficiency: An approach to disease prevention. *The American Journal for Nurse Practitioners, 11*(10), 43–50.

     University of California, San Diego. (2006, November 2). Deficiency in exposure to sunlight linked to ovarian cancer. *ScienceDaily.* Retrieved March 21, 2008, from http://www.sciencedaily.com/releases/2006/11/061102092052.htm

Exercise/Movement

1. Exercise

   a. *Actions/expected responses:* High levels of moderate, recreational exercise is associated with a reduced risk of ovarian cancer. Also, women with jobs that require moderate or strenuous activity experienced a reduction in ovarian cancer risk compared with those who worked in sedentary occupations.

   b. *Routes/dosages/frequencies:* Moderate, but not vigorous, activity is protective.

   c. *Cautions:* Exercise without adequate warming up and cooling down can lead to injury.

   d. *Assessments:* Assess use of exercise, work activity, and inclination to increase movement.

   e. *Tips on use:* For warm-up and cool-down exercises, go to http://www.wellness.ma/adult-fitness/stretching-warmup.htm

   f. *Other considerations:* If women have a job choice, counsel them to choose the more active alternative. Physical activity may decrease ovarian cancer risk by regulating hormone and growth factor levels, and by influencing obesity, which has been shown to increase ovarian cancer risk. Obese women may get more benefit from physical activity against ovarian cancer than will lean women. Regular physical activity also enhances the immune system and the antioxidant defense systems, both of which may help prevent cancer.

g. *References/other sources:*
   Pan, S. Y., Ugnat, A.-M., & Mao, Y. (2005). Physical activity and the risk of ovarian cancer: A case-control study in Canada. *International Journal of Cancer, 117*(2), 300–307.

Herbs/Essential Oils

1. Milk thistle (silymarin)
   a. *Actions/expected responses:* Silymarin, the active substance in milk thistle, stimulates detoxification pathways, inhibits the growth of certain cancer cell lines, exerts direct cytotoxic activity toward certain cancer cell lines, and may increase the efficacy of certain chemotherapy agents. Milk thistle also protects the liver from drug- or alcohol-related injury. Silibinin, a compound of milk thistle, may even prevent the development of liver cancer.
   b. *Routes/dosages/frequencies:* 200 to 400 mg silymarin per day.
   c. *Cautions:* Milk thistle is considered safe and well-tolerated, with gastro-intestinal upset, a mild laxative effect, and rare allergic reaction being the only adverse events reported when taken within the recommended dose range. Counsel pregnant and lactating women or those who are hyper-sensitive (have a known sensitivity to ragweed, marigolds, or chrysanthemums) not to use milk thistle. Avoid taking milk thistle concurrently with antipsychotics, phenytoin, and halothane.
   d. *Assessments:* Assess hypersensitivity to milk thistle.
   e. *Tips on use:* Milk thistle may protect against liver damage from antipsychotics, acetaminophen, phenytoin, and halothane.
   f. *Other considerations:* Preliminary research suggests that silybin may enhance the tumor fighting effects of cisplatin and doxorubicin.
   g. *References/other sources:*
      Bokemeyer, C., Fells, L. M., & Dunn, T. (1996). Silibinin protects against cisplatin-induced nephrotoxicity without compromising cisplatin on isosfamide anti-tumor activity. *British Journal of Cancer, 74,* 2036–2041.
      Lah, J. J., Cui, W., & Hu, K. Q. (2007). Effects and mechanisms of silibinin on human hepatoma cell lines. *World Journal of Gastroenterology, 13*(40), 5299–5305.
      Post-White, J., Ladas, E. J., & Kelly, K. M. (2007). Advances in the use of milk thistle (Silybum marianum). *Integrative Cancer Therapy, 6*(2), 104–109.

Mindset

1. Affirmations
   a. *Actions/expected responses:* Self-affirmation of personal values and beliefs buffers neuroendocrine and psychological stress associated with ovarian cancer.
   b. *Routes/dosages/frequencies:* Repeat aloud or write positive affirmations up to 20 times a day such as, "I balance my creative flow" and "I release whatever it's time to let go of."

c. *Cautions:* Ensure affirmations are positive and acceptable.

d. *Assessments:* Assess anxiety prior to and after completing affirmations for a week.

e. *Tips on use:* Write their favorite affirmations on 3 by 5 cards and place them where they will be read frequently.

f. *Other considerations:* Find more affirmations information at http://www.successconsciousness.com/index_00000a.htm

g. *References/other sources:*

Hay, L. (2000). *Heal your body*. Carlsbad, CA: Hay House.

Schwarzer, R., Babler, J., Kwiatek, P., Schroder, K., & Zang, J. W. (1997). The assessment of optimistic self-beliefs: Assessment of general perceived self-efficacy in thirteen cultures. *World Psychology, 3*(1–2), 177–190.

Nutrition

1. Watercress

a. *Actions/expected responses:* Watercress protects against DNA damage in blood cells, considered an important trigger in cancer development.

b. *Routes/dosages/frequencies:* Eat a bowl of watercress every day for 8 weeks.

c. *Cautions:* None unless sensitive to watercress.

d. *Assessments:* Assess intake of watercress.

e. *Tips on use:* Plasma lutein and beta-carotene increased significantly by 100% and 33%, respectively, after watercress ingestion.

f. *Other considerations:* Watercress can be linked to a reduced risk of cancer via decreased damage to DNA and possible modulation of antioxidant status by increasing carotenoid concentrations.

g. *References/other sources:*

Gill, C. I., Haldar, S., Boyd, L. A., Bennett, R., Whiteford, J., Butler, M., et al. (2007). Watercress supplementation in diet reduces lymphocyte DNA damage and alters blood antioxidant status in healthy adults. *American Journal of Clinical Nutrition, 85*(2), 504–510.

Touch

1. Foot reflexology

a. *Actions/expected responses:* Self-administered foot reflexology can enhance natural killer cells and IgG, strengthening the immune system against cancer and possibly preventing tumor development.

b. *Routes/dosages/frequencies:* Four 40-minute treatments.

c. *Cautions:* None unless the feet have been injured.

d. *Assessments:* Assess knowledge and use of foot self-administered reflexology.

e. *Tips on use:* See http://groups.msn.com/AlternativesToPainandDisease/reflexologyinstructionspg1.msnw and http://groups.msn.com/AlternativesToPainandDisease/reflexologyinstructionspg2.msnw

f. *Other considerations:* Foot reflexology has been shown to significantly improve life satisfaction, the most important predictor of survival for women with advanced cancer.

g. *References/other sources:*

Fox Chase Cancer Center. (2007, November 1). Quality of life is the most important predictor of survival for advanced cancer patients. *Science-Daily.* Retrieved November 12, 2007, from http://www.sciencedaily.com/releases/2007/10/07/071030170208.htm

National Cancer Center. (2006). *Immunity and cancer.* Retrieved February 6, 2008, from http://www.nci.nih.go/cancertopics/understandingcancer/immunesystem/Slide32

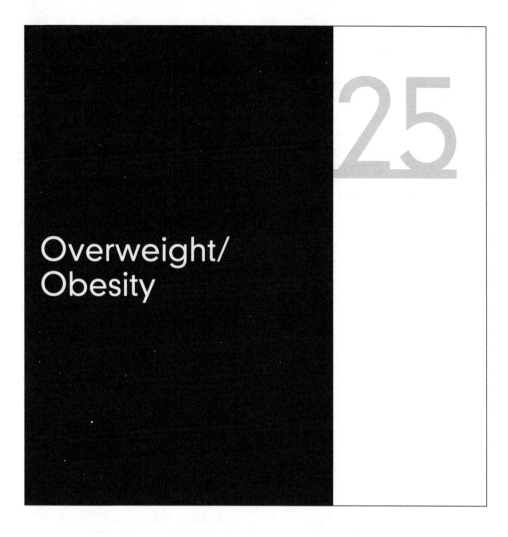

25

Overweight/ Obesity

Although dieting may assist in weight loss, in the long term, it can increase weight. Medical treatment, such as medications and surgery, have negative side effects, while complementary approaches have been shown to be safe and effective.

Environment

1. C-reactive protein (CRP)
    a. *Actions/expected responses:* Studies suggest that CRP is an inflammatory marker that can predict recurrent cardiovascular disease, such as heart attack, stroke and death. Weight loss reduces CRP.
    b. *Routes/dosages/frequencies:* The higher the CRP level, the higher the risk for cardiovascular disease, stroke, and death.
    c. *Cautions:* High CRP levels are associated with low survival rates.
    d. *Assessments:* Assess smoking, weight, blood pressure and sugar intake.
    e. *Tips on use:* Stop smoking, lose weight, and reduce high blood pressure and sugar.

f. *Other considerations:* For information on smoking cessation, go to http://www.helpguide.org/mental/quit_smoking_cessation.htm. For information on cardiovascular risk assessment, go to http://hp2010.nhlbihin.net/at-piii/calculator.asp?usertype=prof.

g. *References/other sources:*

American Heart Association. (2008). *Inflammation, heart disease and stroke: The role of C-reactive protein.* Retrieved August 4, 2008, from http://www.americanheart.org/presenter.jhtml?identifier=4648

Selvin, E., Paynter, N. P., & Erlinger, T. P. (2007). The effect of weight loss on C-reactive protein: A systematic review. *Archives of Internal Medicine, 167*(1), 31–39.

2. Social network

a. *Actions/expected responses:* If a friend becomes obese, friends around them are more apt to become obese.

b. *Routes/dosages/frequencies:* When a person a woman considers a friend becomes obese, the chances of that woman also becoming obese goes up to 57%. Among mutual friends, the effect is even stronger, with chances increasing 171%. Among siblings, if one becomes obese, the likelihood for the other to become obese increases 40%; among spouses, 37% percent.

c. *Cautions:* Distance does not affect weight; a friend who's 500 miles away has just as much impact on a woman's obesity as one who lives next door. People come to think that it is okay to be bigger since those around them are bigger.

d. *Assessments:* Assess family and friends' weight.

e. *Tips on use:* The social network effects extend to a woman's friends' friends' friends. Any intervention should consider the network of a woman's friends.

f. *Other considerations:* When a practitioner helps one woman lose weight, the whole social network could benefit. Not only may obesity be contagious; thinness may be also. Encouraging obese women to find thin friends may be beneficial.

g. *References/other sources:*

University of California—San Diego. (2007, July 26). Obesity is "socially contagious." *ScienceDaily.* Retrieved April 4, 2008, from http://www.sciencedaily.com/releases/2007/07/070725175419.htm

Exercise/Movement

1. Altering fat metabolism and preventing weight gain

a. *Actions/expected responses:* One session of aerobic exercise increases storage of fat in muscle, which improves insulin sensitivity by 25% over their base levels compared to inactivity. Women with increased physical activity can prevent the weight gain associated with aging by at least two times when compared to women who are inactive.

b. *Routes/dosages/frequencies:* 90 minutes at 75% of maximum heart rate. Forty-five minutes on treadmill, followed by 45 minutes on a cycle.

c. *Cautions:* Monitor heart and blood pressure issues.

    d. *Assessments:* Assess exercise levels.

    e. *Tips on use:* Getting a regular dose of exercise may be more important than level of physical fitness.

    f. *Other considerations:* None.

    g. *References/other sources:*

        Kruk, J. (2007). Physical activity in the prevention of the most frequent chronic diseases: An analysis of the recent evidence. *Asian Pacific Journal of Cancer Prevention, 8*(3), 325–338.

        Schenck, S., & Horowitz, J. F. (2007). Dramatic health benefits after just one exercise session. *Journal of Clinical Investigation, 117*(5), 1690–1698. Available online at http://content.jci.org/articles/view/30566

2. Behavioral program results in 100-pound weight loss

    a. *Actions/expected responses:* One in four persons who participated in an intensive weight loss program can go on to lose over 100 pounds.

    b. *Routes/dosages/frequencies:* Intensive 12 week program that included 1,000 to 1,200 calories per day and walking daily.

    c. *Cautions:* Although this program is demanding, it has much lower risks than surgery, which include memory loss and confusion (due to vitamin deficiency) inability to coordinate movement, vomiting, seizures, deafness, psychosis, muscle weakness, and pain or numbness in the feet or hands.

    d. *Assessments:* Assess knowledge of behavioral programs versus weight loss surgery.

    e. *Tips on use:* Evaluate desire to reduce calories and walk daily prior to undertaking such a program.

    f. *Other considerations:* The positive results of the behavioral program went beyond losing 100 pounds. Weight loss was accompanied by improvements in blood pressure, cholesterol levels, diabetes, sleep apnea, and other conditions. Sixty-six percent of participants were able to discontinue medications for high blood lipids, high blood pressure, diabetes, or degenerative joint disease, saving an average of $100 a month.

    g. *References/other sources:*

        American Academy of Neurology. (2007, March 13). Obesity surgery can lead to memory loss, other problems. *ScienceDaily.* Retrieved April 4, 2008, from http://www.sciencedaily.com/releases/2007/03/070312161244.htm

        University of Kentucky. (2007, August 27). 100-pound weight loss possible with behavioral changes. *ScienceDaily.* Retrieved April 2, 2008, from http://www.sciencedaily.com/releases/2007/08/070824180608.htm

3. Dieting without exercise

    a. *Actions/expected responses:* Dieting without exercise causes bone loss.

    b. *Routes/dosages/frequencies:* A 1-year program of calorie restriction, exercise, or no change.

    c. *Cautions:* The diet group lost significant mass in the hip and spine, two common sites of fracture.

    d. *Assessments:* Assess dieting and exercise patterns.

    e. *Tips on use:* Think about risk of bone loss while dieting and not exercising.

    f. *Other considerations:* Combine healthy eating with exercise. For ideas, go to http://www.pueblo.gsa.gov/cic_text/health/fitnexer/fitnexer.htm

   g. *References/other sources:*

     Dieting without exercise causes bone loss. (2007, February). *The Clinical Advisor,* 12.

     Losing weight after pregnancy: Diet and exercise better than diet alone. (2007, July 18). *ScienceDaily.* Retrieved April 9, 2008, from http://www.sciencedaily.com/releases/2007/07/070718002456.htm

4. Focus on health benefits, not appearance

   a. *Actions/expected responses:* Young women reported they enjoyed a step-aerobics class more when the instructor focused on the health-related aspects of the workout, telling them how exercise will make them more fit, as opposed to being told how exercise would tone their legs or other body parts. BMI is not a significant factor in mortality risk, but physical fitness is.

   b. *Routes/dosages/frequencies:* 45-minutes of step aerobics three to four times per week.

   c. *Cautions:* To ward off chronic diseases, all adults should have at least 30 minutes of exercise per day. Anyone with a serious or chronic condition should check with their primary care practitioner.

   d. *Assessments:* Assess preference for exercise focus.

   e. *Tips on use:* Obtain preferred exercise feedback.

   f. *Other considerations:* The presence of mirrors in the exercise room didn't influence how women felt during class.

   g. *References/other sources:*

     Ohio State University. (2007, August 13). Some women benefit more from exercise when emphasis is on health, not appearance. *ScienceDaily.* Retrieved April 5, 2008, from http://www.sciencedaily.com/releases/2007/08/070809125804.htm

5. Splitting up exercise bouts

   a. *Actions/expected responses:* Repeated bouts of exercise burn more fat than one long exercise session.

   b. *Routes/dosages/frequencies:* The American College of Sports Medicine recommends moderate exercise for the duration of 45 to 60 minutes to ensure a sufficient amount of energy is depleted in obese women.

   c. *Cautions:* Go to http://exercise.lifetips.com

   d. *Assessments:* Assess exercise patterns.

   e. *Tips on use:* Break up workout with a 20-minute break after 30-minutes of exercise, followed by another 30 minutes of exercise.

   f. *Other considerations:* To reduce the intimidation of starting an exercise program, walk 15–30 minutes away from home to a friend's house or park, rest for 20 minutes, and then return home. Walking just 30 minutes three times a week can result in a significant reduction in waist and hip girth, overall fitness, and even lowered systolic blood pressure. Other ideas to consider: walk instead of drive, use stairs rather than elevators, and mix aerobic, flexibility, and strength-training exercises to reduce the possibility of being bored.

   g. *References/other sources:*

     American Physiological Society. (2007). *Exercise, exercise, rest, repeat—how a break can help your workout.* Retrieved August 3, 2008, from http://www.the-aps.org/press/journal/07/40.htm

Mindset

1. Affirmations
   a. *Actions/expected responses:* Self-affirmation of personal values and beliefs buffers neuroendocrine and psychological stress. Weight loss is more likely when self-belief in being able to lose weight is high.
   b. *Routes/dosages/frequencies:* Repeat aloud or write positive affirmations up to 20 times a day such as, "I live secure in my spiritual nourishment," "I give myself permission to feel," and "I accept that I am perfect as I am."
   c. *Cautions:* Ensure affirmations are positive and acceptable.
   d. *Assessments:* Assess anxiety prior to and after completing affirmations for a week.
   e. *Tips on use:* Write favorite affirmations on 3 by 5 cards and place them where they will be read frequently.
   f. *Other considerations:* Find more affirmations information at www.success consciousness.com/index_00000a.htm
   g. *References/other sources:*
      Hay, L. (2000). *Heal your body.* Carlsbad, CA: Hay House.
      Queensland University of Technology. (2008, May 2). Weight loss possible when self-belief high. *ScienceDaily.* Retrieved May 12, 2008, from http://www.sciencedaily.com/releases/2008/05/080502082735.htm
      Schwarzer, R., Babler, J., Kwiatek, P., Schroder, K., & Zang, J. W. (1997). The assessment of optimistic self-beliefs: Assessment of general perceived self-efficacy in thirteen cultures. *World Psychology, 3*(1–2), 177–190.
2. Counseling and engagement in weight loss strategies
   a. *Actions/expected responses:* A personal-contact intervention was more effective at preventing or reducing weight regain, but an interactive, Web-based intervention was effective before 30 months.
   b. *Routes/dosages/frequencies:* A personal-contact intervention consisted of monthly person-to-person telephone calls of 5 to 15 minutes and a face-to-face meeting of 45 to 60 minutes every fourth month, without any Internet contact.
   c. *Cautions:* Many behavioral weight loss interventions achieve short-term success, but regain is common.
   d. *Assessments:* Assess need and desire to lose weight. Assess specific types of support needed to continue in a weight loss program.
   e. *Tips on use:* For ideas, go to http://www.thedietchannel.com/General-Dieting-Tips.htm
   f. *Other considerations:* Together overweight and obesity are the second leading cause of preventable death, primarily through effects on cardiovascular disease (CVD) risk factors (hypertension, dyslipidemia, and type 2 diabetes).
   g. *References/other sources:*
      Barclay, L., & Lie, D. (2008). *Behavioral intervention may help overweight, obese patients lose and maintain weight.* Retrieved April 5, 2008, from www.medscape.com/viewarticle/571544
3. Denial about children's weight problems
   a. *Actions/expected responses:* Parents often underestimate their children's weight more often than the children do themselves. Those who

underreported weight were more likely to report a poor diet and exercise than those who correctly reported their weight status.

b. *Routes/dosages/frequencies:* While 87% of the children surveyed were obese according to the most recent Centers for Disease Control and Prevention (CDC) standards, only 41% of parents, and 35% of the children, reported themselves "very overweight." Among parents who reported their child's weight as "about right," 40% had children who actually were at or over the 95th percentile for weight and were considered obese by government standards. Girls were more likely than boys to underestimate their weight.

c. *Cautions:* It may be a challenge to treat obesity if many of the parents of overweight or obese children may not even recognize the problem.

d. *Assessments:* Assess overweight and obesity in families.

e. *Tips on use:* Work on shared communication, using more clear language, goal setting with family members about key behavior changes, identifying barriers to change, and setting realistic goals.

f. *Other considerations:* Obtaining information about the definition of overweight and obesity, evaluating themselves and their family members based on these definitions, and setting reasonable goals for weight loss may be a start.

g. *References/other sources:*

Vanderbilt Medical Center. (2008, March 5). Parents in denial about their children's weight problems, study finds. *ScienceDaily.* Retrieved March 9, 2008, from http://www.sciencedaily.com/releases/2008/03/080304173130.htm

Nutrition

1. Cherries

a. *Actions/expected responses:* Tart cherries may help lose weight.

b. *Routes/dosages/frequencies:* 1.5 cups a day of tart cherries or dried and mixed into a food.

c. *Cautions:* These findings are based on animal studies, but a human trial is underway.

d. *Assessments:* Assess amount of tart cherries consumed.

e. *Tips on use:* For a tasty breakfast, mix 1.5 cups of dried cherries with 1–2 cups lowfat or nonfat plain yogurt, 1 packet of stevia, and 1 banana. Place in blender and blend to preferred consistency.

f. *Other considerations:* None.

g. *References/other sources:*

University of Michigan Health System. (2008, April 10). Tart cherries may reduce factors associated with heart disease and diabetes. *ScienceDaily.* Retrieved April 20, 2008, from http://www.sciencedaily.com/releases/2008/04/080407114647.htm

2. Cinnamon

a. *Actions/expected responses:* Cinnamon slows digestion and steadies blood sugar, reducing the tendency to overeat.

b. *Routes/dosages/frequencies:* 2 1/2 tsp of cinnamon in a bowl of oatmeal or rice can lower blood glucose levels by half.

c. *Cautions:* Until more research is conducted, avoid during pregnancy and lactation in large doses. Can be used safely as a spice.

d. *Assessments:* Assess use of cinnamon and hypersensitivity, including wheezing or rash.

e. *Tips on use:* Store cinnamon in a cool, dry place.

f. *Other considerations:* Sprinkle cinnamon on oatmeal, rice, pears and try it on other foods such as stews, prunes, cereals, plain yogurt and soups.

g. *References/other sources:*

Hlebowicz, J., Darwiche, G., Bjorgell, O., & Almer, L. O. (2007). Effect of cinnamon on postprandial blood glucose, gastric emptying, and satiety in healthy subjects. *American Journal of Clinical Nutrition, 85*(6), 1552–1556.

Skidmore-Roth, L. (2006). Cinnamon. In *Mosby's handbook of herbs and natural supplements* (pp. 302–305). St. Louis, MO: ElsevierMosby.

3. Dairy products and calcium supplements

a. *Actions/expected responses:* Although advertisements claim dairy products and calcium intake promotes weight loss, evidence from 49 clinical trials found no association between calcium or dairy intake and weight loss except in observational studies. In these cases, weight loss may be attributable to other factors, such as exercise, decreased soda intake, lifestyle habits, or increased fiber, fruit, and vegetable intake. In some studies, increasing dairy products increased weight gain.

b. *Routes/dosages/frequencies:* Daily ingestion of dairy foods.

c. *Cautions:* Avoid expecting to lose weight chiefly by eating dairy products.

d. *Assessments:* Evaluate eating dairy foods to lose weight.

e. *Tips on use:* When dairy foods are eaten, eat non-fat or low-fat varieties.

f. *Other considerations:* Avoid using advertisements as a source of health information.

g. *References/other sources:*

Advertisements saying dairy products help you lose weight are misleading, study shows. (2008, May 2). *ScienceDaily.* Retrieved May 14, 2008, from http://www.sciencedaily.com/releases/200805/080502104547.htm

4. Fat and fiber intake

a. *Actions/expected responses:* Decreased fat intake and increased fruit/vegetable/fiber intake is associated with reductions in body mass index (BMI).

b. *Routes/dosages/frequencies:* Daily ingestion of 5–10 fruits or vegetables and a bowl or more of high fiber cereal.

c. *Cautions:* High fiber intake can reduce absorption of valuable minerals.

d. *Assessments:* Assess intake of fiber.

e. *Tips on Use:* A multimineral tablet may need to be taken between high-fiber food meals to ensure that sufficient amounts of zinc, copper, and magnesium are ingested.

f. *Other considerations:* To increase fiber and satiety, add blueberries or strawberries to cereal, mango or peach slices on a slice of bread smothered with peanut butter, or broth-based soup and leafy green salad prior to meal.

g. *References/other sources:*

Knudsen, E., Sandstrom, B., & Solgaard, P. (1996). Zinc, copper and magnesium absorption from a fibre-rich diet. *Journal of Trace Elementary Medical Biology, 10*(2), 68–76.

Linde, J. A., Utter, J., Jeffery, R. W., Sherwood, N. E., Pronk, N. P., & Boyle, R. G. (2006). Specific food intake, fat and fiber intake, and behavioral correlates of BMI among overweight and obese members of a managed care organization. *International Journal of Behavior Nutrition and Physical Activity, 3,* 42.

5. Fructose

a. *Actions/expected responses:* Eating too much fructose causes uric acid levels to spike, blocking the ability of insulin to regulate how body cells use and store sugar and other nutrients for energy, leading to obesity.

b. *Routes/dosages/frequencies:* Processed foods contain a lot of sugar. Probably the biggest source of fructose is soft drinks. The fructose in an apple is as problematic as the high-fructose corn syrup in soda, but the fruit provides necessary fiber and cancer-fighting antioxidants. Fructose has no healthy nutritional properties.

c. *Cautions:* While one apple may be healthy, eating multiple apples in one sitting could send the body over the fructose edge.

d. *Assessments:* Assess number of servings of fructose in foods prepared with high fructose corn syrup and table sugar, such as pastries, ketchup, fruits, and jellies.

e. *Other considerations:* Women often eat more than one serving of fructose-sweetened foods. Check labels of processed foods including sodas (10 1/2 tsp of sugar per serving), low-fat yogurts with fruit (10 tsp of sugar per serving), Mott's applesauce (5 tsp of sugar), 1 tbsp of ketchup (1 tsp of sugar). Use stevia instead of fructose as a sweetener. Stevia is a natural sweetener that contains no calories, has no side effects, and can prevent DNA damage to cells.

f. *References/other sources:*

Ghanta, S., Banerjee, A., Poddar, A., & Chattopadhyay, S. (2007). Oxidative DNA damage preventive activity and antioxidant potential of Stevia rebaudiana (Bertoni) Bertoni, a natural sweetener. *Journal of Agriculture and Food Chemistry, 55*(26), 10962–10967.

University of Florida. (2007, December 14). Too much fructose could leave dieters sugar shocked. *ScienceDaily.* Retrieved December 23, 2007, from http://www.sciencedaily.com/releases/2007/12/071212201311.htm

6. Magnesium

a. *Actions/expected responses:* Eating high amounts of magnesium-rich foods can impose a significant body weight decline.

b. *Routes/dosages/frequencies:* A 10-fold daily increase in magnesium-rich foods.

c. *Cautions:* Choose organic foods whenever possible to avoid untested, genetically modified, and pesticide-laced items.

d. *Assessments:* Assess daily intake of magnesium-rich foods including dry-roasted pumpkin and squash seed kernels, Brazil nuts, halibut, spinach, dry-roasted cashews, cooked soybeans, and pine nuts.

e. *Tips on use:* Use the brands of nuts and seeds that do not contain added oil.

f. *Other considerations:* For more information on magnesium-rich foods, go to www.health.gov/dietaryguidelines/dga2005/document/html/appen dixB.htm

g. *References/other sources:*

Takeda, R., & Nakamura, T. (2008). Effects of high magnesium intake on bone mineral status and lipid metabolism in rats. *Journal of Nutritional Science and Vitaminology, 54*(1), 66–75.

7. Seaweed alginate and pectin

a. *Actions/expected responses:* Foods containing strong-gelling fibers reduce food intake at dinner by signaling satiety in overweight and obese women with low rigid restraint scores.

b. *Routes/dosages/frequencies:* Alginate-pectin (2.8 grams) ingested twice a day, once before breakfast and once mid-afternoon.

c. *Cautions:* To eliminate the dangers of mineral loss from high-fiber diets, a daily multimineral may be necessary.

d. *Assessments:* Assess interest in trying an alginate-pectin beverage to reduce food intake.

e. *Tips on use:* None.

f. *Other considerations:* Women in the lower 50th percentile of rigid restraint consumed 12% less energy during the day and 22% less for the evening snack in the 2.8-gram condition compared with the control condition.

g. *References/other sources:*

Knudsen, E., Sandstrom, B., & Solgaard, P. (1996). Zinc, copper and magnesium absorption from a fibre-rich diet. *Journal of Trace Elementary Medical Biology, 10*(2), 68–76.

Pelkman, C. L., Navia, J. L., Miller, A. E., & Pohle, R. J. (2007). Novel calcium-gelled, alginate-pectin beverage reduced energy intake in nondieting overweight and obese women: Interactions with dietary restraint status. *American Journal of Clinical Nutrition, 86*(6), 1595–1602.

8. Sesame oil

a. *Actions/expected responses:* Use of only sesame oil for 45 days led to a significant reduction in body weight and body mass index (BMI).

b. *Routes/dosages/frequencies:* Daily use as the only oil for foods and cooking.

c. *Cautions:* Oils are calorie-intensive, so 2 tbsp per day may be sufficient to meet needs for body warmth and organ protection.

d. *Assessments:* Assess use of dietary oils.

e. *Tips on use:* Two types of sesame oil are available; one for cooking and the other for salads and noncooking purposes.

f. *Other considerations:* Even during weight loss, oils are needed. For more information, go to http://www.americanheart.org/presenter.jhtml?identi fier=3045789

g. *References/other sources:*

Sankar, D., Rao, M. R., Sanbandam, G., & Pugalendi, K. V. (2006). Effect of sesame oil on diuretics or B-blockers in the modulation of blood pressure, anthrometry, liquid profile and redox status. *Yale Journal of Biological Medicine, 79*(1), 19–26.

9. Targeted dietary advice

a. *Actions/expected responses:* Targeted dietary advice may be given to obese women to increase the intake of vegetables and fruit that contribute to weight reduction.

    b. *Routes/dosages/frequencies:* Women attending a hospital clinic for sleep-related breathing disorders.

    c. *Cautions:* None unless hypersensitive to specific fruits or vegetables.

    d. *Assessments:* Assess intake of vegetables and fruit using a food frequency questionnaire.

    e. *Tips on use:* None.

    f. *Other considerations:* Eat primarily vegetables. See section on fructose earlier in this chapter.

    g. *References/other sources:*

         Svendsen, M., Blomhoff, R., Holme, I., & Tonstad, S. (2007). The effect of an increased intake of vegetables and fruit on weight loss, blood pressure and antioxidant defense in subjects with sleep related breathing disorders. *European Journal of Clinical Nutrition, 61*(11), 1301–1311.

10. Vegetarian diets

    a. *Actions/expected responses:* Vegetarians diets are effective for weight control.

    b. *Routes/dosages/frequencies:* Women adhered to a lacto-ovo (milk and eggs, but no meat or fish) vegetarian diet for 6 months.

    c. *Cautions:* Vegetarians must eat eggs, sea vegetables (dulse, kelp, kombu, and nori), and soybeans and soy products (especially tempeh and miso, which are more easily digestible), or take a B-complex capsule daily to ensure adequate intake of vitamin B12.

    d. *Assessments:* Assess knowledge of lacto-ovo vegetarian principles.

    e. *Tips on use:* For information on vegetarian eating principles, go to http://www.llu.edu/llu/nutrition/vegguide.html

    f. *Other considerations:* None.

    g. *References/other sources:*

         Burke, L. E., Styn, M. A., Steenkiste, A. R., Music, E., Warziski, M., & Choo, J. (2006). A randomized clinical trial testing treatment preference and two dietary options in behavioral weight management: Preliminary results of the impact of diet at 6 months—PREFER study. *Obesity, 14*(11), 2007–2011.

Stress Management

1. Binge-eating

    a. *Actions/expected responses:* Binge-eating is often related to stress and low self-esteem. In a study comparing self-help/bibliotherapy, interpersonal therapy, and behavior weight loss, interpersonal therapy was superior to the two other treatment options. Women with high negative affect (as measured by the Beck Depression Inventory), were more likely to do poorly when the behavioral weight loss approach was used.

    b. *Routes/dosages/frequencies:* 20- to 60-minute therapy sessions over a 24-week period; those in the guided self-help group read *Overcoming Binge Eating* by Fairburn.

    c. *Cautions:* Dieting can also lead to bingeing and weight gain; restricting foods can lead to bouts of overeating; these repeated cycles lead to weight gain.

d. *Assessments:* Assess negative affect and interest in using one of the three methods for weight loss.

e. *Tips on use:* For information on interpersonal therapy, go to http://psych services.psychiatryonline.org/cgi/content/full/51/6/825-a. For information on behavioral weight loss therapy, go to http://www.nhlbi.nih.gov/guide lines/obesity/e_txtbk/txgd/4323.htm. For information on bibliotherapy, go to http://findarticles.com/p/articles/mi_qa4117/is_200312/ai_n9306083

f. *Other considerations:* For a depression self-assement go to http://www. revolutionhealth.com/conditions/mental-behavioral-health/depression/ self-assessment/index?s_kwcid=ContentNetwork|1019680884

g. *References/other sources:*
Fairburn, C. G. (1995). Overcoming binge eating. New York: Guilford Press.
Finn, R. (2003, December). Dieting results in bingeing, weight gain. *Clinical Psychiatry News,* 22.
Lovinger, S. P. (2007, March). Large study of binge-eating disorder is a first. *Clinical Psychiatry News,* 41.

Supplements

1. Pomegranate leaf extract
   a. *Actions/expected responses:* Pomegranate leaf extract can inhibit the development of obesity.
   b. *Routes/dosages/frequencies:* Standardized to 250 mg and one capsule taken daily.
   c. *Cautions:* Avoid during first trimester of pregnancy and when sensitive to pomegranate.
   d. *Assessments:* Assess sensitivity to pomegranate and pregnancy status.
   e. *Tips on use:* None.
   f. *Other considerations:* For more information, go to http://64.233.169.104/ search?q=cache:Sx60RjdNpCgJ:www.rimonest.com/doc/faq1.doc+dosag e+of+pomegranate+seed+oil&hl=en&ct=clnk&cd=12&gl=us
   g. *References/other sources:*
   Lei, F., Zhang, X. N., Wang, W., Xing, D. M., Xie, W. D., Su, H., et al. (2007). Evidence of anti-obesity effects of the pomegranate leaf extract in high-fat diet induced obese mice. *International Journal of Obesity,* *31*(6), 1023–1029.

2. Vinegar
   a. *Actions/expected responses:* Fermented and pickled products reduce postprandial responses and increase the subjective rating of satiety. The rating of satiety is directly related to the acetic acid level.
   b. *Routes/dosages/frequencies:* Daily eating of fermented and pickled products containing acetic acid (vinegar).
   c. *Cautions:* None unless hypersensitive to vinegar.
   d. *Assessments:* Assess use of vinegar, pickles, and other pickled and fermented products containing acetic acid.
   e. *Tips on use:* Ingest pickled and fermented products containing acetic acid.
   f. *Other considerations:* The highest level of vinegar significantly lowers the blood glucose response at 30 and 45 minutes, the insulin responses at 15

and 30 minutes, as well as increases the satiety score at 30, 90, and 120 minutes after meals.

g. *References/other sources:*

Ostman, E., Granfeldt, Y., Persson, L., & Bjorck, I. (2005). Vinegar supplementation lowers glucose and insulin responses and increases satiety after a bread meal in healthy subjects. *European Journal of Clinical Nutrition, 59*(9), 983–988.

3. Water

a. *Actions/expected responses:* Drinking two glasses of water increases metabolic rate by 30% and can aid in weight loss regimens.

b. *Routes/dosages/frequencies:* Daily drinking eight cups of water is recommended to augment energy expenditure.

c. *Cautions:* Drink eight cups of water a day to aid in weight loss.

d. *Assessments:* Assess water intake.

e. *Tips on use:* Drink distilled water or water that has passed through a reverse-osmosis filter to protect against unwanted substances.

f. *Other considerations:* Drink two glasses of water prior to meals to to increase metabolic rate and reduce appetite.

g. *References/other sources:*

Boschmann, M., Steiniger, J., Hille, U., Tank, J., Adams, F., Sharma, A. M., et al. (2003). Water-inducted thermogenesis. *The Journal of Clinical Endocrinology and Metabolism, 88*(12), 6015–6019.

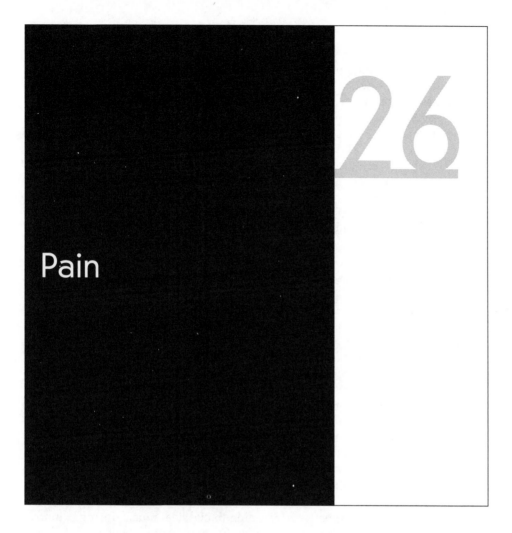

Pain

Medications can work well to reduce acute pain, but they do nothing to address the underlying source of discomfort. Chronic pain requires different measures. Complementary approaches have been shown to be helpful with chronic pain and some acute pain.

Environment

1. Floating
   a. *Actions/expected responses:* Relaxation in large, sound- and light-proof tanks with high-salt water-floating is an effective way to alleviate long-term stress-related pain of fibromyalgia and whiplash.
   b. *Routes/dosages/frequencies:* 12 treatments over 7 weeks activates the body's own system for recuperation and healing.
   c. *Cautions:* Fear of water or darkness may preclude treatment.
   d. *Assessments:* Assess fear of water or darkness.
   e. *Tips on use:* To overcome fears of water or darkness, go to http://www.guidetopsychology.com/sysden.htm

f. *Other considerations:* If no tanks are available, consider filling a large bathtub with warm salty water in a quiet environment and wear an eye mask. Make sure to have someone around to check on your reactions.

g. *References/other sources:*

Swedish Research Council. (2007, November 6). Floating effective for stress and pain, research suggests. *ScienceDaily.* Retrieved November 29, 2007, from http://www.sciencedaily.com/releases /2007/11/071105120604.htm

2. Mirror treatment

a. *Actions/expected responses:* When women who had a foot or leg amputated viewed themselves in a mirror, phantom limb pain was reduced, compared to similar women who practiced mental visualization or viewing a covered mirror.

b. *Routes/dosages/frequencies:* 1 month of viewing a reflective image in a mirror.

c. *Cautions:* None.

d. *Assessments:* Assess for phantom limb pain.

e. *Tips on use:* None.

f. *Other considerations:* 100% of the mirror group reported less phantom pain; in the covered mirror group, only 17% reported a pain decrease, and 50% reported worsening pain; in the mental visualization group, 67% reported worsening pain.

g. *References/other sources:*

Uniformed Services University of the Health Sciences. (2007, November 24). Phantom limb pain may be reduced by simple mirror treatment. *ScienceDaily.* Retrieved November 29, 2007, from http://www. sciencedaily.com/releases/2007/11/071123195218.htm

3. Music

a. *Actions/expected responses:* Listening to classical music during colonoscopy helps reduce the need for sedative medications, as well as anxiety, pain, and dissatisfaction during the procedure. Listening to music during a C-clamp procedure after percutaneous coronary interventions reduces heart rate, respiratory rate, and oxygen saturation, and produces a lower pain score than the control group.

b. *Routes/dosages/frequencies:* During the procedure.

c. *Cautions:* None known.

d. *Assessments:* Assess women's preference for classical music.

e. *Tips on use:* None.

f. *Other considerations:* Listening to music is a simple, inexpensive, and effective way to improve comfort during uncomfortable procedures.

g. *References/other sources:*

Chan, M. F., & Kiang, W. (2007). Effects of music on patients undergoing a C-clamp procedure after percutaneous coronary interventions: A randomized controlled trial. *Heart and Lung, 36*(6), 431–439.

Ovayoulu, N., Ucan, O., Pehlivan, S., Pehlivan, Y., Buyukhatipoglu, H., Savas, M. C., et al. (2006). Listening to Turkish classical music decreases patients' anxiety, pain, dissatisfaction and the dose of sedative and analgesic drugs during colonoscopy: A prospective randomized controlled trial. *World Journal of Gastroenterology, 12*(46), 7532–7536.

4. Sitz baths
   a. *Actions/Expected responses:* Women with anal fissures who received sitz baths and psyllium husk (as opposed to no sitz bath and psyllium husk) scored a lower pain score.
   b. *Routes/dosages/frequencies:* Soaking hips and buttocks in a tub containing plain, lukewarm water for 10 minutes once after defecation in the morning and again at bedtime for 4 weeks.
   c. *Cautions:* No serious adverse effects were noted, but two participants from the sitz bath group developed perianal skin rash.
   d. *Assessments:* Assess pain levels and other reactions to sitz baths.
   e. *Other considerations:* Participants in the sitz bath group reported better satisfaction levels than the control group.
   f. *References/other sources:*
      Gupta, P. (2006). Randomized, controlled study comparing sitz-bath and no-sitz-bath treatments in patients with acute anal fissures. *ANZ Journal of Surgery, 76*(8), 718–721.
5. Vitamin D
   a. *Actions/expected responses:* Vitamin D deficiency is linked with pain. Vitamin D deficiency is a major cause of chronic back pain.
   b. *Routes/dosages/frequencies:* Vitamin D3 is produced in light-skinned women by 4–10 minutes of exposure of face, arms or back to the noonday sun, and by 60–80 minutes of exposure for darker-skinned women. Individuals living at latitudes north of 35 degrees or who may not receive exposure to the sun or who are older than 49 years may need to take a tablespoon of cod liver oil daily.
   c. *Cautions:* Taking amounts over 100,000 IU of vitamin D per day as a supplement may be toxic: signs of toxicity include anorexia, nausea/vomiting, polyuria, polydipsia, weakness, nervousness, and pruritus. Vitamin D supplements can also suppress the proper operation of the immune system.
   d. *Assessments:* Assess level of pain before and after exposure to sun and/or ingesting cod liver oil.
   e. *Tips on use:* Vitamin D2 that is added to so-called fortified foods and many multivitamins and is usually written in prescriptions is inefficiently metabolized in humans; only 20%–40% is metabolized into biologically active vitamin D3.
   f. *Other considerations:* Women using corticosteroids may require additional vitamin D.
   g. *References/other sources:*
      Autoimmunity Research Foundation. (2008, January 27). Vitamin D deficiency study raises new questions about disease and supplements. *ScienceDaily.* Retrieved April 2, 2007, from http://www.sciencedaily.com/releases/2008/01/080125223302.htm.
      Denison, N. (2005, Summer). Easing pain with vitamin D. *On Wisconsin,* 39.
      De Torrente de la Jara, G. P., Picoud, A., & Favrat, B. (2004). Musculoskeletal pain in female asylum seekers and hypovitaminosis D3. *British Medical Journal, 329,* 156–157.
      Plotnikoff, G. A., & Quigley, J. M. (2003). Prevalence of severe hypovitaminosis D in patients with persistent, nonspecific musculoskeletal pain. *Mayo Clinic Proceedings, 78,* 1463–1470.

Exercise/Movement

1. Hydrotherapy versus land-based exercise
   a. *Actions/expected responses:* Hydrotherapy was superior to land-based exercise in relieving pain due to osteoarthritis of the knee before and after walking 50 feet.
   b. *Routes/dosages/frequencies:* Participating in exercises for 18 weeks.
   c. *Cautions:* For more information on water- and land-based exercise, go to http://exercise.lifetips.com
   d. *Assessments:* Assess pain using a visual analog scale for pain. For information, go to http://www.nccn.org/patients/patient_gls/_english/_pain/2_assessment.asp
   e. *Tips on use:* Go to http://ergonomics.about.com/od/ergonomicbasics/ss/painscale_6.htm
   f. *Other considerations:* Land-based exercises also increased knee function and reduced pain, but hydrotherapy was superior.
   g. *References/other sources:*
      Silva, L. E., Valim, V., Pessanha, A. P., Oliveira, L. M., Myamoto, S., Jones, A., et al. (2008). Hydrotherapy versus conventional land-based exercise for the management of pain. *Physical Therapy, 88*(1), 12–21.

2. Supervised exercise versus standard treatment
   a. *Actions/expected responses:* Women with low back pain will do better with supervised exercise than with standard treatment.
   b. *Routes/dosages/frequencies:* 1-hour sessions twice a week for an average of 7 weeks.
   c. *Cautions:* It is important to negotiate graded quotas for gradually increasing amounts of exercise.
   d. *Assessments:* Assess knowledge of ergonomics, prevention, and return-to-work, as needed.
   e. *Tips on use:* Downplay the significance of pain for better results. Pain is benign and it is possible to function with pain; injured athletes demonstrate the point.
   f. *Other considerations:* Women who exercised used half the analgesics that the traditional-care group did. Eighty-five percent of the time it is impossible to determine the cause of back pain. Most of the time the pain goes away without treatment.
   g. *References/other sources:*
      Staal, J. B., Hlobil, H., Twisk, J. W. R., Smid, T., Koke, J. A., & van Mechelen, W. (2004). Graded activity for low back pain in occupational health care: A randomized, controlled trial. *Annals of Internal Medicine, 140*(2), 77–84.

3. Tai chi
   a. *Actions/expected responses:* The sun-style 24 forms of tai chi exercise is effective in decreasing pain.
   b. *Routes/dosages/frequencies:* 60 minutes, twice a week for at least 12 weeks.
   c. *Cautions:* Go to http://nccam.nih.gov/health/taichi/#6
   d. *Assessments:* Assess for pregnancy, hernia, and joint problems prior to suggesting women engage in tai chi.
   e. *Tips on use:* Go to http://nccam.nih.gov/health/taichi/

f. *Other considerations:* Tai chi is also effective for decreasing stiffness and fear of falling, and it improves balance, rising time, and knee joint motion.

g. *References/other sources:*

Lee, H. Y., & Lee, K. J. (2008). Effects of tai chi exercise in elderly with knee osteoarthritis. *Taehan Kanho Hakhoe Chi, 38*(1), 11–18.

4. Yoga during pregnancy

a. *Actions/expected responses:* Pregnant women who participated in a yoga program had a shorter duration of the first stage of labor, shorter total time of labor, and higher levels of maternal comfort outcomes.

b. *Routes/dosages/frequencies:* Six 1-hour sessions.

c. *Cautions:* Go to http://yoga.lifetips.com/cat/56770/yoga-cautions

d. *Assessments:* Assess pregnancy status.

e. *Tips on use:* Go to http://www.santosha.com/asanas/asana.html

f. *Other considerations:* No differences were found in newborn Apgar scores at 1 and 5 minutes.

g. *References/other sources:*

Chuntharapat, S., Petpichetchian, W., & Hatthakit, U. (2008). Yoga during pregnancy: Effects on maternal comfort, labor pain and birth outcomes. *Complementary Therapies in Clinical Practice, 14*(2), 105–115.

5. Yoga versus exercise and a self-care book

a. *Actions/expected responses:* Yoga was superior to the book and exercise groups at 12 weeks. No significant differences in symptoms were found between any two groups at 12 weeks; at 26 weeks, the yoga group was superior to the book group for symptom improvement.

b. *Routes/dosages/frequencies:* 12-week session of yoga or conventional therapeutic exercise classes or a self-care book.

c. *Cautions:* Go to http://yoga.lifetips.com/cat/56770/yoga-cautions

d. *Assessments:* Assess for pregnancy, hypertension, and heavy menstrual flow on yoga days.

e. *Tips on use:* Go to http://www.santosha.com/asanas/asana.html

f. *Other considerations:* Women in the yoga group received motivation from an instructor, while the self-care book group did not. Having instructor motivation could have influenced the outcome of this study. If using only a book, engage a significant other to provide motivation, for example, a daily call inquiring about progress, problems, and so forth.

g. *References/other sources:*

Sherman, K. J., Cherkin, D. C., Erro, J., Miglioretti, D. L., & Deyo, R. A. (2005). Comparing yoga, exercise, and a self-care book for chronic low back pain: A randomized, controlled trial. *Annals of Internal Medicine, 143*(12), 849–856.

Herbs/Essential Oils

1. Peppermint oil for intractable postherpetic pain

a. *Actions/expected responses:* Peppermint oil on herpes zoster (shingles) may work better than any offerings from a pain clinic to relieve pain.

b. *Routes/dosages/frequencies:* Two to three drops of essential peppermint oil massaged into the affected skin three to four times a day.

c. *Cautions:* Peppermint oil should not be used on the face, especially near the eyes, mucuous membranes, and abrasions.

d. *Assessments:* Assess for redness or other skin reactions to undiluted oil.

e. *Tips on use:* Dilute peppermint oil in almond oil (1:5 ratio) if any redness occurs at treatment sites. Dilution of essential oil may reduce pain relief. An occasional supplement of full-strength oil is recommended.

f. *Other considerations:* Topical peppermint essential oil produces immediate relief.

g. *References/other sources:*

Davis, S., Harding, L., & Baranowski, A. P. (2002). A novel treatment of post herpetic neuralgia using peppermint oil. *Clinical Journal of Pain, 18*(3), 200–202.

Mindset

1. Affirmations

a. *Actions/expected responses:* Self-affirmation of personal values and beliefs buffers neuroendocrine and psychological stress.

b. *Routes/dosages/frequencies:* Repeat aloud or write positive affirmations up to 20 times a day such as, "I have no need for punishment, only joy," "Life flows easily through me," and "I release the past and live in the joyful present."

c. *Cautions:* Ensure affirmations are positive and acceptable.

d. *Assessments:* Assess anxiety prior to and after completing affirmations for a week.

e. *Tips on use:* Write favorite affirmations on 3 by 5 cards and place them where they will be read frequently.

f. *Other considerations:* Find more affirmations information at http://www.successconsciousness.com/index_00000a.htm

g. *References/other sources:*

Hay, L. (2000). *Heal your body.* Carlsbad, CA: Hay House.

Schwarzer, R., Babler, J., Kwiatek, P., Schroder, K., & Zang, J. W. (1997). The assessment of optimistic self-beliefs: Assessment of general perceived self-efficacy in thirteen cultures. *World Psychology, 3*(1–2), 177–190.

Nutrition

1. Cherry juice

a. *Actions/expected responses:* Pain and strength loss were significantly less in the cherry juice trial (versus placebo) for muscle damage.

b. *Routes/dosages/frequencies:* 12 fluid ounces of cherry juice blend twice a day for 8 consecutive days.

c. *Cautions:* None unless hypersensitive to cherry juice.

d. *Assessments:* Assess pain prior to and after drinking cherry juice.

e. *Tips on use:* None.

f. *Other considerations:* Numerous antioxidant and anti-inflammatory agents have been identified in tart cherries.

g. *References/other sources:*

Connolly, D. A., McHugh, M. P., Padilla-Zakour, O. I., Carlson, L., & Sayres, S. P. (2006). Efficacy of a tart cherry juice blend in preventing the symptoms of muscle damage. *British Journal of Sports Medicine, 40*(8), 679–683.

Stress Management

1. Breathing therapy

   a. *Actions/expected responses:* Women suffering from chronic low back pain improved significantly (over physical therapy) with breath therapy.

   b. *Routes/dosages/frequencies:* 6 to 8 weeks (12 sessions) of breath therapy.

   c. *Cautions:* Breath therapy is safe according to the researcher.

   d. *Assessments:* Assess pain prior to and after breath therapy sessions.

   e. *Tips on use:* Go to http://www.painsupport.co.uk/newsletter/2002win_01 .html

   f. *Other considerations:* Go to http://marks.on.ufanet.ru/PSY/BRE6.HTM

   g. *References/other sources:*

   Mehling, W. E., Hamel, K. A., Acree, M., Byl, N., & Hecht, F. M. (2005). Randomized controlled trial for breath therapy for patients with chronic low-back pain. *Alternative Therapies in Health and Medicine, 11*(4), 44–52.

2. Guided imagery with relaxation

   a. *Actions/expected responses:* Using guided imagery, women disabled by osteoarthritis significantly reduced pain and increased quality of life and mobility.

   b. *Routes/dosages/frequencies:* Using guided imagery with relaxation for 12 weeks.

   c. *Cautions:* Go to http://www.minddisorders.com/Flu-Inv/Guided-imagery-therapy.html

   d. *Assessments:* Assess pain prior to and after using guided imagery and relaxation.

   e. *Tips on use:* Go to http://www.minddisorders.com/Flu-Inv/Guided-imag ery-therapy.html

   f. *Other considerations:* None.

   g. *References/other sources:*

   Baird, C. L., & Sands, L. P. (2006). Effect of guided imagery with relaxation on health-related quality of life in older women with osteoarthritis. *Research in Nursing and Health, 29*(5), 442–451.

3. Hypnotherapy

   a. *Actions/expected responses:* The hypnotherapy group showed significantly lower pain ratings than the control group and reported a significant reduction in pain from baseline for burn participants. A significant reduction in trauma re-experience scores occurred in the hypnotherapy group but not in the control group.

b. *Routes/dosages/frequencies:* Direct and indirect hypnotic suggestions were used to reduce pain and re-experiencing of trauma.

c. *Cautions:* Go to http://www.lifehealinghypnosis.com/health_wellness.php

d. *Assessments:* Quantify pain by asking women to use a self-report numeric rating scale ranging from 0 to 5 prior to and after participating in hypnotherapy.

e. *Tips on use:* Go to http://www.lifehealinghypnosis.com/hypnosis_faq.php

f. *Other considerations:* The number of recalled vivid, troubling events of the trauma in 24-hour intervals was used for rating the re-experiencing of trauma.

g. *References/other sources:*

Jensen, M., & Patterson, D. R. (2006). Hypnotic treatment of chronic pain. *Journal of Behavioral Medicine, 29*(1), 95–124.

Shakibaei, F., Harandi, A. A., Gholamrezaei, A., Samoei, R., & Salehi, P. (2008). Hypnotherapy in management of pain and reexperiencing of trauma in burns. *International Journal of Clinical Experimental Hypnosis, 56*(2), 185–197.

4. Mindfulness-based and cognitive-behavioral stress reduction

a. *Actions/expected responses:* Mindfulness-based stress reduction (MBSR) is more effective in reducing pain than is cognitive-behavioral stress reduction.

b. *Routes/dosages/frequencies:* 8-week course using meditation, gentle yoga, and body scanning exercises to increase mindfulness.

c. *Cautions:* Go to http://www.lifetips.com/cat/56770/yoga-cautions/

d. *Assessments:* Assess pain prior to and after mindfulness meditation practice.

e. *Tips on use:* Go to http://www.stjohn.org/InnerPage.aspx?PageID=1779

f. *Other considerations:* None.

g. *References/other sources:*

Smith, B. W., Shelley, B. M., Dalen, J., Wiggins, K., Tooley, E., & Bernard, J. (2008). A pilot study comparing the effects of mindfulness-based and cognitive-behavioral stress reduction. *Journal of Alternative Complementary Medicine, 14*(3), 251–258.

Supplements

1. Lysine

a. *Actions/expected responses:* Taking lysine can reduce the pain of herpes simplex (both mouth and genital lesions), episiotomy (especially when combined with anti-inflammatory medication), migraine headaches, and painful periods.

b. *Routes/dosages/frequencies:* Women with herpes simplex can take 3,000–9,000 mg per day in divided doses. To prevent recurrences, take 500–1,500 mg a day.

c. *Cautions:* A diet that contains pastries, doughnuts, cookies, and cereals and other simple sugars can make it difficult to absorb lysine. A small study with chicks found elevated cholesterol and/or triglyceride levels when fed with L-lysine. Vegetarians are at special risk for low lysine levels.

d. *Assessments:* Assess for symptoms of lysine deficiency: kidney stones, fatigue, nausea, dizziness, loss of appetite, agitation, bloodshot eyes, slow growth, anemia, and reproductive disorders. Healthy foods rich in lysine include poultry, cod and sardines, nuts, eggs, tofu, chickpeas, and dried beans (black, kidney, etc.).

e. *Tips on use:* Women with cardiovascular conditions should consider increasing dietary sources of lysine (as should vegetarians), and discuss taking lysine with their primary health care practitioner prior to doing so.

f. *Other considerations:* Lysine plays an essential role in the production of carnitine, a nutrient responsible for lowering cholesterol. Lysine also improves the absorption of calcium and may help prevent bone loss associated with osteoporosis.

g. *References/other sources:*

University of Maryland Medical Center Complementary Medicine. (2002). *Lysine.* Retrieved August 4, 2008, from http://www.umm.edu/altmed/articles/lysine-000312.htm

2. Peppermint oil

a. *Actions/expected responses:* Taking enteric-coated peppermint oil for irritable bowel syndrome pain resulted in a 50% reduction of symptoms.

b. *Routes/dosages/frequencies:* Two enteric-coated capsules twice a day for 4 weeks.

c. *Cautions:* Peppermint should not be used by women with hypersensitivity to it or by those with gallbladder inflammation, severe hepatic disease, gastro-esophageal reflux disease, or obstruction of bile ducts. Avoid during pregnancy or lactation.

d. *Assessments:* Assess for hypersensitivity reactions (flushing, rash, headache, heartburn, mucous membrane irritation, itching).

e. *Tips on use:* Store peppermint capsules in a cool, dry place.

f. *Other considerations:* Peppermint oil internally also reduced diarrhea, constipation, feeling of incomplete evacuation, or urgency at defecation.

g. *References/other sources:*

Cappello, G., Spezzaferro, M., Grossi, L., Manzoli, L., & Marzio, L. (2007). Peppermint oil (Mintoil) in the treatment of irritable bowel syndrome: A prospective double blind placebo-controlled randomized trial. *Digestion and Liver Disease, 39*(6), 530–536.

Skidmore-Roth, L. (2006). Peppermint. In *Mosby's handbook of herbs and natural supplements* (pp. 821–825). St. Louis, MO: ElsevierMosby.

Touch

1. Acupressure for dysmenorrhea

a. *Actions/expected responses:* Acupressure to the Sanyinjiao point effectively reduced menstrual pain for 94% of the women treated as compared to the control group (who rested for 20 minutes).

    b. *Routes/dosages/frequencies:* Acupressure to the Sanyinjiao point, above the ankle, for 20 minutes.

    c. *Cautions:* No adverse events reported.

    d. *Assessments:* Assess menstrual pain prior to and after massaging the Sanyinjiao point.

    e. *Tips on use:* Massage the Sanyinjiao point.

    f. *Other considerations:* Acupressure can be an effective, cost-free self-care intervention for relieving menstrual pain. For more information on acupressure, go to http://209.85.207.104/search?q=cache:LgHf2iXhNSkJ: acupuncture.rhizome.net.nz/acupressure/Acupressure.pdf+Sanyinjiao+ acupressure+point&hl=en&ct=clnk&cd=3&gl=us

    g. *References/other sources:*

        Chen, H. M., & Chen, C. H. (2004). Effects of acupressure at the Sanyin-jiao point on primary dysmenorrhoea. *Journal of Advanced Nursing, 48*(4), 380–387.

2. Acupressure for labor pain

    a. *Actions/expected responses:* Acupressure on L14 and BL67 points produced a significant difference (over a light skin stroking and control conversation group) in decreased labor pain.

    b. *Routes/dosages/frequencies:* One parturient treatment.

    c. *Cautions:* Caution should be used in clients vulnerable to psychotic decompensation.

    d. *Assessments:* Assess labor pain prior to and after acupressure.

    e. *Tips on Use:* The Chih-yin point (Bladder 67) is located approximately 1/10" behind the lateral corner of the smallest toe's nail of either foot. The Adjoining Valley (L4) point affects the large intestine, which surrounds a portion of the uterus. It is located in the webbing between the thumb and forefinger; the right spot will be tender to firm pressure.

    f. *References/other sources:*

        Chung, U. L., Kuo, S. C., & Huang, C. L. (2003). Effects of L14 and BL 67 acupressure on labor pain and uterine contractions in the first stage of labor. *Journal of Nursing Research, 11*(4), 251–260.

3. Acupressure for lower back pain

    a. *Actions/expected responses:* Women who received acupoint stimulation followed by acupressure with aromatic lavender oil had 39% greater reduction in pain intensity than a control group.

    b. *Routes/dosages/frequencies:* Eight-session relaxation acupoint stimulation followed by acupressure with lavender oil over a 3-week period.

    c. *Cautions:* No adverse effects were reported.

    d. *Assessments:* Assess pain level prior to and after acupressure.

    e. *Tips on use:* None.

    f. *Other considerations:* The control group received usual care only. The treatment group also showed significantly improved walking time and greater lateral spine flexion range.

    g. *References/other sources:*

        Yip, Y. B., & Tse, S. H. (2004). The effectiveness of relaxation acupoint stimulation and acupressure with aromatic lavender essential oil for non-specific low back pain. *Complementary Therapies in Medicine, 12*(1), 28–37.

4. Acupressure presurgery
   a. *Actions/expected responses:* Acupressure in the prehospital setting effectively reduces pain and anxiety in women with distal radial trauma as compared to sham treatment to the wrong points.
   b. *Routes/dosages/frequencies:* Acupressure was performed at Baihui and Hegu points: GV 20 on the head and L14 on the hand.
   c. *Cautions:* Care must be taken not to harm the injured wrist.
   d. *Assessments:* Assess pain prior to and after applying acupressure.
   e. *Tips on use:* Go to http://www.stressreliefproducts.com/charts/large-chart.htm and http://www.eclecticenergies.com/acupressure/howto.php
   f. *Other considerations:* None.
   g. *References/other sources:*
      Lang, T., Hager, H., Funovits, V., Barker, R., Steinlechner, B., Hoerauf, K., et al. (2007). Prehospital analgesia with acupressure at the Baihui and Hegu points in patients with radial fractures: A prospective, randomized, double-blind trial. *The American Journal of Emergency Medicine, 25*(8), 887–893.

5. Acupressure Relief Brief
   a. *Actions/expected responses:* 90% of women wearing an acupressure garment obtained at least a 25% reduction in menstrual pain severity compared to only 8% of the control group.
   b. *Routes/dosages/frequencies:* Relief Brief is a cotton Lycra panty brief with a fixed number of lower abdominal and lower back latex foam acupads that provide pressure to dysmenorrheal-relieving Chinese acupressure points. The Relief Brief is worn during menstruation.
   c. *Cautions:* None known.
   d. *Assessments:* Assess menstrual pain prior to and after wearing the Relief Brief.
   e. *Tips on use:* None.
   f. *Other considerations:* Pain medication dropped to two pills per day for the Relief Brief group but remained at six pills for the control group. For more information on the Relief Brief, contact Diana.Taylor@nursing.ucsf.edu
   g. *References/other sources:*
      Taylor, D., Miakowski, C., & Kohn, J. (2002). A randomized clinical trial of the effectiveness of an acupressure device (Relief Brief) for managing symptoms of dysmenorrhea. *Journal of Alternative and Complementary Medicine, 8*(3), 357–370.

6. Aromatherapy
   a. *Actions/expected responses:* Topically applied lavender, clary sage, and rose is effective in decreasing menstrual pain (cramps).
   b. *Routes/dosages/frequencies:* Abdominal massage using two drops of lavender, one drop of clary sage and one drop of rose in 5 cc of almond oil.
   c. *Cautions:* Avoid use if hypersensitive to any of the essential oils.
   d. *Assessments:* Assess for hypersensitivity reactions such as contact dermatitis.
   e. *Tips on use:* Store essential oils in a cool, dry place.
   f. *Other considerations:* Lavender, when inhaled, produces a sedative effect.

    g. *References/other sources:*

Han, S. H., Hur, M. H., Buckle, J., Choi, J., & Lee, M. S. (2006). Effect of aromatherapy on symptoms of dysmenorrheal in college students. *Journal of Alternative and Complementary Medicine, 12*(6), 535–541.

7. Healing touch, music, and guided imagery
    a. *Actions/expected responses:* 55% of women treated by healing touch practitioners with more training reported pain relief (with or without music and guided imagery), and showed a statistically significant reduction in sIgA, a measure of stress, as opposed to a control group.
    b. *Routes/dosages/frequencies:* One healing touch treatment in either practitioner office or client's home.
    c. *Cautions:* None known if practiced by an experienced practitioner.
    d. *Assessments:* Assess pain prior to and after healing touch.
    e. *Tips on use:* Go to http://www.healingtouchinternational.org/index.php?option=com_content&task=view&id=2&Itemid=239
    f. *Other considerations:* None.
    g. *References/other sources:*

Wilkinson, D. S., Knox, P. L., Chatman, J. E., Johnson, T. L., Barbour, N., Myles, Y., et al. (2002). The clinical effectiveness of healing touch. *Journal of Alternative and Complementary Medicine, 8*(1), 33–47.

8. Massage for acute postoperative pain
    a. *Actions/expected responses:* Massage therapy improves pain management and postoperative anxiety among women who experience unrelieved postoperative pain.
    b. *Routes/dosages/frequencies:* 20 minutes of back massage every evening for up to 5 postoperative days.
    c. *Cautions:* Go to http://www.mjbovo.com/AltMed/Massage.htm#cautions
    d. *Assessments:* Assess pain prior to and after massage.
    e. *Tips on use:* Health care providers, especially nurses, can reduce pain at the bedside by using massage techniques.
    f. *Other considerations:* Pharmacological interventions alone may not address all of the factors involved in the experience of pain. With pain now being emphasized as the fifth vital sign and with renewed concerns for treatment safety, less dangerous approaches to pain, such as back massage, must be reintegrated into care.
    g. *References/other sources:*

Barclay, L., & Murata, P. (2007). Massage may help relieve acute postoperative pain. *Archives of Surgery, 142,* 1158–1167.

9. Massage for lower back pain
    a. *Actions/expected responses:* Compared to relaxation therapy sessions, massage therapy is more effective in reducing pain, stress hormones, and symptoms associated with chronic lower back pain.
    b. *Routes/dosages/frequencies:* 30-minute sessions, twice a week for 5 weeks.
    c. *Cautions:* Go to http://www.mjbovo.com/AltMed/Massage.htm#cautions
    d. *Assessments:* Assess pain prior to and after massage and/or relaxation therapy sessions.
    e. *Tips on use:* Go to http://www.easyvigour.net.nz/backpain/h_BackMassage.htm
    f. *Other considerations:* None.

g. *References/other sources:*

Hernandez-Reif, M., Field, T., Krasnegor, J., & Theakston, H. (2001). Lower back pain is reduced and range of motion increased after massage therapy. *International Journal of Neuroscience, 106*(3–4), 131–145.

10. Static magnet for dysmenorrhea

a. *Actions/expected responses:* Women who wore a magnet device showed a significant reduction in menstrual pain.

b. *Routes/dosages/frequencies:* Magnet device of 2,700 gauss attached over the pelvic area during the menstrual period.

c. *Cautions:* None reported.

d. *Assessments:* Assess menstrual pain prior to and while wearing the magnet device.

e. *Tips on use:* Assessment is made by telephone before and after random allocation to use of either the static magnet device (2700 gauss) or an identical, weaker magnetic placebo device (140 gauss). Use the McGill Pain and Visual Analogue Scales to rate associated symptoms such as irritability, restriction of usual activities, and painkiller consumption.

f. *Other considerations:* A reduction in irritability symptoms in the magnet group approached statistical significance ($p = 0.056$).

g. *References/other sources:*

Eccles, N. K. (2005). A randomized, double-blinded, placebo-controlled pilot study to investigate the effectiveness of a static magnet to relieve dysmenorrhea. *Journal of Alternative and Complementary Medicine, 11*(4), 681–687.

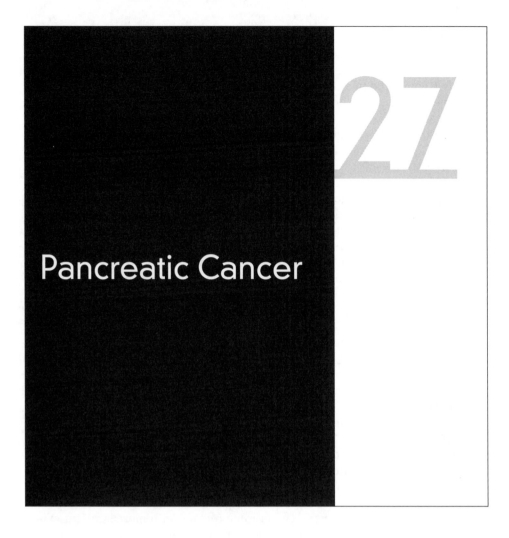

Pancreatic Cancer

Medical treatment for pancreatic cancer includes surgery, chemotherapy, and radiation. All these approaches have negative side effects. Evidence supports the use of complementary approaches, which have been shown to be safe and effective for some women.

Environment

1. Computed Tomography (CT) scans
   a. *Actions/expected responses:* CT scans could be responsible for raising the risk of cancer.
   b. *Routes/dosages/frequencies:* A typical CT scan delivers 50 to 100 times more radiation than a conventional X-ray.
   c. *Cautions:* Brenner and Hall (2007) estimate that one-third of all CT scans might not be necessary.
   d. *Assessments:* Assess number of CT scans.
   e. *Tips on use:* Suggest using the safer options of ultrasound and magnetic resonance imaging, which do not expose women to radiation.

f. *Other considerations:* An estimated 62 million CT scans were performed in 2006 compared to only 3 million in 1980.

g. *References/other sources:*

Brenner, D., & Hall, E. J. (2007). Computed tomography, an increasing source of radiation exposure. *New England Journal of Medicine, 357* (22), 2277–2284.

2. Organochlorines

a. *Actions/expected responses:* Survival of women with high concentrations of persistent organic pollutants in their adipose tissue was significantly less than those with low concentrations.

b. *Routes/dosages/frequencies:* High concentrations of persistent organic pollutants in adipose tissue may reduce survival time from pancreatic cancer.

c. *Cautions:* Organic pollutants include motor vehicle emissions, exposure to petroleum and chemical industries, emissions from waste incinerators and service stations, domestic solid fuel and gas combustion, spray painting, dry-cleaning and other solvent usage, pesticide use, and cigarette smoke.

d. *Assessments:* Assess exposure to organic pollutants.

e. *Tips on use:* Go to http://www.epa.qld.gov.au/environmental_manage ment/air/air_quality_monitoring/air_pollutants/organic_pollutants/

f. *Other considerations:* Counsel women to eliminate sources of organochlorides in their daily life and to lose weight if overweight. See Overweight/ Obesity for ideas.

g. *References/other sources:*

Hardell, L., Carlberg, M., Hardell, K., Bjornfoth, H., Wickbom, G., Ionescu, M., et al. (2007). Decreased survival in pancreatic cancer patients with high concentrations of organochlorines in adipose tissue. *Biomedical Pharmacotherapy,* 61(10), 659–664.

3. Sunlight/vitamin D

a. *Actions/expected responses:* Geographic regions with more sunlight exposure have lower incidences and mortality for cancer. Women who met the U.S. Recommended Daily Allowance of vitamin D (400 IU a day) had a 43% lower risk of pancreatic cancer (see "Other considerations").

b. *Routes/dosages/frequencies:* Vitamin D3 is produced in light-skinned women by 4–10 minutes of exposure of face, arms, or back to the noonday sun, and by 60–80 minutes of exposure for darker-skinned women. Individuals living at latitudes north of 35 degrees or who may not receive exposure to the sun or who are older than 49 years may need to take a tablespoon of cod liver oil daily.

c. *Cautions:* Vitamin D supplements can suppress the proper operation of the immune system (see "Other considerations").

d. *Assessments:* Assess exposure to sun and/or ingestion of cod liver oil.

e. *Tips on use:* Vitamin D2 that is added to so-called fortified foods and many multivitamins and is usually written in prescriptions is inefficiently metabolized in humans; only 20%–40% is metabolized into biologically active vitamin D3.

f. *Other considerations:* Women using corticosteroids may require additional vitamin D. Ingested vitamin D can block VDR (immune system) activation, the opposite effect to that of sunshine, and can be immunosuppressive. Low blood levels of vitamin D may be actually a result of the disease process. Supplementation may make the disease worse.

g. *References/other sources:*

Autoimmunity Research Foundation. (2008, January 27). Vitamin D deficiency study raises new questions about disease and supplements. *ScienceDaily*. Retrieved February 13, 2008, from http://www.sciencedaily.com/releases/2008/01/080125223302.htm

Jockers, B. S. (2007). Vitamin D sufficiency: An approach to disease prevention. *The American Journal for Nurse Practitioners, 11*(10), 43–50.

Skinner, H. G., Michaud, D. S., Giovannucci, E., Willett, W. C., Colditz, G. A., & Fuch, C. S. (2006). Vitamin D intake and the risk for pancreatic cancer in two cohort studies. *Cancer Epidemiology Biomarkers and Prevention, 15,* 1688–1695.

Exercise/Movement

1. Physical inactivity and obesity
   a. *Actions/expected responses:* By virtue of their influence on insulin resistance, obesity and physical inactivity may increase risk of pancreatic cancer.
   b. *Routes/dosages/frequencies:* Obesity significantly increased the risk of pancreatic cancer. Physical activity appears to decrease the risk of pancreatic cancer among those who are overweight.
   c. *Cautions:* Being inactive and overweight may increase risk for pancreatic cancer.
   d. *Assessments:* Assess activity and overweight status.
   e. *Tips on use:* Overweight women should increase their activity level and lose weight to reduce their risk for pancreatic cancer.
   f. *Other considerations:* For exercise tips, go to http://exercise.lifetips.com. For obesity/overweight suggestions, see pages 287–298.
   g. *References/other sources:*

Inoue, M., Tajimi, K., Takezaki, T., Hamajima, N., Hirose, K., Ito, H., et al. (2003). Epidemiology of pancreatic cancer in Japan: A nested case-control study from the Hospital-based Epidemiologic Research Program at Aichi Cancer Center (HERPACC). *International Journal of Epidemiology, 32*(2), 257–262.

Rodriguez, C., Bernstein, L., Chao, A., Thun, M. J., & Calle, E. E. (2005). Obesity, recreational physical activity, and risk of pancreatic cancer in a large U.S. cohort. *Cancer Epidemiological Biomarkers and Prevention, 14*(2), 459–466.

University of Missouri-Columbia. (2008, March 21). Killer stairs? Taking the elevator could be worse for your body. *ScienceDaily*. Retrieved March 25, 2008, from http://www.sciencedaily.com/releases/2008/03/08031812741.htm

Herbs/Essential Oils

1. Aromatherapy foot soak and reflexology
   a. *Actions/expected responses:* Combined modality treatments consisting of aromatherapy foot soak and reflexology appears to be effective for alleviating fatigue in the terminally ill.

   b. *Routes/dosages/frequencies:* Feet are soaked in warm water containing lavender essential oil for 3 minutes, followed by reflexology treatment with jojoba oil containing lavender essential oil for 10 minutes.

   c. *Cautions:* No adverse effects were reported, but to ensure safety, perform a patch test to avoid hypersensitivity to lavender essential oil.

   d. *Assessments:* Assess fatigue prior to and after aromatherapy treatment.

   e. *Tips on use:* Fatigue can be evaluated using the Cancer Fatigue Scale, 1 hour before, 1 hour after, and 4 hours after treatment.

   f. *Other considerations:* None.

   g. *References/other sources:*

       Kohara, H., Miyauchi, T., Suehiro, Y., Ueoka, H., Takeymana, H., & Morita, T. (2004). Combined modality treatment of aromatherapy footsoak and reflexology relieves fatigue in patients with cancer. *Journal of Palliative Medicine, 7*(6), 791–796.

2. Curcumin (turmeric)

   a. *Actions/expected responses:* Curcumin has antiproliferative and antiangiogenic activities that make it therapeutically efficacious for pancreatic cancer. It has been shown to stabilize, reduce tumor size, and provide partial remission in survivors.

   b. *Routes/dosages/frequencies:* 8 grams by mouth daily for 2 months.

   c. *Cautions:* No toxicities were found.

   d. *Assessments:* Assess for hypersensitivity reactions including dermatitis, and monitor coagulant studies for long-term use of the herb.

   e. *Tips on use:* Store curcumin in a cool, dry place. Do not take on an empty stomach. Turmeric/curcumin can be sprinkled on food as a spice. Indian curry is another good source.

   f. *Other considerations:* None.

   g. *References/other sources:*

       Anand, P., Kunnumakkara, A. B., Newman, R. A., & Aggarwal, B. B. (2007). Bioavailability of curcumin: Problems and promises. *Molecular Pharmacology, 4*(6), 807–818.

       Dhillon, N., Wolff, R. A., Abbruzzese, J. L., Hong, D.S., Camacho, H., Li, L., et al. (2006). Phase II clinical trial of curcumin in patients with advanced pancreatic cancer. *Journal of Clinical Oncology, 24*(18S Suppl.), ASCO Annual Meeting Proceedings (Post-Meeting Edition), 14151.

       Novak Kujundzic, R., Grbesa, I., Ivkic, M., Katdare, M., & Gall-Troselj, K. (2008). Curcumin downregulates H19 gene transcription in tumor cells. *Journal of Cell Biochemistry, 104*(5), 1781–1792.

3. Milk thistle (silymarin)

   a. *Actions/expected responses:* Silymarin, the active substance in milk thistle, stimulates detoxification pathways, inhibits the growth of certain cancer cell lines, exerts direct cytotoxic activity toward certain cancer cell lines, and may increase the efficacy of certain chemotherapy agents. Milk thistle also protects the liver from drug or alcohol-related injury. Silibinin, a compound of milk thistle, may even prevent the development of liver cancer.

   b. *Routes/dosages/frequencies:* 200–400 mg silymarin per day.

   c. *Cautions:* Milk thistle is considered safe and well-tolerated, with gastrointestinal upset, a mild laxative effect, and rare allergic reaction being the only adverse events reported when taken within the recommended dose range. Pregnant and lactating women or those who are hypersensitive (have a known sensitivity to ragweed, marigolds, or chrysanthemums) should not use milk thistle. Avoid taking milk thistle concurrently with antipsychotics, phenytoin, and halothane.

d. *Assessments:* Assess hypersensitivity to milk thistle.

e. *Tips on use:* Milk thistle may protect against liver damage from antipsychotics, acetaminophen, phenytoin, and halothane.

f. *Other considerations:* Preliminary research suggests that silybin may enhance the tumor fighting effects of cisplatin and doxorubicin.

g. *References/other sources:*

Bokemeyer, C., Fells, L. M., & Dunn, T. (1996). Silibinin protects against cisplatin-induced nephrotoxicity without compromising cisplatin on isosfamide anti-tumor activity. *British Journal of Cancer, 74,* 2036–2041.

Lah, J. J., Cui, W., & Hu, K. Q. (2007). Effects and mechanisms of silibinin on human hepatoma cell lines. *World Journal of Gastroenterology, 13*(40), 5299–5305.

Post-White, J., Ladas, E. J., & Kelly, K. M. (2007). Advances in the use of milk thistle (Silybum marianum). *Integrative Cancer Therapy, 6*(2), 104–109.

Mindset

1. Affirmations

a. *Actions/expected responses:* Self-affirmation of personal values and beliefs buffers neuroendocrine and psychological stress.

b. *Routes/dosages/frequencies:* Repeat aloud or write positive affirmations up to 20 times a day such as, "My life is sweet," "I love and approve of myself," and "I create sweetness and joy."

c. *Cautions:* Ensure affirmations are positive and acceptable.

d. *Assessments:* Assess anxiety prior to and after completing affirmations for a week.

e. *Tips on use:* Write favorite affirmations on 3 by 5 cards and place them in places where they will be read frequently.

f. *Other considerations:* Find more affirmations information at http://www.successconsciousness.com/index_00000a.htm

g. *References/other sources:*

Hay, L. (2000). *Heal your body.* Carlsbad, CA: Hay House.

Schwarzer, R., Babler, J., Kwiatek, P., Schroder, K., & Zang, J. W. (1997). The assessment of optimistic self-beliefs: Assessment of general perceived self-efficacy in thirteen cultures. *World Psychology, 3*(1–2), 177–190.

Nutrition

1. Flavonols

a. *Actions/expected responses:* A diet rich in flavonols from foods such as onions, apples, and berries may cut the risk of developing pancreatic cancer by about 25%, a multiethnic study reported.

    b. *Routes/dosages/frequencies:* Daily ingestion of kaempferols (spinach and cabbage) are associated with the largest risk reduction (22% across all participants), while quercetin (found in onions and applies) and myricetin (found in red onions and berries) also reduce pancreatic cancer risk.

    c. *Cautions:* None unless sensitive to foods.

    d. *Assessments:* Assess intake of flavonols.

    e. *Tips on use:* Strive for organic, local produce.

    f. *Other considerations:* The advantages for smokers may be even more profound—a risk reduction of 59%.

    g. *References/other sources:*

      Nothings, U., Murphy, S. P., Wilkens, L. R., Henderson, B. E., & Kolonel, L. N. (2007). Flavonols and pancreatic cancer risk—the Multiethnic Cohort Study. *American Journal of Epidemiology, 166*(8), 924–931.

2. Folate

    a. *Actions/expected responses:* Results of a large study found that increased intake of folate from food sources was statistically significantly inversely associated with risk of pancreatic cancer.

    b. *Routes/dosages/frequencies:* Eating folate-rich foods daily may reduce risk for pancreatic cancer.

    c. *Cautions:* Avoid folate-rich foods for which hypersensitivity exists.

    d. *Assessments:* Assess intake of folate-rich foods, especially leafy green vegetables (like spinach and turnip greens), fruits (citrus fruits and juices), and dried beans and peas that can help meet the suggested amount of 1,000 micrograms (mcg) a day. Women on diets who do not eat breads, cereals, or pasta, who abuse alcohol, or who take medications that interfere with folate absorption may not receive sufficient amounts of the nutrient.

    e. *Tips on use:* None.

    f. *Other considerations:* Folate from supplements was not associated with pancreatic cancer protection.

    g. *References/other sources:*

      Larsson, S. C., Hakansson, N., Giovannucci, E., & Wolk, A. (2006). Folate intake and pancreatic cancer incidence: A prospective study of Swedish women and men. *Journal of National Cancer Institute, 98*(6), 407–413.

3. Green tea

    a. *Actions/expected responses:* Green tea is protective against pancreatic cancer before disease occurs and after onset, possibly by creating a detoxifying effect.

    b. *Routes/dosages/frequencies:* Two to five cups of decaffeinated tea daily (1 tsp tea leaves in 8 ounces of hot water).

    c. *Cautions:* May decrease iron absorption, so separate iron-rich foods or iron pills by at least 2 hours from green tea ingestion.

    d. *Assessments:* Assess for hypersensitivity reactions. Also assess for cardiovascular (increased blood pressure, palpitations, and irregular heartbeat), central nervous system (anxiety, nervousness, insomnia), and gastrointestinal (nausea, heartburn, increased stomach acid) reactions.

    e. *Tips on use:* Caffeinated green tea can interact with MAOIs and lead to a hypertensive crisis. Do not take green tea with anticoagulants/antiplatelets (may increase risk of bleeding), beta-adrenergic blockers (can lead to increased inotropic effects), or benzodiazepines (may increase sedation). Store green tea in a cool, dry place.

f. *Other considerations:* Dairy products may decrease the therapeutic effects of green tea, so separate their intake by several hours. Digestive process affects anticancer activity of tea in gastrointestinal cells; add citrus (such as lemon juice) or take ascorbic acid (vitamin C) to protect the catechins in green tea from digestive degradation.

g. *References/other sources:*

American Association for Cancer Research. (2007, August 12). Green tea boosts production of detox enzymes, rendering cancerous chemicals harmless. *ScienceDaily.* Retrieved December 20, 2007, from http://www.sciencedaily.com/releases/2007/08/070810194923.htm

Federation of American Societies for Experimental Biology (2008, April 10). Digestive process affects anti-cancer activity of tea in gastrointestinal cells. *ScienceDaily.* Retrieved April 20, 2008, from http://www.sciencedaily.com/releases/2008/04/080407172713.htm

Pettit, J. L. (2001). Green tea. *Clinician Reviews, 11*(1), 71–72.

Skidmore-Roth, L. (2006). Green tea. In *Mosby's handbook of herbs and natural supplements* (pp. 535–539). St. Louis, MO: ElsevierMosby.

4. Omega-3 fatty acids

a. *Actions/expected responses:* Omega-3 fatty acids may inhibit proliferation of pancreatic cancer cells.

b. *Routes/dosages/frequencies:* Eat fish, dried beans, winter squash, walnuts, and flax. For specific amounts, go to http://www.whfoods.com/genpage.php?tname=george&dbid=75

c. *Cautions:* Farmed fish contains more PCBs, and 11 other environmental toxins are present at higher levels than in wild fish. Farmed fish may also be less nutritious.

d. *Assessments:* Assess intake of omega-rich foods.

e. *Tips on use:* The following fish contain the most omega-3 fatty acids and are the least tainted: 6 ounces of wild Atlantic salmon (3.1 grams), 3 ounces of sardines in sardine oil (2.8 grams), 6 ounces of wild rainbow trout (1.7 grams), 3 ounces of mackerel (1.0 grams), 6 ounces of specialty or gourmet Pacific Albacore tuna canned in water (1.35 grams).

f. *Other considerations:* Smaller, family-owned tuna fisheries fresh-freeze their fish and only cook it once, preserving their natural juices and fats. The larger commercial canneries cook their fish twice, during which time natural juices and fats are lost.

g. *References/other sources:*

Hering, J., Garrean, S., Dekoj, T. R., Razzak, A., Saied, A., Trevino, J., et al. (2007). Inhibition of proliferation by omega-3 fatty acids in chemoresistant pancreatic cancer cells. *Annals of Surgical Oncology, 14,* 3620–3628.

Indiana University. (2004, January 9). Farmed salmon more toxic than wild salmon, study finds. *ScienceDaily.* Retrieved February 3, 2008, from http://www.sciencedaily.com/releases/2004/01/040109072244.htm

Norwegian School of Veterinary Science. (2008, February 28). Farmed fish fed cheap food may be less nutritious for humans. *ScienceDaily.* Retrieved March 9, 2008, from http://www.sciencedaily.com/releases/2008/02/080226164105.htm

5. Starchy diet
   a. *Actions/expected responses:* A diet high in starchy foods (high glycemic index) may increase the risk of pancreatic cancer in women who are over-weight and sedentary.
   b. *Routes/dosages/frequencies:* Eating fructose and foods such as potatoes, rice, and white bread daily is associated with pancreatic cancer.
   c. *Cautions:* Women who are obese and inactive tend to be insulin resistant, causing them to produce large amounts of insulin to compensate and putting themselves at great risk for pancreatic cancer.
   d. *Assessments:* Assess intake of starchy foods and fructose.
   e. *Tips on use:* Substitute less starchy vegetables such as broccoli for pota-toes and rice, and snack on fruit to reduce pancreatic cancer risk.
   f. *Other considerations:* None.
   g. *References/other sources:*
      Dana-Farber Cancer Institute. (2002, September 4). Study suggests a possible link between high-starch diet and pancreatic cancer. *ScienceDaily.* Retrieved April 9, 2008, from http://www.sciencedaily.com/releases/2002/09/020904073950.htm

6. Sugar and sugar-sweetened foods
   a. *Actions/expected responses:* Emerging evidence indicates that hyperglyce-mia and hyperinsulinemia may be implicated in the development of pan-creatic cancer.
   b. *Routes/dosages/frequencies:* Adding sugar to coffee, tea, cereals, and so forth and eating high-sugar foods.
   c. *Cautions:* Frequent consumption of sugar and high-sugar foods may in-crease the risk of pancreatic cancer by inducing frequent postprandial hy-perglycemia, increasing insulin demand, and decreasing insulin sensitivity.
   d. *Assessments:* Assess intake of sugar.
   e. *Tips on use:* Use safer sweeteners such as stevia or molasses.
   f. *Other considerations:* Stevia, an herb, is an alternative sweetener that pre-vents DNA damage, can be used by women diagnosed with diabetes or hypoglycemia, and acts like a general tonic. Counsel women to use this herb in either liquid or powder form.
   g. *References/other sources:*
      Ghanta, S., Banerjee, A., Poddar, A., & Chattopadyay, S. (2007). Oxidative potential of Stevia rebaudiana (Bertoni) Bertoni, a natural sweetener. *Journal of Agricultural and Food Chemistry, 55*(26), 10962–10967.
      Larsson, S. C., Bergkvist, L., & Wolk, A. (2006). Consumption of sugar and sugar-sweetened foods and the risk of pancreatic cancer in a prospec-tive study. *American Journal of Clinical Nutrition, 84*(5), 1171–1176.

7. Watercress
   a. *Actions/expected responses:* Watercress can be linked to a reduced risk of cancer via decreased damage to DNA and possible modulation of antioxi-dant status by increasing carotenoid concentrations.
   b. *Routes/dosages/frequencies:* Eating a bowlful of watercress every day for 8 weeks resulted in blood triglyceride levels being reduced by 10% and blood levels of the antioxidants lutein and beta-carotene to increase by 100% and 33%, respectively.
   c. *Cautions:* None known unless women are hypersensitive to watercress.
   d. *Assessments:* Assess intake of watercress.

e. *Tips on use:* Seek out watercress at produce stands and supermarkets and ask managers to order this vegetables.

f. *Other considerations:* Cruciferous vegetable consumption is associated with a reduced risk of several cancers in epidemiologic studies.

g. *References/other sources:*

Gill, C. I., Haldar, S., Boyd, L. A., Bennett, R., Whiteford, J., Butler, M., et al. (2007). Watercress supplementation in diet reduces lymphocyte DNA damage and alters blood antioxidant status in healthy adults. *American Journal of Clinical Nutrition, 85*(2), 504–510.

8. Western diet

a. *Actions/expected responses:* Epidemiological evidence on the relationship between nutrition and pancreatic cancer found consistently positive associations between the intakes of meat, carbohydrates, and dietary cholesterol and pancreatic cancer.

b. *Routes/dosages/frequencies:* Nutrition and food patterns explain 35% of all cases in the etiology of pancreatic cancer.

c. *Cautions:* Meat, carbohydrates, dietary cholesterol, are correlated with increased risk for pancreatic cancer.

d. *Assessments:* Assess intake of meat, carbohydrates, and dietary cholesterol.

e. *Tips on use:* There are good carbs and bad carbs and good and bad sources of dietary fats.

f. *Other considerations:* Good carbs include whole grain breads, cereals, brown rice, bulgur wheat, berries, millet, hulled barley, whole wheat pasta, dried beans (e.g., black, pinto, kidney), and lots of fruits and vegetables. Eat potatoes only occasionally, and steer clear of processed cereals, breads, and white rice. Good oils include olive oil, sesame oil, peanut oil, cashews, almonds, peanuts and most other nuts, avocados, and up to 1 egg a day. Bad oils include whole milk, butter, cheese, ice cream, red meat, chocolate, coconuts, coconut milk and oil, poultry skin, palm oil and palm kernel oil, most margarines, vegetable shortening, partially hydrogenated vegetable oil, deep fried chips, many fast foods, and most commercial baked goods.

g. *References/other sources:*

Harvard School of Public Health. (2007). *Fats and cholesterol—the good, the bad and the healthy diet.* Retrieved April 16, 2008 from http://www.hsph.harvard.edu/nutritionsource/fats.html

Harvard School of Public Health. (2007). *Good carbs guide the way.* Retrieved April 16, 2008, from http://www.hsph.harvard.edu/nutrition sources/carbohydrates.html

Wang, L., & Li, H. (2006). Advances in research on genetic epidemiology of pancreatic cancer. *Acta Academiae Medicinae Sinicae, 28*(2), 289–293.

Stress Management

1. Stress management

a. *Actions/expected responses:* A weak immune system is one of the major factors that promotes cancer metastases after an operation, chemotherapy, or radiation therapy. Fear and stress weaken the immune system.

b. *Routes/dosages/frequencies:* Regular stress management practice prior to and after medical treatment may help to prevent metastases.

   c. *Cautions:* Go to http://www.mindtools.com/stress/RelaxationTechniques/Yoga.htm

   d. *Assessments:* Assess stress management skills.

   e. *Tips on use:* Go to http://www.mindtools.com/pages/main/newMN_TCS.htm

   f. *Other considerations:* None.

   g. *References/other sources:*

      Tel Aviv University. (2008, February 29). Stress and fear can affect cancer's recurrence. *ScienceDaily.* Retrieved March 9, 2008, from http://www.sciencedaily.com/releases/2008/02/080227142656.htm

Supplements

1. Aloe

   a. *Actions/expected responses:* Animal studies have shown that aloe prevents pancreatic neoplasia.

   b. *Routes/dosages/frequencies:* By mouth, 3 ounces of aloe following meals.

   c. *Cautions:* None unless hypersensitive to aloe (see http://www.mindtools.com/stress/RelaxationTechniques/Yoga.htm). Do not use aloe plants; diarrhea can result if aloe is taken from the wrong leaf area.

   d. *Assessments:* Assess sensitivity to aloe.

   e. *Tips on use:* Refrigerate aloe to enhance taste.

   f. *Other considerations:* None.

   g. *References/other sources:*

      Furukawa, F., Nishikawa, A., Chihara, T., Shimpo, K., Beppu, H., Kuzuya, H., et al. (2002). Chemopreventive effects of Aloe arborescens on N-nitrosobis (2-oxopropyl) amine-induced pancreatic carcinogenesis in hamsters. *Cancer Letter, 178*(2), 117–122.

2. Pycnogenol and ginkgo biloba extract

   a. *Actions/expected responses:* Either pycnogenol or ginkgo biloba extract can protect against antimutagenic activity in animal studies. They have potential as antimutagenic agents for lung cancer.

   b. *Routes/dosages/frequencies:* 5–100 microgram/mL.

   c. *Cautions:* Until more research is completed, pregnant and lactating women should not use these supplements, nor should they be given to children. Ginkgo should not be taken concurrently with anticoagulants.

   d. *Assessments:* Assess reaction to pycnogenol and ginkgo.

   e. *Tips on use:* Store supplements in a cool, dry place.

   f. *Other considerations:* Pycnogenol has also been found useful in preventing venous thrombosis, thrombophlebitis, gingival bleeding and plaque, inflammatory bowel disease, venous insufficiency, digestive conditions, and menopause symptoms.

   g. *References/other sources:*

      Krizkova, L., Chovanova, Z., Durackova, Z., & Krajcovic, J. (2008). Antimutagenic in vitro activity of plan polyphenols: Pycnogenol and ginkgo biloba extract. *Phytotherapy Research, 22*(3), 384–388.

3. Vitamins A, C, and E

   a. *Actions/expected responses:* Dietary intake of foods high in vitamins A, C, and E and/or vitamin supplementation may decrease the risk of pancreatic cancer. When derived from plant sources, all three vitamins show an inverse relationship to this type of cancer. Dietary intake of animal-origin nutrients was correlated with a high risk for pancreatic cancer.

b. *Routes/dosages/frequencies:* By mouth. The best way to obtain vitamins is via food. See "Assessments" section for food sources. If women are extremely ill, stressed, or can't or don't eat well, a multivitamin or juices made from fresh vegetables and fruits may be the best approach for this population.

c. *Cautions:* If supplements are chosen, choose brands that do not contain additional herbs, fillers, dyes, and so forth. Strive for the least processed form available. Vitamin C should not be taken when fat resides in the stomach because at this time it can promote, rather than prevent, the formation of certain cancer-causing chemicals.

d. *Assessments:* Assess intake of vitamin A foods (animal livers, apricots, asparagus, beet greens, broccoli, cantaloupe, carrots, collards, dandelion greens, papaya, peaches, red peppers, spinach, sweet potatoes, Swiss chard, turnip greens, watercress, yellow squash), vitamin C foods (asparagus, avocadoes, beet greens, black currants, broccoli, Brussels sprouts, cantaloupe, collards, dandelion greens, grapefruit, kale, lemons, mangos, mustard greens, onions, oranges, papayas, green peas, sweet peppers, persimmons, pineapple, radishes, spinach, strawberries, Swiss chard, tomatoes, turnip greens, and watercress), and vitamin E foods (brown rice, cold-pressed vegetable oils, cornmeal, dark green leafy vegetables, eggs, legumes, nuts, oatmeal, organ meats, seeds, soybeans, wheat germ, and whole grains).

e. *Tips on use:* Store supplements in a cool, dry place. Follow directions on the bottle.

f. *Other considerations:* Juicers are available online and at health food stores. Making juices may be especially useful for women who have lost their appetite or have digestion issues.

g. *References/other sources:*

Balch, J. F., & Balch, P. A. (1997). *Prescription for nutritional healing.* Garden City Park, NY: Avery Publishing Group.

Combet, E., Paterson, S., Iijama, K., Winter, J., Mullen, W., Crozier, A., et al. (2007). Fat transforms ascorbic acid from inhibiting to promoting acid-catalyzed N. nitrosation. *Gut, 56,* 1678–1684.

McCarroll, J. A., Phillips, P. A., Santucci, N., Pirola, R. C., Wilson, J. S., & Apte, M. V. (2006). Vitamin A inhibits pancreatic stellate cell activation: Implications for treatment of pancreatic fibrosis. *Gut, 55*(1), 9–89.

Sylvester, P. W. (2007). Vitamin E and apoptosis. *Vitamins and Hormones, 76,* 329–356.

Zhongguo, Y., Xue, K., Xue, Y., & Xue, B. (2006). Advances in research on genetic epidemiology of pancreatic cancer. *Acta Academiae Medicinai Senicae, 28*(2), 289–293.

Touch

1. Acupressure

a. *Actions/expected responses:* Acupressure can relieve nausea, vomiting, and retching associated with chemotherapy.

b. *Routes/dosages/frequencies:* Finger acupressure treatment is given bilaterally at the acupressure points P6 and ST36, located on the forearm and by the knee, every 2–3 hours.

c. *Cautions:* Use gentle acupressure if knee or forearm conditions are apparent.

d. *Assessments:* Collect baseline and posttreatment questions about amount of nausea, vomiting, and retching, and keep a daily log of the intensity of these symptoms.

e. *Tips on use:* Gentle acupressure means holding the spot with middle three fingers until a strong pulsation is felt (signaling a blockage has opened), and then moving to the next spot. For more information on using acupressure, go to http://www.eclecticenergies.com/acupressure/howto.php

f. *Other considerations:* Changes will begin to occur immediately and will continue for several days. Gentle acupressure points that can strengthen the pancreas are all on the right side of the body and include the inside of the ankle, the instep, bottom of big toe, back of knee, and halfway between outside of elbow and shoulder.

g. *References/other sources:*

Dayton, B. R. (1998). *High touch jin shin workbook 1.* Friday Harbor, WA: High Touch Network.

Dribble, S. L., Luce, J., Cooper, B. A., Israel, J., Cohen, M., Nussey, B., et al. (2007). Acupressure for chemotherapy-induced nausea and vomiting: A randomized clinical trial. *Oncology Nursing Forum, 34*(4), 813–820.

Gardani, G., Cerrone, R., Biella, C., Mancini, L., Proserpio, E., Casiraghi, M., et al. (2006). Effect of acupressure on nausea and vomiting induced by chemotherapy in cancer patients. *Minerva Medicine, 97*(5), 391–394.

2. Foot reflexology

a. *Actions/expected responses:* Self-administered foot reflexology enhances natural killer cells and IgG, strengthening the immune system against cancer and possibly preventing tumor development.

b. *Routes/dosages/frequencies:* Four 40-minute treatments.

c. *Cautions:* None unless the feet have been injured.

d. *Assessments:* Obtain a baseline for immune responses prior to and after reflexology

e. *Tips on use:* Go to http://groups.msn.com/AlternativesToPainandDisease/ reflexologyinstructionspg1.msnw and http://groups.msn.com/Alternatives ToPainandDisease/reflexologyinstructionspg2.msnw

f. *Other considerations:* Foot reflexology has been shown to significantly improve life satisfaction, the most important predictor of survival for women with advanced cancer.

g. *References/other sources:*

Fox Chase Cancer Center. (2007, November 1). Quality of life is the most important predictor of survival for advanced cancer patients. *Science-Daily.* Retrieved November 12, 2007, from http://www.sciencedaily. com/releases/2007/10/07/071030170208.htm

National Cancer Center. (2006). *Immunity and cancer.* Retrieved February 6, 2008, from http://www.nci.nih.go/cancertopics/understandingcan cer/immunesystem/Slide32

28

PMS

Medical treatment for PMS includes medications. Complementary approaches for PMS are evidence based and can be effective while effecting no or few side effectives.

Environment

1. Tobacco smoke
   a. *Actions/expected responses:* Women who smoke are twice as likely to experience dysmenorrheal (painful menstruation) as nonsmokers and smoking prolongs the symptoms of this condition. Cramped quarters and indoor exposure to environmental tobacco smoke (ETS) may triple a woman's risk of menstrual pain. The researchers estimated that for each day that two or more cigarettes were smoked by the woman or in cramped quarters, the risk of dysmenorrheal climbs by 30%.
   b. *Routes/dosages/frequencies:* The more ETS a woman is exposed to daily, the higher her risk for dysmenorrhea.

   c. *Cautions:* Smoking or being in a room with others who do can increase menstrual pain.
   d. *Assessments:* Assess exposure to tobacco smoke. Keep a diary of menstrual pain and tobacco exposure.
   e. *Tips for use:* Stop smoking and/or avoid being in close quarters with smokers prior to and during menstrual periods. For tips on how to stop smoking go to Office of the Surgeon General (2008).
   f. *Other considerations:* Request family and friends do not smoke around you.
   g. *References/other sources:*
      Office of the Surgeon General. (2008). *Tobacco cession: You can quit smoking now.* Retrieved August 4, 2008, from http://www.surgeongeneral. gov/tobacco/
      Potera, C. (2000). Smoke-filled rooms. ETS causes menstrual pain. *Environmental Health Perspectives, 108*(11), A520.

Exercise/Movement

1. Qiqong
   a. *Actions/expected responses:* The slow, gentle movements of qiqong can reduce negative feeling, pain, water retention, and total PMS symptoms, compared to placebo controls.
   b. *Routes/dosages/frequencies:* Each intervention was completed eight times during the second and third cycles with women completing a PMS diary.
   c. *Cautions:* None identified.
   d. *Assessments:* Assess PMS symptoms prior to and after performing qiqong.
   e. *Tips on use:* For a gentle movement exercise that can help with PMS, go to http://valternativehealthcare.com/category/qi-qongchi-kong
   f. *Other considerations:* None.
   g. *References/other sources:*
      Jang, H. S., & Lee, M. S. (2004). Effects of qi therapy (external qigong) on premenstrual syndrome: A randomized placebo-controlled study. *Journal of Alternative and Complementary Medicine, 10*(3), 456–462.

Herbs/Essential Oils

1. Chaste tree (Vitex agnes-castus)
   a. *Actions/expected responses:* Extracts of the fruits of the chaste tree were shown in double-blind, placebo-controlled studies to have beneficial effects on premenstrual breast tenderness and possibly other symptoms of the premenstrual syndrome (headache, edema, constipation, and tension).
   b. *Routes/dosages/frequencies:* 2 ml fluid extract a day, or 175–225 mg powdered extract or 20 mg capsules daily.
   c. *Cautions:* Avoid if pregnant or breast feeding until additional studies focusing on these populations are completed. Avoid if hypersensitive to chaste tree.
   d. *Assessments:* Assess breast pain and other premenstrual symptoms prior to and after taking chaste tree.

e. *Tips on use:* Store chaste tree in a cool, dry place.

f. *Other considerations:* Dopaminergic action via opioid receptors was identified.

g. *References/other sources:*

Berger, D., Schaffner, W., Schrader, E., Meier, B., & Brattstrom, A. (2000). Efficacy of Vitex agnus castus L. extract Ze 440 in patients with premenstrual syndrome (PMS). *Archives of Gynecology and Obstetrics, 264*(3), 150–153.

Loch, E. G., Selle, H., & Boblitz, N. (2000). Treatment of premenstrual syndrome with a phytopharmaceutical formulation containing Vitex agnur castus. *Journal of Women's Health and Gender Based Medicine, 9*(3), 315–320.

Wuttke, W., Jarry, H., Christoffel, V., Spengler, B., & Seidlova-Wuttke, D. (2003). Chaste tree (Vitex agnus-castus)—pharmacology and clinical indications. *Phytomedicine, 10*(4), 348–357.

Mindset

1. Affirmations
   a. *Actions/expected responses:* Self-affirmation of personal values and beliefs buffers neuroendocrine and psychological stress.
   b. *Routes/dosages/frequencies:* Repeat aloud or write positive affirmations up to 20 times a day such as, "All is well," "I accept that I am a beautiful woman," and "I accept all my body processes as normal and perfect."
   c. *Cautions:* Ensure affirmations are positive and acceptable.
   d. *Assessments:* Assess anxiety prior to and after completing affirmations for a week.
   e. *Tips on use:* Write favorite affirmations on 3 by 5 cards and place them in places where they will be read frequently.
   f. *Other considerations:* Find more affirmations information at http://www. successconsciousness.com/index_00000a.htm
   g. *References/other sources:*

Hay, L. (2000). *Heal your body.* Carlsbad, CA: Hay House.

Schwarzer, R., Babler, J., Kwiatek, P., Schroder, K., & Zang, J. W. (1997). The assessment of optimistic self-beliefs: Assessment of general perceived self-efficacy in thirteen cultures. *World Psychology, 3*(1–2), 177–190.

Nutrition

1. Calcium and vitamin D
   a. *Actions/expected responses:* Blood calcium and vitamin D levels are lower in women with PMS, and the intake of calcium and vitamin D from food is inversely related to PMS.
   b. *Routes/dosages/frequencies:* Women need between 1,000 and 1500 mg of calcium daily and 400 IU to 2,000 (or more) IU of vitamin D daily.
   c. *Cautions:* Vitamin D supplements can suppress the proper operation of the immune system.

d. *Assessments:* Assess PMS before and after exposure to sun (15 minutes for fair-skinned women and up to 40 minutes three times a week for darker-skinned women) and/or ingesting cod liver oil and high-calcium foods.

e. *Tips on use:* Vitamin D2 that is added to so-called fortified foods and many multivitamins and is usually written in prescriptions is inefficiently metabolized in humans; only 20%–40% is metabolized into biologically active vitamin D3. Foods high in calcium that may be more easily metabolized include sardines in oil including bones, canned pink salmon including bones, boiled soybeans, cooked collards, cooked turnip greens, tofu, and dried figs. Besides spending time in the sun, women can be counseled to eat egg yolks, saltwater fish, and/or take a tablespoon of cod liver oil every day.

f. *Other considerations:* Women using corticosteroids may require additional vitamin D. For more high calcium and vitamin D foods, go to http://www.niams.nih.gov/Health_Info/Bone/Bone_Health/Nutrition/default.asp

g. *References/other sources:*

Autoimmunity Research Foundation. (2008, January 27). Vitamin D deficiency study raises new questions about disease and supplements. *ScienceDaily.* Retrieved February 13, 2008, from http://www.sciencedaily.com/releases/2008/01/080125223302.htm

Bertone-Johnson, E. R., Hankinson, S. E., Bendich, A., Johnson, S. R., Willett, W. C., & Manson, J. E. (2005). Calcium and vitamin D intake and risk of incident premenstrual syndrome. *Archives of Internal Medicine, 165*(11), 1246–1252.

2. Fat, carbohydrate, simple sugars, protein and alcohol

a. *Actions/expected responses:* Overweight women with PMS showed a significant increase in fat, simple sugars, and alcohol premenstrually, and a decrease in protein (as compared to women without PMS). One study found a significant increase in premenstrual episodes of eating.

b. *Routes/dosages/frequencies:* Women with PMS ingest significantly greater amounts premenstrually of cereals, cakes and desserts, and high-sugar foods.

c. *Cautions:* Eating significantly greater amounts of high-sugar foods and less protein may contribute to PMS symptoms.

d. *Assessments:* Assess intake of high-sugar foods and protein premenstrually.

e. *Tips on use:* Women who increase their nutrient intake during the premenstrual phase may benefit from more frequent reminders from self or others to eat more protein and fewer sugary foods premenstrually. Sweeten drinks and foods with stevia, a non-nutrient, safe and effective sweetener that also repairs DNA.

f. *Other considerations:* Eat more protein during the premenstrual period. Refer women to sugar alternatives, for example, http://www.marthastewart.com/portal/site/mslo/menuitem.3a0656639de62ad593598e10d373a0a0/?vgnextoid=3ecbcec294688110VgnVCM1000003d370a0aRCRD&rsc=related

g. *References/other sources:*

Bryant, M., Truesdale, K. P., & Dye, L. (2006). Modest changes in dietary intake across the menstrual cycle: Implications for food intake research. *British Journal of Nutrition, 96*(5), 888–894.

Cross, G. B., Marley, J., Miles, H., & Willson, K. (2001). Changes in nutrient intake during the menstrual cycle of overweight women with premenstrual syndrome. *British Journal of Nutrition, 85*(4), 475–482.

Ghanta, S., Banerjee, A., Poddar, A., & Chattopadhyay, S. (2007). Oxidataive DNA damage preventive activity and antioxidant potential of Stevia rebaudiana (Bertoni) Bertoni, a natural sweetener. *Journal of Agriculture and Food Chemistry 55*(26), 10952–10967.

3. Obesity
   a. *Actions/expected responses:* Obesity is a risk factor for PMS.
   b. *Routes/dosages/frequencies:* Obese women had a three-fold increased risk for PMS as compared to nonobese women.
   c. *Cautions:* None. Reducing obesity will also reduce risk factors for heart disease, cancer, and other conditions.
   d. *Assessments:* Assess obesity (about 30 pounds overweight).
   e. *Tips on use:* Go to pp. 287–298.
   f. *Other considerations:* None.
   g. *References/other sources:*

   Masho, S. W., Adera, T., & South-Paul, J. (2005). Obesity as a risk factor for premenstrual syndrome. *Journal of Psychsomatics and Obstetric Gynaecology, 26*(1), 33–39.

4. Soy isoflavones
   a. *Actions/expected responses:* The beneficial effect of dietary soy isoflavones on certain menstrual symptoms was established.
   b. *Routes/dosages/frequencies:* 25 grams daily.
   c. *Cautions:* Hypersensitivity to soy.
   d. *Assessments:* Assess hypersensitivity to soy.
   e. *Tips on use:* Eat up to 25 grams daily, including several of the following: 4 ounces firm tofu = 13 grams soy protein; 4 ounces soft or silken tofu = 9 grams soy protein; 1 soy-based burger = 10 to 12 grams soy protein; 8 ounces plain soy milk = 10 grams soy protein; 1 soy protein bar = 14 grams soy protein; 1/2 cup cooked soybeans = 16 grams soy protein. Fermented soy products (miso, tempeh) are more digestible than other forms.
   f. *Other considerations:* None.
   g. *References/other sources:*

   Kim, H. W., Kwon, M. K., Kim, N. S., & Reame, N. E. (2006). Intake of dietary soy isoflavones in relation to perimenstrual symptoms of Korean women living in the USA. *Nursing Health Science, 8*(2), 108–113.

Stress Management

1. Cognitive-behavioral therapy (CBT)
   a. *Actions/expected responses:* Compared to relaxation or hormone therapy, women who participated in CBT achieved significant positive benefits after the first treatment month that continued throughout and were maintained at follow-up 3 months later.
   b. *Routes/dosages/frequencies:* Weekly sessions of up to an hour.
   c. *Cautions:* The therapist must be an expert in CBT, and women must be willing and persistent to benefit.

    d. *Assessments:* Assess PMS symptoms prior to and after participating in CBT.

    e. *Tips on use:* For more information, go to http://www.mind.org.uk/Informa tion/Booklets/Making+Sense/MakingSenseCBT.htm

    f. *Other considerations:* None.

    g. *References/other sources:*

        Morse, C. A., Dennerstein, L., Farrell, E., & Varnavides, K. (1991). A comparison of hormone therapy, coping skills training, and relaxation for the relief of premenstrual syndrome. *Journal of Behavioral Medicine, 14*(5), 469–489.

Supplements

1. Pycnogenol (pine bark)

    a. *Actions/expected responses:* After 60 mg a day of pycnogenol women with dysmenorrheal (menstrual cramps) had a significantly lower pain score and required statistically significantly less analgesic medication both during and even after supplementation ended.

    b. *Routes/dosages/frequencies:* 60 mg a day as a capsule.

    c. *Cautions:* None unless hypersensitive to pine bark.

    d. *Assessments:* Assess intake of analgesic medication and pain level prior to and after taking pycnogenol.

    e. *Tips on use:* Take with or right after meals.

    f. *Other considerations:* None.

    g. *References/other sources:*

        Suzuki, N., Uebaba, K., Kohama, T., Moniwa, N., Kanayama, N., & Koike, K. (2008). French maritime pine bark extract significantly lowers the requirement for analgesic medication in dysmenorrheal: A multicenter, randomized, double-blind, placebo-controlled study. *Journal of Reproductive Medicine, 53*(5), 338–346.

2. Pyridoxine (vitamin B6)

    a. *Actions/expected responses:* Compared to placebo, pyridoxine significantly reduced PMS symptoms of depression, irritability, and tiredness.

    b. *Routes/dosages/frequencies:* 50 mg a day of pyridoxine.

    c. *Cautions:* Go to http://www.drugs.com/cdi/pyridoxine-vitamin-b6.html

    d. *Assessments:* Assess depression, irritability, and fatigue prior to and after taking vitamin B6.

    e. *Tips on use:* Counsel women to keep pyridoxine in a cool, dry spot.

    f. *Other considerations:* None.

    g. *References/other sources:*

        Doll, H., Brown, S., Thuston, A., & Vessey, M. (1989). Pyridoxine (vitamin B6) and the premenstrual syndrome: A randomized crossover trial. *The Journal of the Royal College of General Practitioners, 39*(326), 364–368.

3. Vitamin E

    a. *Actions/expected responses:* Compared to placebo, vitamin E resulted in greater relief of symptoms.

    b. *Routes/dosages/frequencies:* 200 units twice a day taken 2 days before the expected start of menstruation.

c. *Cautions:* None unless hypersensitive to vitamin E.

d. *Assessments:* Assess symptoms prior to and after taking vitamin E.

e. *Tips on use:* Keep vitamin E capsules in a cool, dry place.

f. *Assessments:* Assess symptoms prior to and after taking vitamin E.

g. *References/other sources:*

Rasgon, N. L., & Yargin, K. N. (2005). Vitamin E for treatment of dysmenorrhea. *British Journal of Gynecology, 112*(8), 466–469.

Touch

1. Ear, hand, and foot reflexology

   a. *Actions/expected responses:* Women treated by ear, hand, and foot reflexology experienced a significantly greater decrease in premenstrual symptoms than the women in a control group.

   b. *Routes/dosages/frequencies:* 30-minute sessions once a week for 8 weeks.

   c. *Cautions:* Those with ear, hand, or foot problems, gout, arthritis, and vascular conditions such as varicose veins should be careful using these procedures.

   d. *Assessments:* Assess PMS symptoms on a scale of 1 (none) to 10 (or more) prior to and after ear, hand, and foot reflexology sessions.

   e. *Tips on use:* For more information on ear, hand, and foot reflexology, go to http://reflexology.suite101.com/article.cfm/foot_hand_ear_reflexology

   f. *Other considerations:* None.

   g. *References/other sources:*

   Kesselring, A. (1994). Foot reflex zone massage. *Schweizerische Medizinische Wochenschrift, 62,* 88–93.

   Lee, Y. M. (2006). Effect of self-foot reflexology massage on depression, stress response and immune functions of middle aged women. *Taehan Kanho Hakkoe Chi, 36*(1), 179–188.

   Oleson, T., & Flocco, W. (1993). Randomized controlled study of premenstrual symptoms treated with ear, hand, and foot reflexology. *Obstetrics and Gynecology, 82*(6), 906–911.

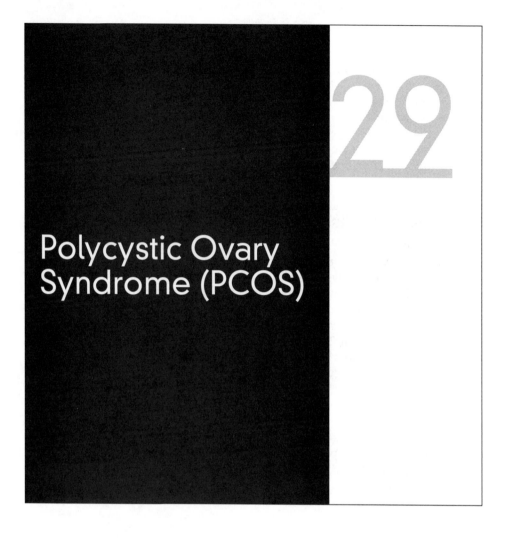

Polycystic Ovary Syndrome (PCOS)

29

Medication and surgery are traditional medical approaches for polycystic ovary syndrome (PCOS). Both have negative side effects. Complementary approaches are evidence based with few or no side effects.

Exercise/Movement

1. Exercise
   a. *Actions/expected responses:* Endurance and exercise plus nutritional counseling may benefit the metabolic and reproductive abnormalities associated with PCOS.
   b. *Routes/dosages/frequencies:* Daily exercise and nutritional counseling for at least 12 weeks.
   c. *Cautions:* Always do warm-ups before and cool-downs after exercising. For suggestions, go to http://www.medicinenet.com/fitness_exercise_for_a_healthy_heart/page3.htm
   d. *Assessments:* Assess weight loss prior to and after exercise and changing nutritional habits.

    e. *Tips on use:* For more information on exercise, go to http://exercise.life
       tips.com
    f. *Other considerations:* None.
    g. *References/other sources:*
       Bruner, B., Chad, K., & Chizen, D. (2006). Effects of exercise and nutritional
          counseling in women with polycystic ovary syndrome. *Applied Physi-*
          ological Nutrition and Metabolism, 31(4), 384–391.

Herbs/Essential Oils

1. Chinese herbs
    a. *Actions/expected responses:* Chinese herbs for nourishing yin to reduce
       fire can significantly reduce the serum levels of testosterone and insulin
       in PCOS women. Chinese herbs for invigorating spleen and replenishing
       qi can significantly reduce the serum level of insulin in PCOS women.
    b. *Routes/dosages/frequencies:* Consult a Chinese medicine practitioner.
    c. *Cautions:* Consult a Chinese medicine practitioner.
    d. *Assessments:* Assess PCOS symptoms prior to and after taking Chinese
       herbs.
    e. *Tips on use:* Store Chinese herbs in a cool, dry place.
    f. *Other considerations:* None.
    g. *References/other sources:*
       Jia, L. N., & Wang, X. J. (2006). Clinical observation on treatment of
          43 women with polycystic ovary syndrome based on syndrome differ-
          entiation. *Zhong Xi Yhi Jie He Xue Bao, 4*(6), 585–588.

Mindset

1. Affirmations
    a. *Actions/expected responses:* Self-affirmation of personal values and be-
       liefs buffers neuroendocrine and psychological stress.
    b. *Routes/dosages/frequencies:* Repeat aloud or write positive affirmations up
       to 20 times a day such as, "I create beautiful movies in my mind and act on
       them" and "I love me and my life."
    c. *Cautions:* Ensure chosen affirmations are positive and acceptable.
    d. *Assessments:* Assess anxiety prior to and after completing affirmations for
       a week.
    e. *Tips on use:* Write favorite affirmations on 3 by 5 cards and place them in
       places where they will be read frequently.
    f. *Other considerations:* Find more affirmations information at http://www.
       successconsciousness.com/index_00000a.htm
    g. *References/other sources:*
       Hay, L. (2000). *Heal your body.* Carlsbad, CA: Hay House.
       Schwarzer, R., Babler, J., Kwiatek, P., Schroder, K., & Zang, J. W. (1997).
          The assessment of optimistic self-beliefs: Assessment of general per-
          ceived self-efficacy in thirteen cultures. *World Psychology, 3*(1–2),
          177–190.

Nutrition

1. Healthy diet
   a. *Actions/expected responses:* Women diagnosed with PCOS were found to consume significantly more white bread and fried potatoes than a control group. Several different scenarios of diets appear to work well with PCOS: (a) 1,200–1,400 calories per day (25% protein, 25% fat, 50% carbohydrates) plus 25–30 grams of fiber per week ameliorated hyperinsulinemia and hyperandrogenemia; a moderate reduction in dietary carbohydrates (43%) reduced the fasting and postchallenge insulin concentrations, which over time may improve reproductive/endocrine outcomes; an eating pattern similar to the type 2 diabetes diet including a decrease in refined carbohydrates, as well as a decrease in trans and saturated fats and an increase in anti-inflammatory compounds (omega-3 fatty acids, vitamin E, fiber, and red wine) can improve the androgen profile of PCOS women.
   b. *Routes/dosages/frequencies:* Daily eating patterns.
   c. *Cautions:* None unless hypersensitive to particular foods.
   d. *Assessments:* Assess PCOS symptoms prior to and after dietary changes.
   e. *Tips on use:* For information, go to http://www.helpguide.org/life/healthy_eating_diet.htm
   f. *Other considerations:* None.
   g. *References/other sources:*

   Douglas, C. C., Gower, B. A., Darnell, B. E., OValle, F., Oster, R. A., & Azziz, R. (2006). Role of diet in the treatment of polycystic ovary syndrome. *Fertility and Sterility, 85*(3), 679–688.

   Liepa, G. U., Sengupta, A., & Karsie, D. (2008). Polycystic ovary syndrome (PCOS) and other androgen excess-related conditions: Can changes in dietary intake make a difference? *Nutrition in Clinical Practice, 23*(1), 63–71.

   Qublan, H. S., Yannakoula, E. K., Al-Qudah, M. A., & El-Uri, F. I. (2007). *Saudi Medical Journal, 28*(11), 1694–1699.

Supplements

1. Inositol
   a. *Actions/expected responses:* Inositol improves ovarian function in women with oligomenorrhea and polycystic ovaries. As opposed to a control group, significant weight loss (and leptin reduction) was recorded in the inositol group.
   b. *Routes/dosages/frequencies:* 100 mg twice a day.
   c. *Cautions:* None, unless a woman is hypersensitive to the form in which inositol is given.
   d. *Assessments:* Assess weight loss prior to and after taking inositol.
   e. *Tips on use:* Store inositol in a cool, dry spot.
   f. *Other considerations:* This substance is found in many foods including whole grain cereals, nuts, beans, and fruit, especially cantaloupe melons and oranges. Inositol is not considered a vitamin because it can be synthesized by the body.

g. *References/other sources:*

Gerli, S., Mignosa, M., & Di Renzo, G. C. (2003). Effects of inositol on ovarian function and metabolic factors in women with PCOS: A randomized double blind placebo-controlled trial. *European Review of Medical Pharmacology and Science, 7*(6), 151–159.

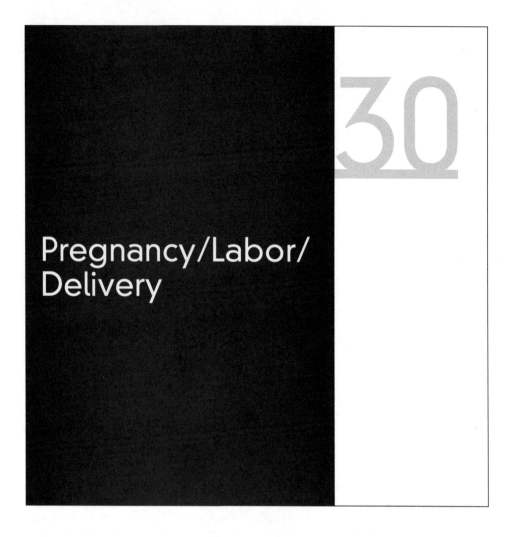

30 Pregnancy/Labor/

Pregnancy/Labor/Delivery

Pregnancy is a normal process, although medications (to reduce pain) or surgery (to assist delivery) may be used. Complementary approaches are evidence based and have few, if any, side effects.

Environment

1. Air pollution
   a. *Actions/expected responses:* Air pollution is linked to premature birth in pregnant women.
   b. *Routes/dosages/frequencies:* Being exposed to vehicle traffic can increase the likelihood of having a preterm baby by 10%–25% more than women who lived in less polluted areas. This is especially true for women who breathed polluted air during the first trimester or during the last months and weeks of pregnancy.
   c. *Cautions:* Pregnant women who live in regions with high carbon monoxide or fine-particle levels are at risk.
   d. *Assessments:* Assess exposure to vehicle traffic.

e. *Tips on use:* Choose living arrangements away from high carbon monoxide or fine-particle areas.

f. *Other considerations:* None.

g. *References/other sources:*

University of California, Los Angeles. (2007, August 27). Air pollution linked to premature birth in pregnant women. *ScienceDaily*. Retrieved April 19, 2008, http://www.sciencedaily.com/releases/2007/080708231503 43.htm

2. Breastfeeding-friendly practices in hospitals

a. *Actions/expected responses:* Breast milk and breastfeeding are recognized as the ideal choices of nutrition and feeding for infants. Breastfeeding-friendly practices in hospitals following birth can significantly improve long-term breastfeeding success.

b. *Routes/dosages/frequencies:* Nearly two-thirds of mothers who followed available supportive practices were still breastfeeding 4 months after going home: (a) initiating breastfeeding within 1 hour of delivery, (b) keeping infants in the mother's hospital room (rooming in), (c) feeding infants only breast milk in the hospital, (d) prohibiting pacifier use in the hospital, (e) providing a telephone number to call for breastfeeding help after hospital discharge.

c. *Cautions:* None known.

d. *Assessments:* Assess inclination to breast-feed and whether the chosen delivery hospital practices the five supportive guidelines for breastfeeding.

e. *Tips on use:* Go to www.nursingmothers.org/tips.htm

f. *Other considerations:* In addition to receiving essential nutrients, breastfed infants have lower rates of ear infections, gastroenteritis, asthma, obesity, and diabetes. Benefits for mothers include decreased incidence of breast and ovarian cancer. National goals in the United States are a breastfeeding initiation rate of 75% (with an exclusive breastfeeding rate for the first 3 months of 60%), and continuation of 50% at 6 months of age (with 25% exclusively breastfeeding).

g. *References/other sources:*

Blackwell Publishing Ltd. (2007, August 30). Hospital practices affect long-term breastfeeding success. *ScienceDaily*. Retrieved April 21, 2008, from http://www.sciencedaily.com/releases/2007/08/070828 154929.htm

3. CenteringPregnancy for pregnant adolescents

a. *Actions/expected responses:* This holistic approach toward prenatal care is well suited to adolescents because it also considers their developmental need for socializing and peer support. This program is associated with an improvement in birth outcomes when compared with traditional or adult-focused care.

b. *Routes/dosages/frequencies:* This approach to adolescent pregnancy includes 20 contact hours over approximately 28 weeks and is comprehensive, incorporating essential risk assessments, education, and support. The class sections are divided into two parts: formal education and a discussion period.

c. *Cautions:* Teens in a traditional, hospital-based program are 1.5 times less likely to receive comprehensive care. Teen clinics, though significantly less likely to lead to threatened preterm labor, preterm prelabor, prolonged rupture of membranes, or preterm delivery, often lack funding. Many health departments lack special funding for adolescent programs, making it difficult to improve birth outcomes. Traditional programs usually provide individual counseling without peer support.

d. *Assessments:* Assess age and availability of a CenteringPregnancy program.

e. *Tips on use:* This approach is most useful to teens because it allows them to express their concerns and listen to other participants' descriptions of their pregnancy experience. Many pregnant teenagers are relieved to learn that other pregnant teens are having the same problems. This normalizes the experience, is reassuring, and builds confidence.

f. *Other considerations:* CenteringPregnancy programs focus on adjustment to pregnancy, fetal development, nutrition, exercise, dangers of substance abuse and appropriate referral, preparation for childbirth (including relaxation and breathing methods), infant breastfeeding, baby care and coping techniques, parenting techniques and self-esteem building, contraception and postpartum depression, physical or sexual abuse, sexuality, and communication.

g. *References/other sources:*

Grady, M. A. J., & Bloom, K. C. (2004). Pregnancy outcomes of adolescents enrolled in a CenteringPregnancy program. *Journal of Midwifery and Women's Health, 49,* 412–420.

Moeller, A. H., Vezeau, T. M., & Carr, K. C. (2007). CenteringPregnancy: A new program for adolescent prenatal care. *The American Journal for Nurse Practitioners, 11*(5), 48–56.

Quinlivan, J. A., & Evans, S. F. (2004). Teenage antenatal clinics may reduce the rate of preterm birth: A prospective study. *British Journal of Gynecology, 111*(6), 571–578.

4. C-sections

a. *Actions/expected responses:* Turning fetuses that are in a breech presentation can prevent unnecessary C-sections, which increase the risk for potentially fatal complications.

b. *Routes/dosages/frequencies:* A physician or midwife uses their hands to manipulate the mother's abdomen and help the baby turn in a somersault-like motion (external cephalic version or ECV) at 34–36 week's gestation.

c. *Cautions:* Turning a breech baby at 37–38 weeks (the current procedure) is less successful. Except in breech births, women having a nonemergency caesarean birth have double the risk of illness or even death compared to a vaginal birth. Overweight pregnant women have greater risk for infection (including death due to wound infection), delayed wound healing, and blood clots. All pregnant women who undergo c-section have a greater risk of infection, hemorrhage, reaction to anesthesiology, and other surgical risks.

d. *Assessments:* Assess for breech presentation and knowledge of c-section risks.

e. *Tips on use:* A fetus is in breech position about once in every 25–30 full-term births. Women with fetuses in breech position can ask for ECV at 34–36 weeks. For more information on ECV and alternative procedures, go to http://www.babycenter.com/0_breech-birth_158.bc

f. *Other considerations:* A pilot study conducted in 2002 showed that earlier ECV was about 10% more successful in turning breech babies than later ECV. A large clinical trial is now underway. Investigate the availability of midwives, doulas, and pain management technologies, which can make natural birth more tolerable and cesarean delivery less desirable.

g. *References/other sources:*

> *British Medical Journal.* (2007, November 1). Caesarean births pose higher risks for mother and baby, study finds. *ScienceDaily.* Retrieved November 12, 2007, from http://www.sciencedaily.com/releases/2007/10/071031095716.htm

> Chettle, C. C. (2008, April 21). Shocking high rates: Surgical site infections remain a constant threat. *Nurse.com,* 24–28.

> Huiras, R. (2008, April 21). Maternal death rate increases. *Nursing.com,* 20–21.

> McMaster University. (2007, June 20). When to turn breech babies. *ScienceDaily.* Retrieved April 22, 2008, from http://www.sciencedaily.com/releases/2007/06/070614151740.htm

5. Dental X-rays

   a. *Actions/expected responses:* Dental X-rays during pregnancy are associated with low-birth-weight infants at term.

   b. *Routes/dosages/frequencies:* Both high- and low-dose radiation exposure in women have been associated with low-birth-weight offspring.

   b. *Cautions:* Exposure higher than 0.4GY was associated with an increased risk (about double) of low-birth-weight infants.

   d. *Assessments:* Assess pregnancy status.

   e. *Tips on use:* Counsel women to avoid dental X-rays during pregnancy.

   f. *Other considerations:* None.

   g. *References/other sources:*

   > Hujoel, P. P., Bollen, A. M., Noonan, C. J., & del Aguila, M. A. (2004). Antepartum dental radiography and infant low birth weight. *Journal of the American Medical Association, 28*(16), 1987–1993.

6. Dioxin

   a. *Actions/expected responses:* Intrauterine dioxin exposure can disrupt the develop of mammary glands and predispose offspring to mammary cancer.

   b. *Routes/dosages/frequencies:* Women are exposed to dioxin primarily through consumption of animal products: meat, poultry, dairy products, and human breast milk.

   c. *Cautions:* Dioxin is formed by the incineration of products containing PVC (polyvinyl chloride), PCBs, and other chlorinated compounds. Dioxin also comes from industrial processes that use chlorine and from the combustion of diesel and gasoline, which contain chlorinated additives.

   d. *Assessments:* Assess exposure to dioxin.

e. *Tips on use:* Counsel pregnant or lactating women to avoid eating animal products, pumping gasoline into their vehicles, or being near vehicle exhaust whenever possible.

f. *Other considerations:* Dioxins are known human carcinogens and hormone mimickers. Very low levels are found in the air and plants. Encourage pregnant and lactating women to eat more vegetables, fruits, dried beans, and whole grains and less or no animal products.

g. *References/other sources:*

Warner, M. B., Eskenazi, B., Mocarelli, P., Gerthoux, P. M., Samuels, S., & Needham, L. (2002). Serum dioxin concentrations and breast cancer risk in the Seveso Women's Health Study. *Environmental Health Perspectives, 110,* 625–628.

World Health Organization. (2007). *Dioxins and their effect on human health.* Retrieved December 17, 2007, from http://www.who.int/mediacentre/factsheets/fs225/en/print.html

7. Household exposure to pesticides

a. *Actions/expected responses:* Maternal exposure to household pesticides during pregnancy was significantly associated with childhood hematopoietic malignancies, the most common childhood cancers (leukemia, Hodgkin's lymphoma, and non-Hodgkin's lymphoma).

b. *Routes/dosages/frequencies:* The use of professional pest control services at any time from 1 year before birth to 3 years after was associated with a significantly increased risk of childhood leukemia. Pesticides used at home, on pets or for garden crops, were also significantly associated with childhood cancers.

c. *Cautions:* Caution women not to use professional pest control services and not to use pesticides themselves in the home, on pets, or in the garden if pregnant or contemplating becoming pregnant.

d. *Assessments:* Assess use of pesticides.

e. *Tips on use:* For information on safe alternatives to pesticides, go to http://www.pesticide.org/factsheets.html

f. *Other considerations:* None.

g. *References/other sources:*

Rudant, J., Menegaux, F., Leverger, G., Baruchel, A., Nelken, B., Bertrand, Y., et al. (2007). Household exposure to pesticides and risk of childhood hematopoietic malignancies: The ESCALE Study (SFCE). *Environmental Health Perspectives, 115*(12), 1787–1793. Retrieved April 25, 2008, from http://www.ehponline.org/docs/2007/10596/abstract.html

Xiaomei, M., Buffler, P. A., Gunier, R. B., Dahl, G., Smith, M. T., Reinier, K., et al. (2002). Critical windows of exposure to household pesticides and risk of childhood leukemia—Children's Health Articles. *Environmental Health Perspectives, 110*(9), 955–960.

8. Kneeling for pregnancy

a. *Actions/expected responses:* Compared to sitting position, lateral position (kneeling) was associated with reduced duration of second stage of labor, a small reduction in assisted delivery, a reduction in episiotomies, less reporting of severe pain during second-stage labor, fewer instances of abnormal fetal heart rate pattern, and significantly reduced feelings of discomfort, vulnerability, exposure, difficulty, and postpartum perineal pain.

b. *Routes/dosages/frequencies:* Kneeling toward the head of the delivery bed or cushion versus sitting position with the head of bed raised at least 60 degrees in the second stage of labor until the child's head crowns.

c. *Cautions:* Kneeling position may increase risk of blood loss and perineal tears.

d. *Assessments:* Assess preferred method of labor.

e. *Tips on use:* Encourage women to give birth in the position they find most comfortable. Based on a systematic review of 19 trials of variable quality with 5,674 women, no clear benefits or risks of various delivery positions have been demonstrated in methodologically stringent trials.

f. *Other considerations:* None.

g. *References/other sources:*

Gupta, J. K., Hofmeyr, G. J., & Smyth, R. (2004). Position in the second stage of labour for women without epidural anaesthesia. *Cochrane Database of Systematic Reviews.* Retrieved from http://www.mrw.interscience. wiley.com/cochrane/clsysrev/articles/CD002006/frame.html

Ragnar, I., Altman, D., Tyden, T., & Olsson, S. E. (2006). Comparison of the maternal experience and duration of labour in two upright delivery positions—a randomized controlled trial. *British Journal of Gynecology, 113*(2), 165–170.

9. Methylmercury and PCBs

a. *Actions/expected responses:* When women eat freshwater fish, methylmercury and PCBs may interact when they cross the placenta and enter the developing brain of the fetus to create cell damage.

b. *Routes/dosages/frequencies:* It is best to avoid eating any freshwater fish.

c. *Cautions:* Human health studies indicate that: (a) reproductive function may be disrupted by exposure to PCBs, (b) neurobehavioral and developmental deficits occur in newborns and continue through school-aged children who had in utero exposure to PCBs, (c) other systemic effects (e.g., self-reported liver disease and diabetes, and effects on the thyroid and immune systems) are associated with elevated serum levels of PCBs, and (d) increased cancer risks (e.g., non-Hodgkin's lymphoma) are associated with PCB exposures.

d. *Assessments:* Assess intake of freshwater fish.

e. *Tips on use:* Eat saltwater fish only. (See "Nutrition" section below.)

f. *Other considerations:* None.

g. *References/other sources:*

The Environmental Protection Agency. (2008, July 23). *Basic information on the national forum on contaminants in fish.* Retrieved August 4, 2008, from http://www.epa.gov/fishadvisories/forum/basic.htm

10. Nonstick Chemicals

a. *Actions/expected responses:* Fetuses exposed to chemicals used in nonstick cookware were born at significantly lower body weight.

b. *Routes/dosages/frequencies:* Intrauterine exposure when mother uses nonstick cookware.

c. *Cautions:* The chemicals (high perfluorooctanoate, or PFOA, and perfluo-rooctane sulfonate, or PFOS) have a long half-life in the human body. Even low exposure can result in a low-birth-weight baby.

d. *Assessments:* Assess pregnant women's exposure to nonstick cookware.

e. *Tips on use:* Advise women not to use nonstick cookware.

f. *Other considerations:* None.

g. *References/other sources:*

> Vanderbilt University. (2007, August 24). Non-stick chemicals linked to low birth weight. *ScienceDaily.* Retrieved April 25, 2008, from http://www.sciencedaily.com/releases/2007/08/070823171709.htm

11. Power-frequency fields

a. *Actions/expected responses:* Power-frequency fields are associated with modified brain activity due to electromagnetic fields (EMFs).

b. *Routes/dosages/frequencies:* Current levels of long-term exposure to some kinds of electromagnetic fields are not protective of public health.

c. *Cautions:* Scientific evidence raises concerns about the health impacts of mobile or cell phone radiation, power lines, interior wiring and grounding of buildings, and appliances such as microwaves, wireless technologies, and electric blankets.

d. *Assessments:* Assess exposure to EMFs listed in "Cautions."

e. *Tips on use:* Until new public safety limits and limits on further deploy-ment of risky technologies are warranted, avoid exposure to EMFs.

f. *Other considerations:* An international working group of renowned scientists, researchers, and public health policy professionals (The Bioinitiative Working Group) has released its report on electromag-netic fields and health. It raises serious concerns about the safety of existing public limits that regulate how much EMF is allowable from power lines, cell phones, and many other EMF sources of exposure in daily life.

g. *References and other sources:*

> Hardell, L., & Sage, C. (2007). Biological effects from electromagnetic field exposure and public exposure standards. *Biomedical Pharmacotherapy, 62*(2), 104–109.

12. Smoking

a. *Actions/expected responses:* Pregnant women who suffer from the high-risk condition preeclampsia, which leads to the death of hundreds of babies every year, may be putting the lives of their unborn children at significantly increased risk if they continue to smoke during preg-nancy.

b. *Routes/dosages/frequencies:* If women give up smoking before or even during pregnancy they can significantly reduce these risks.

c. *Cautions:* Preeclampsia and eclampsia cause an estimated 70,000 deaths worldwide among pregnant women each year. Smokers are five times more likely to develop eclampsia.

d. *Assessments:* Assess for smoking.

e. *Tips on use:* Support women in quitting at every stage of pregnancy.

f. *Other considerations:* For smoking cessation information, go to: http://www.helpguide.org/mental/quit_smoking_cessation.htm

g. *References/other sources:*

University of Nottingham. (2008, February 23). Smoking during pregnancy can put mothers and babies at risk. *ScienceDaily.* Retrieved
February 28, 2008, from http://www.sciencedaily.com/releases/
2008/02/080111095354.htm

13. SSRIs linked with birth defects

a. *Actions/expected responses:* Maternal use of selective serotonin reuptake
inhibitors (SSRIs) during pregnancy may be associated with an increased
risk of major birth defects, such as tetralogy of Fallot.

b. *Routes/dosages/frequencies:* The risk was highest with paroxetine (Paxil).

c. *Cautions:* Counsel pregnant women about the potential dangers of taking SSRIs. An overdose or an interaction with other drugs can lead to
hallucinations, agitation, confusion, fluctuating blood pressure, seizures,
fever, stiffness, and irregular heartbeats. A withdrawal syndrome can
occur when stopping Paxil, including dizziness, nausea, headaches, fatigue, poor concentration, mental fogginess, and moodiness. Clinical trials
on Paxil were only conducted for 5 to 16 weeks, so there is no way to know
the longer-term effects of taking this drug.

d. *Assessments:* Assess women's intake of SSRIs.

e. *Tips on use:* Use safer approaches to insomnia, anxiety, depression, and
stress. See "Nutrition," "Exercise/Movement," and "Stress Management"
below for ideas.

f. *Other considerations:* The data were derived from the National Birth Defects Prevention Study, a multisite study of birth defects risk factors based
on standardized telephone interviews with mothers.

g. *References/other sources:*

Alwan, S. (2005). *Use of SSRIs linked with birth defects.* Annual meeting of
the Teratology Society, September 5, St. Petersburg Beach, FL.

14. Vitamin D deficiency

a. *Actions/expected responses:* Vitamin D deficiency early in pregnancy is
associated with a five-fold increased risk of preeclampsia, marked by
soaring blood pressure and swelling of the hands and feet. Preeclampsia,
also known as toxemia, is the leading cause of premature delivery and
maternal and fetal illness and death worldwide.

b. *Routes/dosages/frequencies:* Even a small decline in vitamin D concentration more than doubled the risk of preeclampsia. Because newborn's
vitamin D stores are completely reliant on vitamin D from the mother,
low vitamin levels also were observed in the umbilical cord blood of newborns from mothers with preeclampsia.

c. *Cautions:* Vitamin D deficiency early in life is associated with rickets, as
well as increased risk for type 1 diabetes, asthma, and schizophrenia.

d. *Assessments:* Assess intake of vitamin D.

e. *Tips on use:* Daily sensible sun exposure (4–10 minutes with face and
arms exposed for light-skinned women and 60–80 minutes for dark skin)
can most often provide the needed amount of vitamin D. Sun exposure
should be at solar noon when UVB rays are most directly penetrating.

f. *Other considerations:* Women residing at latitudes north of 35 degrees may
have a difficult time obtaining sufficient sunshine in the wintertime. They
may need to take a tablespoon of cod liver oil daily, eat fatty fish several

times a week, eat eggs several times a week (the yolks are the portion that contain vitamin D), and/or take fish oil supplements.

g. *References/other sources:*

Autoimmunity Research Foundation. (2008, January 27). Vitamin D deficiency study raises new questions about disease and supplements. *ScienceDaily.* Retrieved February 13, 2008, from http://www.science daily.com/releases/2008/01/080125223302.htm

Jocker, B. S. (2007). Vitamin D sufficiency: An approach to disease prevention. *The American Journal for Nurse Practitioners, 11*(10), 43–60.

University of Pittsburgh Schools of the Health Sciences. (2007, September 11). Low vitamin D during pregnancy linked to pre-eclampsia. *ScienceDaily.* Retrieved April 25, 2008, from http://www.sciencedaily. com/releases/2007/09/070907102114.htm

Exercise/Movement

1. Aerobic exercise
   a. *Actions/expected responses:* Significantly lower heart rates occur among fetuses exposed to maternal exercise.
   b. *Routes/dosages/frequencies:* Moderate-to-heavy intensity aerobic activity for 30 minutes per session three times per week.
   c. *Cautions:* Go to yourfitnessguide.blogspot.com/2008/05/exercise-cau tions-for-pregnancy.html.
   d. *Assessments:* Assess exercise participation.
   e. *Tips on use:* Go to http://exercise.lifetips.com.
   f. *Other considerations:* None.
   g. *References/other sources:*

   American Physiological Society. (2008, April 10). Exercise during pregnancy leads to a healthier heart in moms and babies-to-be. *ScienceDaily.* Retrieved April 20, 2008, from http://www.sciencedaily.com/ releases/2008/04/080407114630.htm

2. Kegels for urinary incontinence
   a. *Actions/expected responses:* Carrying the increasing weight of a baby in the pelvis floor, as does childbirth; after a vaginal delivery, nerves around the pelvic floor usually become stretched and bruised and may be unable to make the muscles respond as well. Being overweight or obese, smoking, insufficient fluid intake, caffeine, carbonated drinks, and alcohol also increase the risk of urinary incontinence. Kegel exercises strengthen the pelvic floor and can calm an overactive bladder or stress incontinence.
   b. *Routes/dosages/frequencies:* Teach women to empty their bladder and then hold the muscle that voluntarily stops the stream of urine for a count of 10 seconds then relax for another count of 10 seconds to a daily total of 35 seconds. The bladder can be trained by resisting a premature signal to void and holding urine 5 minutes longer, adding 5 minutes each week until 4 hours elapse between urinations. Vaginal weights can also be purchased to help identify and use the correct muscles.
   c. *Cautions:* Ask women to avoid holding their breath or tightening stomach or leg muscles, and to focus on the muscles of their pelvic floor. Also teach

women to avoid starting and stopping the urine flow when urinating; this can lead to incomplete bladder emptying and bladder infection.

d. *Assessments:* Assess urinary incontinence prior to and after completing Kegels and bladder training.

e. *Tips on use:* Start a 2-day diary of urination history, including incontinence and what triggered each event, and voiding into a measured container to keep track of amounts passed. For information on vaginal weights, see Johnson (2000). If Kegels are unsuccessful, go to http://www.massageto day.com/mpacms/mt/article.php?id=13515

f. *Other considerations:* None.

g. *References/other sources:*

Dallosso, H. M., McGrother, C. W., Matthews, R. J., & Donaldson, M. M. K. (2003). Association of diet and other lifestyle factors with overactive bladder and stress incontinence: A longitudinal study in women. *British Journal of Urology International, 92*(1), 69.

Johnson, S. T. (2000). From incontinence to confidence. *American Journal of Nursing, 100*(2), 69–75.

Shamliyan, T. A., Kane, R. L., Wyman, J., & Wilt, T. J. (2008). Systematic review: Randomized, controlled trials of nonsurgical treatments for urinary incontinence in women. *Annals of Internal Medicine, 148*(6), 459–473.

3. Yoga

a. *Actions/expected responses:* Compared to a control group, pregnant women who participated in yoga had higher levels of maternal comfort during labor and 2 hours postlabor, experienced less subject-evaluated labor pain, a shorter first stage of labor, and a shorter total time of labor.

b. *Routes/dosages/frequencies:* Six 1-hour sessions at prescribed weeks during pregnancy.

c. *Cautions:* Go to http://yoga.lifetips.com/cat/56770/yoga-cautions/

d. *Assessments:* Assess pregnant women's participation in yoga. Assess effect of engaging in yoga on labor.

e. *Tips on use:* Go to http://www.santosha.com/asanas/asana.html

f. *Other considerations:* None.

g. *References/other sources:*

Chuntharapat, S., Petpichetchian, W., & Hatthakit, U. (2008). Yoga during pregnancy: Effects on maternal comfort, labor pain and birth outcomes. *Complementary Therapies in Clinical Practice, 14*(2), 105–115.

Herbs/Essential Oils

1. Aromatherapy

a. *Actions/expected responses:* Aromatherapy can optimize a woman's coping skills during labor, helping to release endorphins, and reducing the use of oxytocin to help with contractions. Women who used aromatherapy were significantly less likely to have an epidural, irrespective of parity and labor onset. Aromatherapy also altered the culture of the maternity unit, making people more kind to each other.

b. *Routes/dosages/frequencies:* A drop of essential oil was placed on a pillow or T-shirt, in a footbath, in a massage oil, or in a compress.

c. *Cautions:* Counsel women to use essential oils cautiously and avoid using larger than therapeutic doses (see "Routes/dosages/frequencies.")

d. *Assessments:* Assess labor difficulties prior to and after using aromatherapy.

e. *Tips on use:* Drops of essential oils are used as needed. Lavender, frankincense, rose, jasmine, and chamomile essential oils can be used for anxiety, peppermint for nausea and vomiting, and clary sage to assist contractions and enhance labor.

f. *Other considerations:* None.

g. *References/other sources:*

Liptak, E. (2002). Aromatherapy in childbirth: Lightening the labor. *Integrative Nursing, 1*(1), 10.

2. Ginger

a. *Actions/expected responses:* Effectively treats stomach upset and nausea and vomiting at least as effectively as the medical treatment (central nervous system anticholinergics) and without any side effects.

b. *Routes/dosages/frequencies:* Fresh ginger, available in supermarkets, is recommended by the American College of Obstetricians and Gynecologists.

c. *Cautions:* Allergic reactions are rare and ginger is as safe as placebo.

d. *Assessments:* Assess level of nausea, vomiting, and stomach upset. Assess symptoms prior to and after taking ginger.

e. *Tips on use:* Fresh ginger can be scraped into stews, soups, salads, oatmeal, and other cereals, even sandwiches.

f. *Other considerations:* The new antiemetics for nausea and vomiting are very costly; ginger is a very inexpensive, safe, healthy, and tasty alternative.

g. *References/other sources:*

Niebyl, I. R., & Goodwin, T. M. (2002). Overview of nausea and vomiting of pregnancy with an emphasis on vitamins and ginger. *American Journal of Obstetrics and Gynecology, 186*(5 Suppl.), S253–S255.

Sego, S. (2007, April). Alternative meds update: Ginger. *The Clinical Advisor,* 159–160.

Mindset

1. Affirmations

a. *Actions/expected responses:* Self-affirmation of personal values and beliefs buffers neuroendocrine and psychological stress.

b. *Routes/dosages/frequencies:* Repeat aloud or write positive affirmations up to 20 times a day such as, "I lovingly carry life inside me" and "My baby is perfect in every way."

c. *Cautions:* Ensure affirmations are positive and acceptable.

d. *Assessments:* Assess anxiety prior to and after completing affirmations for a week.

e. *Tips on use*: Write favorite affirmations on 3 by 5 cards and place them where they will be read frequently.

f. *Other considerations:* Find more affirmations information at http://www.successconsciousness.com/index_00000a.htm

g. *References/other sources:*

Hay, L. (2000). *Heal your body*. Carlsbad, CA: Hay House.

Schwarzer, R., Babler, J., Kwiatek, P., Schroder, K., & Zang, J. W. (1997). The assessment of optimistic self-beliefs: Assessment of general perceived self-efficacy in thirteen cultures. *World Psychology, 3*(1–2), 177–190.

2. Parental identity

a. *Actions/expected responses:* Early relationships color pregnant women's views of what to expect from their pregnancy.

b. *Routes/dosages/frequencies:* Women whose early childhood relationships with their parents were fraught with rejection and unresolved conflicts expected their child to be more demanding of them and to need more boundaries. Women who described their childhood relationships with their parents as rejecting but had difficulty recalling many of the representative events expected to develop a less warm and close relationship with their baby. Women who had a balanced view of their early experiences with their parents had the most optimal expectations toward impending motherhood. Women who had goals they wanted to reach were more positive than those concerned with self-defense, security, and responsibility.

c. *Cautions:* If concerned about parental role, go to http://www.perinatal project.com/links_women.php

d. *Assessments:* Assess thoughts, perceptions and feelings about parental identity.

e. *Tips on use:* Choose tools from "Cautions" and "Other considerations" to help adapt better to the transition to motherhood.

f. *Other considerations:* For more tools, go to http://www.mindtools.com/smpage.html

g. *References/other sources:*

University of Haifa. (2008, February 27). What women think during their first pregnancy. *ScienceDaily*. Retrieved March 9, 2008, from http://www.sciencedaily.com/releases/2008/02/080226092744.htm

Nutrition

1. Caffeine

a. *Actions/expected responses:* Caffeinated coffee, tea, soda, or hot chocolate are associated with an increased risk of miscarriage.

b. *Routes/dosages/frequencies:* Women who consumed two or more cups of regular coffee or five 12-ounce cans per day of caffeinated soda had twice the miscarriage risk as women who consumed no caffeine.

c. *Cautions:* Women should stop caffeine consumption during pregnancy to reduce the risk of miscarriage.

d. *Assessments:* Assess caffeine intake.

e. *Tips on use:* To reduce caffeine intake, counsel women to mix 1/2 coffee with 1/2 decaffeinated coffee and slowly reduce to decaffeinated coffee only and then switch to a cereal beverage such as Cafix; even decaffein-ated coffee contains caffeine, and the beans have been sprayed with toxic pesticides.

f. *Other considerations:* Because caffeine is a drug, it is best to slowly de-crease tea, caffeinated soda, or chocolate from the diet. Teach women to use natural energy boosts like a brisk walk, yoga stretches, or snacking on dried fruits and nuts.

g. *References/other sources:*

Kaiser Permanente Division of Research. (2008, January 22). Caffeine is linked to miscarriage risk, new study shows. *ScienceDaily.* Re-trieved January 30, 2008, from http://www.sciencedaily.com/releases/2008/01/080121080402.htm

2. Calcium

a. *Actions/expected responses:* In 12 studies comparing at least 1 gram of cal-cium daily during pregnancy with placebo, calcium reduced the rate of preeclampsia and reduced the rare occurrence of the outcome of maternal death or serious morbidity. Adequate dietary calcium before and in early pregnancy may be needed to prevent underlying pathology responsible for preeclampsia.

b. *Routes/dosages/frequencies:* 1,500 mg per day.

c. *Cautions:* Without adequate daily calcium, high blood pressure, maternal death, and serious morbidity can result.

d. *Assessments:* Assess daily intake of calcium.

e. *Tips on use:* Eat high-calcium foods daily. For foods high in calcium, go to www.health.gov/dietaryguidelines/dga2005/document/html/appendixB.htm and scroll to calcium.

f. *Other considerations:* Some of the highest sources of nondairy calcium in-clude soy beverages, sardines, tofu, and pink salmon with bones.

g. *References/other sources:*

Hofmeyr, G. J., Duley, L., & Atallah, A. (2007). Dietary calcium supplemen-tation for prevention of pre-eclampsia and related problems: A sys-tematic review and commentary. *British Journal of Gynecology, 114*(8), 933–934.

3. Copper

a. *Actions/expected responses:* Copper within certain enzymes in the brain help form key neurotransmitters that allow brain cells to talk to one an-other. Adequate amounts of copper are critical to the fetus during preg-nancy but 8%–12% of childbearing-age women have inadequate copper intakes.

b. *Routes/dosages/frequencies:* Eating a balanced diet containing a variety of nutritious foods is the best approach to getting adequate copper, including beef liver, mushrooms, trail mix, barley, and canned tomato puree.

c. *Cautions:* Without adequate copper, the fetus brain may not develop.

d. *Assessments:* Assess intake of copper.

e. *Tips on use:* Add high copper foods to daily diet.

f. *Other considerations:* The areas of the brain most affected by low-copper diets are the gyrus and hippocampal areas, most important to high brain functions, such as learning.

g. *References/other sources:*

U.S. Department of Agriculture. (2007, October 9). Copper: An important nutrient for fetal brain development. *ScienceDaily*. Retrieved April 26, 2008, from http://www.sciencedaily.com/releases/2007/10/071006084704.htm

4. Eating and weight patterns prior to pregnancy
   a. *Actions/expected responses:* Eating junk food while pregnant and breastfeeding may lead to obese offspring. Maternal obesity prior to pregnancy is associated with birth defects, greater risk of having hyperactive children, and difficulty breastfeeding.
   b. *Routes/dosages/frequencies:* Losing weight prior to becoming pregnant and changing to healthier eating patterns can have significant effects on women and their offspring.
   c. *Cautions:* Maintaining a normal healthy weight before, during, and after pregnancy is important. Gaining weight between pregnancies can lead to preeclampsia, diabetes, pregnancy-induced high blood pressure and high birth weight. Losing weight between pregnancies can lead to giving birth prematurely.
   d. *Assessments:* Assess weight prior to becoming pregnant.
   e. *Tips on use:* Attain a healthy weight prior to first pregnancy. Avoid junk food while pregnant. For more information, go to http://www.weightlossresources.co.uk/diet/diet_tips.htm
   f. *References/other sources:*
      British Medical Journal. (2007, July 30). Weight gain or weight loss can affect unborn baby. *ScienceDaily*. Retrieved April 27, 2008, from http://www.sciencedaily.com/releases/2007/07/070726193820.htm
      JAMA and Archives Journals. (2007, August 9). Maternal obesity prior to pregnancy associated with birth defects. *ScienceDaily*. Retrieved April 27, 2008, from http://www.sciencedaily.com/releases/2007/08/070806164539.htm
      Jevitt, C., Hernandez, I., & Groer, M. (2007). Lactation complicated by overweight and obesity: Supporting the mother and newborn. *Journal of Midwifery and Women's Health, 52*(6), 606–613.
      Upsala University. (2007, November 1). Overweight mothers run greater risk of having hyperactive children. *ScienceDaily*. Retrieved November 12, 2007, from http://www.sciencedaily.com/releases/2007/11/071101092754.htm
      Wellcome Trust. (2007, August 15). Eating junk food while pregnant and breastfeeding may lead to obese offspring. *ScienceDaily*. Retrieved April 27, 2008, from http://www.sciencedaily.com/releases/2007/08/070814212154.htm

5. Fiber
   a. *Actions/expected responses:* Exposure to whole wheat during pregnancy may reduce offspring's breast cancer risk by improving DNA damage repair mechanisms.
   b. *Routes/dosages/frequencies:* Daily ingestion of whole wheat products.
   c. *Cautions:* Some women are hypersensitive to wheat and should use rolled oats.
   d. *Assessments:* Assess for hypersensitivity to wheat.

e. *Tips on use:* Whole wheat foods include whole wheat breads, whole wheat cereals, whole wheat muffins, whole wheat pasta, and whole wheat cookies.

f. *Other considerations:* None.

g. *References/other sources:*

Yu, B., Khan, G., Foxworth, A., Huang, K., & Hilakivi-Clarke, L. (2006). Maternal dietary exposure to fiber during pregnancy and mammary tumorigenesis among rat offspring. *International Journal of Cancer, 119*(10), 2279–2286.

6. Fish

a. *Actions/expected responses:* More than 90% of women consume less than the FDA recommended amount of fish. This leads to an inadequate intake of omega-3 fatty acids resulting in risks to their health and the health of their unborn children. Some data show a connection with reduced preterm labor and postpartum depression in mothers who ate ocean fish when pregnant. A fish-rich diet in pregnancy can help to protect children from asthma and allergies.

b. *Routes/dosages/frequencies:* A minimum of 12 ounces per week of fish like salmon, tuna, sardines, and Spanish mackerel.

c. *Cautions:* Avoid fresh-water fish.

d. *Assessments:* Assess intake of fish.

e. *Tips on use:* Although fish may contain some mercury, they also contain selenium, an essential mineral, that appears to protect against the toxicity from trace amounts of mercury.

f. *Other considerations:* None.

g. *References/other sources:*

Mediterranean diet in pregnancy helps ward off childhood asthma and allergy. (2008). *ScienceDaily.* Retrieved April 27, 2008, from http://www.sciencedaily.com/releases/2008/01/080115170113.htm

National Healthy Mothers, Healthy Babies Coalition. (2007, October 5). Pregnant women should eat fish after all, experts urge. *ScienceDaily.* Retrieved April 26, 2008, from http://www.sciencedaily.com/releases/2007/10/071004133313.htm

7. Folate

a. *Actions/expected responses:* Folic acid reduces the risk of recurrent early pregnancy loss, birth defects in newborns, preeclampsia in pregnant women, and may protect offspring from colorectal cancer. Low-carb diets take a toll on women's folate levels.

b. *Routes/dosages/frequencies:* 400 micrograms (mcg) a day. Leafy green vegetables (like spinach and turnip greens), fruits (citrus fruits and juices), and dried beans and peas are all natural sources of folate that can help meet the suggested amount per day.

c. *Cautions:* Women on diets who do not eat breads, cereals, or pasta, who abuse alcohol, or who take medications that interfere with folate absorption may not receive sufficient amounts of the nutrient and may need additional amounts. Medications and medical conditions that increase the need for folate or result in an increased excretion of folate include: anticonvulsant medications, metformin, sulfasalazine, triamterene, methotrexate, barbiturates, pregnancy and lactation, alcohol abuse, malabsorption, kidney dialysis, liver disease, and certain anemias. Because folate is a water-soluble B-vitamin, unneeded amounts will be eliminated in the urine.

d. *Assessments:* Assess for signs of folate deficiency: anemia, diarrhea, loss of appetite, weight loss, weakness, sore tongue, headaches, heart palpitations, irritability, forgetfulness, behavioral disorders, and an elevated level of homocysteine.

e. *Tips on use:* Avoid flour-fortified foods as a source of folic acid; new research has shown the introduction of flour fortified with folic acid into common foods has been linked to colon cancer. Folate can be lost from foods during cooking, so counsel women to serve fruits and vegetables raw whenever possible and to store vegetables in the refrigerator. Eat whole grain cereals, breads, and pasta to avoid fortified flours.

f. *Other considerations:* Exceeding 1,000 micrograms (mcg) per day of folate may trigger vitamin B12 deficiency. To compensate, take a multivitamin that contains B12 or eat at least one food daily that contains B12: nutritional yeast (unless susceptible to candida), clams, eggs, herring, kidney, liver, Spanish mackerel, seafood, milk, or dairy products.

g. *References/other sources:*

American Association for Cancer Research. (2008, April 16). Folic acid supplementation provided in utero, but not after birth, may protect offspring from colorectal cancer. *ScienceDaily*. Retrieved April 24, 2008, from http://www.sciencedaily.com/releases/2008/04/08041 3183000. htm

Low carb, low folate? (2007). *Clinician Reviews, 17*(2), 14.

Murphy, M. (2004). *Folate fact sheet.* Retrieved April 16, 2007, from http://ohioline.osu.edu/hyg-fact/5000/5533.html

University of Ottawa. (2008, January 24). Large study links folic acid supplementation with reduced risk of preeclampsia during pregnancy. *ScienceDaily*. Retrieved January 30, 2008, from http://www.science daily.com/releases/2008/01/080123113752.htm

Willianne, L., Nelen, D. M., Blom, H. J., Steegers, E. A. P., Heijer, M. D., Thomas, C., et al. (2000). Homocysteine and folate levels as risk factors for recurrent early pregnancy loss. *Obstetrics and Gynecology, 95*, 519–524.

Wright, J., Dainty, J., & Fingles, P. (2007). Folic acid metabolism in human subjects: Potential implications for proposed mandatory folic acid fortification in the UK. *British Journal of Nutrition, 98*, 667–675.

8. Trans fat, sugar, and fertility

a. *Actions/expected responses:* Women who ate less trans fat and sugar from carbohydrates, consumed more protein from vegetables (not animals), ate more fiber and iron, took more multivitamins, weighed less, exercised for longer periods of time each day, and consumed more high-fat dairy products (not low-fat) were 89% more fertile. A six-fold difference in ovulatory infertility risk occurred between women following five or more low-risk dietary and lifestyle habits and those following none.

b. *Routes/dosages/frequencies:* Daily adherence to a fertility lifestyle.

c. *Cautions:* Merely changing one lifestyle factor is probably not sufficient to increase fertility. The more fertility factors followed, the more infertility risk drops.

d. *Assessments:* Assess infertility.

e. *Tips on use:* For tips on lowering trans fat use, go to http://www.hsph.harvard.edu/nutritionsource/nutrition-news/transfats/

f. *Other considerations:* None.

g. *References/other sources:*

Harvard School of Public Health. (2007, November 4). Diet and lifestyle changes may help prevent infertility from ovulatory disorders. *ScienceDaily*. Retrieved November 29, 2007, from http://www.sciencedaily.com/releases/2007/10/071031114319.htm

Stress Management

1. Anxious or depressed mothers-to-be

a. *Actions/expected responses:* Anxious or depressed mothers-to-be are at increased risk of having children who will experience sleep problems or cerebral palsy.

b. *Routes/dosages/frequencies:* Mothers classified as clinically anxious or depressed 18 weeks into pregnancy, compared to their nondepressed or nonanxious counterparts, were about 40% more likely to have an 18-month-old who refused to go to bed, woke up early, and kept crawling out of bed. The child's behavior often persisted until age 30 months. Chronic mild stress in pregnant mothers may increase the risk that their offspring will develop cerebral palsy.

c. *Cautions:* Limit stress to help reduce sleep disorders and/or cerebral palsy in offspring.

d. *Assessments:* Assess stress level.

e. *Tips on use:* Go to http://www.mindtools.com for ways to help pregnant women reduce their stress.

f. *Other considerations:* None.

g. *References/other sources:*

Society for Neuroscience. (2007, July 12). Mild stress in the womb may worsen risk of cerebral palsy. *ScienceDaily*. Retrieved April 27, 2008, from http://www.sciencedaily.com/releases/2007/07/070711105828.htm

University of Rochester Medical Center. (2007, July 30). Prenatal stress keeps infants, toddlers up at night, study says. *ScienceDaily*. Retrieved April 27, 2008, from http://www.sciencedaily.com/releases/2007/07/070727122926.htm

2. Hypnotherapy for labor

a. *Actions/expected responses:* Hypnosis has been shown to reduce labor length and pain levels, increase enjoyment of labor, and stop preterm labor.

b. *Routes/dosages/frequencies:* As needed.

c. *Cautions:* Go to http://www.ncpamd.com/medical_hypnosis.htm#Contraindications_for_Hypnosis

d. *Assessments:* Assess need for hypnotherapy.

e. *Tips on use:* Go to http://psychceu.com/peterson/hypnosis.html

f. *Other considerations:* None.

    g. *References/other sources:*

> Brown, D. C., & Hammond, D. C. (2007). Evidence-based clinical hypnosis for obstetrics, labor and delivery, and preterm labor. *International Journal of Clinical Hypnosis, 55*(3), 355–371.

Supplements

1. Multivitamin
   a. *Actions/expected responses:* Women taking a multivitamin before conception through week 12 of pregnancy significantly reduced nausea and vomiting.
   b. *Routes/dosages/frequencies:* One tablet or capsule per day.
   c. *Cautions:* Choose products without additional fillers, dyes, iron, and unnecessary ingredients.
   d. *Assessments:* Assess multivitamin use.
   e. *Tips on use:* None.
   f. *Other considerations:* Lifestyle actions that can reduce nausea and vomiting, include: eat frequently and in small amounts; eat high-carbohydrates (fruits, vegetables, dried beans and dried peas, whole grains) and low-fat, except for 1–2 tablespoons of extra virgin olive oil on salads or to use in low-heat cooking; eat high protein, especially nonanimal foods (soy burgers, soy chips, soy milk, soy cheese, tempeh, beans and rice); avoid spicy foods and any offensive smells; drink clear liquids such as lemonade and ginger ale; lie down and rest as needed; change position slowly, especially when rising; get outside and breathe in fresh air; brush teeth an hour after eating to avoid nausea and vomiting due to excess salivation or smell of toothpaste.
   g. *References/other sources:*

   > Ahn, E., Pairaudeau, N., Pairaudeau, N., Jr., Cerat, Y., Couturier, B., Fortier, A., et al. (2006). A randomized cross over trial of tolerability and compliance of a micronutrient supplement with low iron separated from calcium vs high iron combined with calcium in pregnant women. *BiomedCentral, 4*(6), 10.
   >
   > Hunter, L. P., Sullivan, C. A., Young, R. E., & Weber, C. E. (2007). Nausea and vomiting of pregnancy: Clinical management. *The American Journal for Nurse Practitioner, 11*(8), 57–67.

2. Probiotics
   a. *Actions/expected responses:* Listeria monocytogenes is particularly dangerous during pregnancy. A probiotic taken during pregnancy could provide protection in a form that would be acceptable to expectant mothers.
   b. *Routes/dosages/frequencies:* Lactobacillus salivarius is available as a supplement at health foods stores. One to ten billion organisms by mouth.
   c. *Cautions:* A nondairy form should be used by women hypersensitive to milk.
   d. *Assessments:* Assess for lactose intolerance.
   e. *Tips on use:* Keep probiotics in the refrigerator. Follow directions on bottle.

f. *Other considerations:* The probiotic kills Listeria monocytogenes by producing an antibiotic-like compound called a bacteriocin.

g. *References/other sources:*

Corr, S. C., Li, Y., Riedel, C. U., O'Toole, P. W., Hill, C., & Gahan, C. G. M. (2007). Bacteriocin production as a mechanism for the antiinfective activity of Lactobacillus salivarius UCC118. *Proceedings of the National Academy of Sciences, 104*(18), 7617–7621.

3. Pycnogenol

a. *Actions/expected responses:* Thrombotic events (blood clots in the legs) are the leading cause of death in pregnant women. Pycnogenol has been shown to prevent venous thrombosis and thrombophlebitis in moderate-to high-risk women.

b. *Routes/dosages/frequencies:* Two to three 100-mg capsules per day with a glass of water.

c. *Cautions:* Can cause reduced blood platelet aggregation (clotting). Otherwise this supplement is safe except for women who are hypersensitive to pine.

d. *Assessments:* Assess for previous thrombotic events, smoking, and alcohol use.

e. *Tips on use:*. Follow directions on bottle.

f. *Other considerations:* Pycnogenol is a mixture of bioflavonoids found in pine bark.

g. *References/other sources:*

Belcaro, G., Cesarone, M. R., Rohdewald, P., Ricci, A., Ippolito, E., Dugall, M., et al. (2004). Prevention of venous thrombosis and thrombophlebitis in long-haul flights with pycnogenol. *Clinical Applications of Thrombosis/Hemostasis, 10*(4), 373–377.

James, A. Jamison, M., Brancazio, L., & Myers, E. (2006). Venous thromboembolism during pregnancy and the postpartum period: Incidence, risk factors, and mortality. *American Journal of Obstetrics and Gynecology, 194*(5), 1311–1315.

Risk factors that develop in pregnancy: Thromboembolic events. (2003). Retrieved April 28, 2008, from http://www.merck.com/mmhe/sec22/ch258/ch258c.html

4. Vitamin B6

a. *Actions/expected responses:* Vitamin B6 can create a significant reduction in vomiting and severe nausea.

b. *Routes/dosages/frequencies:* 10–25 mg three times a day.

c. *Cautions:* Avoid exceeding 75 mg a day.

d. *Assessments:* Assess intake of vitamin B6

e. *Tips on use:* Store vitamin B6 in a cool, dry place.

f. *References/other sources:*

Hunter, L. P., Sullivan, C. A., Young, R. E., & Weber, C. E. (2007). Nausea and vomiting of pregnancy: Clinical management. *The American Journal for Nurse Practitioner, 11*(8), 57–67.

Niebyl, I. R., & Goodwin, T. M. (2002). Overview of nausea and vomiting of pregnancy with an emphasis on vitamins and ginger. *American Journal of Obstetrics and Gynecology, 186*(5 Suppl.), S253–S255.

Sripramote, M., & Lekhyananda, N. (2003). A randomized comparison of ginger and vitamin B6 in the treatment of nausea and vomiting of pregnancy. *Journal of Medical Association Thailand, 86*(9), 846–853.

Touch

1. Acupressure on labor pain during first stage of labor
   a. *Actions/expected responses:* Compared to light skin stroking or no treatment/conversation only, acupressure showed a significant difference in decreased labor pain during the active phase of the first stage of labor.
   b. *Routes/dosages/frequencies:* Use: L14 (at the midpoint radial side) and BL67 (just behind small toe).
   c. *Cautions:* Force must not be applied. Use body weight to lean into a point or meridian when applying pressure. For contraindications, go to http://www.kemh.health.wa.gov.au/development/manuals/sectionb/4/8275.pdf
   d. *Assessments:* Assess labor pain prior to and after acupressure.
   e. *Tips on use:* Another point that may bring relief is acupoint pericardium 8. It is located in the center of the palm where the middle finger touches the palms when the hand is bent forward.
   f. *Other considerations:* Go to http://www.kemh.health.wa.gov.au/development/manuals/sectionb/4/8275.pdf
   g. *References/other sources:*
      Chung, U. L., Hung, L. C., Kuo, S. C., & Huang, C. L. (2003). Effects of L14 and BL 67 acupressure on labor pain and uterine contractions in the first stage of labor. *Journal of Nursing Research, 11*(4), 251–260.
2. Acupressure on nausea and vomiting during pregnancy
   a. *Actions/expected responses:* Acupressure to P6 acupoint reduced the symptoms of nausea and vomiting during pregnancy, as compared to acupressure to a sham point on the top of the wrist.
   b. *Routes/dosages/frequencies:* Applying acupressure bands to P6 point on the inside of the wrists all day.
   c. *Cautions:* None known.
   d. *Assessments:* Assess nausea and vomiting prior to and after applying the acupressure bands.
   e. *Tips on use:* According to customers at Amazon.com, at least two types are available, but the bell-shape style may be uncomfortable for some women. The model with elastic bands and a disk shape may be more comfortable; it stays in place and is not as tight. http://www.amazon.com/review/product/B0007DHMZG/ref=cm_cr_dp_hist_3?%5Fencoding=UTF8&filterBy=addThreeStar
   f. *Other considerations:* None.
   g. *References/other sources:*
      Gurkan, O., & Arslan, H. (2008). Effect of acupressure on nausea and vomiting during pregnancy. *Complementary Therapies in Clinical Practice, 14*(1), 46–52.
3. Massage therapy for depressed pregnant women
   a. *Actions/expected responses:* Immediately after massage therapy sessions, pregnant women reported lower levels of anxiety and depressed mood

and less leg and back pain, as compared to a progressive muscle relaxation group and a control group that received standard prenatal care.

b. *Routes/dosages/frequencies:* 20-minute sessions by their significant others each week for 16 weeks of pregnancy, starting during the second trimester.

c. *Cautions:* Go to http://nccam.nih.gov/health/massage/

d. *Assessments:* Teach significant other to assess levels of anxiety, depression, and leg and back pain prior to and after massage.

e. *Tips on use:* Go to http://www.ehow.com/how_2044911_give-massage.html

f. *Other considerations:* None.

g. *References/other sources:*

Field, T., Diego, M. A., Hernandez-Reif, M., Schanberg, S., & Kuhn, C. (2004). Massage therapy effects on depressed pregnant women. *Journal of Psychosomatic and Obstetrical Gynaecology, 25*(2), 115–132.

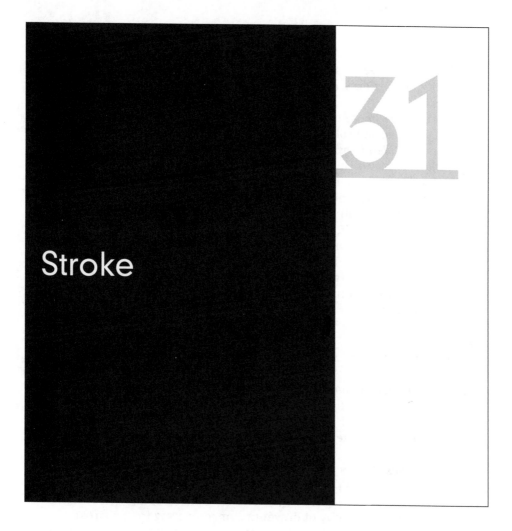

31

Stroke

Medical treatment for stroke includes antiplatelets, anticoagulants, salicylates, thrombolytic agents and surgery, all of which carry negative side effects. Evidence-based complementary approaches are available and have few, if any, side effects.

Environment

1. Music
   a. *Actions/expected responses:* In recovery from a stroke, members of a music-listening group improved verbal memory by 60% (as compared to 18% in audio book listeners and 29% in nonlisteners), improved ability to control and perform mental operations and resolve conflicts among responses by 17% (as compared to zero for the other two groups), and experienced less depressed and confused moods than the control group.
   b. *Routes/dosages/frequencies:* Starting within the first weeks of recovery, and listening daily to music in a self-chosen genre.
   c. *Cautions:* None known.

    d. *Assessments:* Assess preference for music genre. Assess memory and ability to perform mental operations prior to and after listening to music.

    e. *Tips on use:* Choose music with lyrics. Research suggests it is the combination of music and voice that plays a crucial role in improved recovery.

    f. *Other considerations:* Other ways that listening to music can help with stroke recovery include enhanced arousal (alertness), attention, and mood, mediated by dopaminergic mesocorticolimbic system that gives feelings of reward, pleasure, and arousal; directly stimulating damaged areas of the brain; and stimulating general areas of brain plasticity and helping the brain to repair itself.

    g. *References/other sources:*

        University of Helsinki. (2008, February 21). Listening to music improves stroke patients' recovery, study shows. *ScienceDaily*. Retrieved February 28, 2008, from http://www.sciencedaily.com/releases/2008/02/08021920 3554.htm

2. Social network

    a. *Actions/expected responses*: Having many friends and family members appears to be associated with a dramatically lower risk of suffering a stroke.

    b. *Routes/dosages/frequencies:* This can be an intense relationship with one or two other close friends or significant others and can be developed in church groups, work groups, or recreational groups.

    c. *Cautions:* Encourage women to think of disease as more than a physical condition.

    d. *Assessments:* Assess psychological and environmental characteristics that make women more prone to be socially isolated.

    e. *Tips on use:* Encourage women to spend time developing friends and a social network as a way of preventing or recovering from a stroke.

    f. *Other considerations:* Some theories include the idea that socioeconomic factors, such as the possibility that being socially isolated feeds into worse health outcomes. Women who cannot afford a bus pass and are relatively tied to their home can't go out to lunch with friends for financial reasons and can become more socially isolated. This can lead to not having friends check on them or be available to bring them for care when their health fails.

    g. *References/other sources:*

        Ross, M. F. (2005). *Size, strength of social networks influence heart disease risk.* Press release, University of Florida, Gainesville, Office of the Senior Vice President for Health Affairs, Office of News and Communications.

3. Water

    a. *Actions/expected responses:* Water replaces lost fluids, while caffeinated beverages or alcohol increase fluid output, leeching out needed liquids, minerals, and vitamins. Dehydration has been linked to stroke.

    b. *Routes/dosages/frequencies:* At least 8–10 glasses a day.

    c. *Cautions:* Tap water and even bottled water can contain parasites, weed killers, nitrates (correlated with spontaneous miscarriage and so-called blue-baby syndrome), salmonella, E. coli, chlorine, fluoride, and other potentially dangerous substances.

    d. *Assessments:* Assess type and quantity of water women drink.

e. *Tips on use:* Drink (and cook with) only distilled water or reverse-osmosis filtered water.

f. *Other considerations:* Fluid intake is probably adequate when thirst is rarely experienced and when urine is colorless or slightly yellow. As women age, they may experience less thirst. Drink water before thirst sets in because by that time dehydration may already have taken over.

g. *References/other sources:*

Doull, J., Boekelheide, K., Farishian, B. G., Isaacson, R. L., Klotz, J. B., Limeback. H., et al. (2006). *Committee on Fluoride in Drinking Water Board on Environmental Studies and Toxicology, Division of Earth and Life Sciences, National Research Council of the National Academies. Fluoride in drinking water: A scientific review of EPA's standards.* Washington, DC: National Academies Press.

Manz, F. (2007). Hydration and disease. *Journal of American College of Nutrition, 26*(5 Suppl.), 535S–541S.

Exercise/Movement

1. Exercise
   a. *Actions/expected responses:* A high level of leisure time physical activity reduces the risk of all subtypes of stroke. Daily active commuting also reduces the risk of ischemic stroke.
   b. *Routes/dosages/frequencies:* 20–30 minutes of leisure time high physical activity and daily active commuting.
   c. *Cautions:* See http://www.webmd.com/fitness-exercise/exercise-precautions
   d. *Assessments:* Assess exercise patterns.
   e. *Tips on use:* Go to http://exercise.lifetips.com
   f. *Other considerations:* None.
   g. *References/other sources:*

   Chong, L., Folson, A. R., & Blair, S. N. (2003). Physical activity and stroke risk: A meta-analysis. *Stroke, 34*(10), 2475–2481.

   Hu, G., Sarti, C., Jousilahti, P., Silventoinen, K., Barengo, N. C., & Tuomilehto, J. (2005). Leisure time, occupational, and commuting physical activity and the risk of stroke. *Stroke, 36*(9), 1994–1999.

2. Occupational therapy
   a. *Actions/expected responses:* In nine randomized trials, occupational therapy reduced poststroke deterioration in eating, dressing, bathing, toileting, and moving about in social activities, when compared to usual care.
   b. *Routes/dosages/frequencies:* Not yet known.
   c. *Cautions:* None known.
   d. *Assessments:* Assess need for occupational therapy poststroke.
   e. *Tips on use:* None.
   f. *Other considerations:* For more information about occupational therapy, go to http://stroke.about.com/b/2006/10/26/occupational-therapy-in-stroke-rehabilitation.htm.
   g. *References/other sources:*

   Alper, B. S. (2008, April). Evidence-based medicine: Occupational therapy reduces post-stroke deterioration in ADLs. *The Clinical Advisor,* 129–130.

Herbs/Essential Oils

1. Garlic
   a. *Actions/expected responses:* Aged garlic extract (AGE) exerts inhibition on platelet aggregation and adhesion that may be important in the development of stroke.
   b. *Routes/dosages/frequencies:* 3/4 tsp daily AGE or one to three cloves of garlic.
   c. *Cautions:* Avoid concurrent use with anticoagulants. Should not be used during pregnancy or lactation, but dietary amounts are acceptable. AGE should not be used by women with stomach inflammation or hypersensitivity to this herb.
   d. *Assessments:* Assess the items listed under "Cautions."
   e. *Tips on use:* Use dietary garlic if possible to eliminate cautions.
   f. *Other considerations:* None.
   g. *References/other sources:*
      Steiner, M., & Li, W. (2001). Aged garlic extract, a modulator of cardiovascular risk factors: A dose-finding study on the effects of AGE on platelet functions. *Journal of Nutrition, 131*(3S), 980S–984S.

Mindset

1. Affirmations
   a. *Actions/expected responses:* Self-affirmation of personal values and belief buffers neuroendocrine and psychological stress.
   b. *Routes/dosages/frequencies:* Repeat aloud or write positive affirmations up to 20 times a day such as, "I easily adapt to the new" and "I accept change and life joyfully."
   c. *Cautions:* Ensure affirmations are positive and acceptable.
   d. *Assessments:* Assess anxiety prior to and after completing affirmations for a week.
   e. *Tips on use:* Write favorite affirmations on 3 by 5 cards and place them where they will be read frequently.
   f. *Other considerations:* Find more affirmations information at http://www.successconsciousness.com/index_00000a.htm
   g. *References/other sources:*
      Hay, L. (2000). *Heal your body.* Carlsbad, CA: Hay House.
      Schwarzer, R., Babler, J., Kwiatek, P., Schroder, K., & Zang, J. W. (1997). The assessment of optimistic self-beliefs: Assessment of general perceived self-efficacy in thirteen cultures. *World Psychology, 3*(1–2), 177–190.

Nutrition

1. DASH Diet
   a. *Actions/expected responses:* Greater intake of fruits, vegetables, whole grains, nuts, and legumes is associated with a lower risk for stroke. Greater intake of red and processed meats, sweetened beverages, and sodium is associated with increased risk for stroke.

b. *Routes/dosages/frequencies:* Daily ingestion.

c. *Cautions:* Reduce or eliminate intake of red and processed meats, sweetened beverages, and sodium to reduce risk for stroke.

d. *Assessments:* Assess intake of foods associated with stroke.

e. *Tips on use:* For nutritional ideas, go to http://nutrition.about.com/od/change yourdiet/Diet.htm

f. *Other considerations:* None.

g. *References/other sources:*

JAMA and Archives Journals. (2008, April 15). Blood pressure-lowering diet also may be associated with lower risk for heart disease, stroke. *ScienceDaily.* Retrieved April 24, 2008, from http://www.sciencedaily. com/releases/2008/04/080414161540.htm

2. Flavonoids and quercetin

a. *Actions/expected responses:* High intakes of flavonoids and quercetin are associated with decreased risk of stroke.

b. *Routes/dosages/frequencies:* Eating foods high in flavonoids daily, especially fruits and vegetables, and quercetin-rich foods (especially apples, berries, and onions).

c. *Cautions:* Avoid foods that produce a negative reaction.

d. *Assessments:* Assess intake of fruits and vegetables and food sensitivities.

e. *Tips on use:* For foods high in flavonoids, go to http://www.nal.usda.gov/ fnic/foodcomp/Data/Flav/flav.pdf

f. *Other considerations:* None.

g. *References/other sources:*

Edwards, R. L., Lyon, T., Litwin, S. E., Rabovsky, A., Symons, J. D., & Jalili, T. (2007). Quercetin reduces blood pressure in hypertensive subjects. *The Journal of Nutrition, 137*(11), 2405–2411.

Mursu, J., Voutilainen, S., Tuomainen, T. P., Kurl, S., & Salonen, J. T. (2008). Flavonoid intake and the risk of ischaemic stroke and CVD mortality in middle-aged Finnish men: The Kuopio Ischaemic Heart Disease Risk Factor study. *British Journal of Nutrition, 1,* 1–6.

3. Green tea

a. *Actions/expected responses:* Green tea consumption is associated with a reduced risk for stroke.

b. *Routes/dosages/frequencies:* By mouth, daily. Available in capsules, extract, or tea.

c. *Cautions:* Should not be used by women with hypersensitivity to green tea or by those with kidney inflammation, gastrointestinal ulcers, insomnia, cardiovascular disease, or increased intraocular pressure. High doses of green tea can result in palpitations and irregular heartbeat, anxiety, nervousness, insomnia, nausea, heartburn, and increased stomach acid. The decaffeinated form may be a better choice for these reasons.

d. *Assessments:* Assess women for hypersensitivity prior to and after they drink green tea.

e. *Tips on use:* Store green tea in a cool, dry place.

f. *Other considerations:* Antacids may decrease the therapeutic effects of green tea, and green tea may interact with anticoagulants/antiplatelets, increasing risk of bleeding. Avoid drinking green tea while taking MAOIs or bronchodilators.

g. *References/other sources:*
   Kuriyama, S., Shimazu, T., Ohmori, K., Kikuchi, N., Nakaya, N., Nishino, Y., et al. (2006). Green tea consumption and mortality due to cardiovascular disease, cancer, and all causes in Japan: The Ohsaki Study. *Journal of the American Medical Association, 296*(10), 1255–1265.

4. Overweight/obesity
   a. *Actions/expected responses:* Obesity is linked to stroke increase among middle-aged women.
   b. *Routes/dosages/frequencies:* The women in the NHANES nutritional survey were significantly more obese than women a decade prior, with an average BMI of 28.67 kg/m^2 versus 27.11 kg/m^2 the decade prior. (A BMI of 25 to 30 is considered overweight; 30.1 or more is considered obese.)
   c. *Cautions:* The more overweight a woman is, the greater her risk for stroke.
   d. *Assessments:* Assess weight.
   e. *Tips on use:* Go to http://weightloss.about.com/library/100tips/bltip6.htm
   f. *Other considerations:* None.
   g. *References/other sources:*
      America Heart Association. (2008, February 22). Obesity linked to stroke increase among middle-aged women. *ScienceDaily.* Retrieved February 28, 2008, from http://www.sciencedaily.com/releases/2008/02/080221080606.htm

5. Salt
   a. *Actions/expected responses:* Reduction of salt intake in women over 65 years of age can help prevent stroke.
   b. *Routes/dosages/frequencies:* Ingesting salty foods or adding salt to meals.
   c. *Cautions:* High salt intake can increase stroke risk.
   d. *Assessments:* Assess salt intake.
   e. *Tips on use:* Go to http://library.thinkquest.org/13799/html/reduce_sodium.html or http://dietbites.com/Sodium-In-Foods/index.html
   f. *Other considerations:* None.
   g. *References/other sources:*
      Cook, N. R., Cutler, J. A., Obarzanek, E., Buring, J. E., Rexrode, K. M., Kumanyika, S., et al. (2007). Long term effects of dietary sodium reduction on cardiovascular disease outcomes: Observational follow-up of the trials of hypertension prevention. *British Medical Journal, 334*(7599), 855.

6. Soybean lecithin
   a. *Actions/expected responses:* Soybean lecithin is effective in treatment of acute cerebral infarction.
   b. *Routes/dosages/frequencies:* 10-gram soybean lecithin capsules three times a day.
   c. *Cautions:* Assess for gastrointestinal upset and sensitivity to lecithin.
   d. *Assessments:* Assess for reactions listed in "Cautions" when using lecithin.
   e. *Tips on use:* Store lecithin in a cool, dry place.
   f. *Other considerations:* None.
   g. *References/other sources:*
      Shi, F., Zhou, J., & Meng, D. (2001). Curative effect of soybean lecithin on cerebral infarction. *Zhonghua Yi Xue Za Zhi, 81*(21), 1301–1313.

7. Vitamin C
   a. *Actions/expected responses:* Low levels of vitamin C may serve as a biological marker of lifestyle or other factors associated with reduced stroke risk. Eating more fruits and vegetables is associated with lower prevalence of stroke.
   b. *Routes/dosages/frequencies:* Daily intake of fruits and vegetables high in vitamin C.
   c. *Cautions:* Insufficient intake of vitamin C may lead to stroke.
   d. *Assessments:* Assess vitamin C intake.
   e. *Tips on use:* Foods rich in vitamin C include guava, red bell pepper, papaya, orange juice, orange, broccoli, green bell pepper, kohlrabi, strawberries, and grapefruit. For more foods and ways to preserve vitamin C in meal production, go to http://ohioline.osu.edu/hyg-fact/5000/5552.html
   f. *Other considerations:* None.
   g. *References/other sources:*
      Myint, P. K., Luben, R. N., Welch, A. A., Bingham, S. A., Wareham, N. J., & Khaw, K. T. (2008). Plasma vitamin C concentrations predict risk of incident stroke over 10 y in 20 649 participants of the European Prospective Investigation in Cancer Norfolk prospective population study. *American Journal of Clinical Nutrition, 87*(1), 64–69.

Stress Management

1. Faith
   a. *Actions/expected responses:* Emotional distress is common in the aftermath of stroke and can impact negatively on the outcome.
   b. *Routes/dosages/frequencies:* The strength of religious beliefs influences the ability to cope after a stroke event, with stronger religious beliefs acting as a possible protective factor against emotional distress.
   c. *Cautions:* None.
   d. *Assessments:* Assess need for religious support.
   e. *Tips on use:* Find needed support.
   f. *Other considerations*: To find a local support group, go to http://www.strokeassociation.org/presenter.jhtml?identifier=3030354
   g. *References/other sources:*
      Giaquinto, S., Spiridigliozzi, C., & Caracciolo, B. (2007). Can faith protect from emotional distress after stroke? *Stroke, 38*(3), 993–997.

Touch

1. Aromatherapy acupressure
   a. *Actions/expected responses:* Aromatherapy acupressure exerts positive effects on hemiplegic shoulder pain, compared to acupressure alone, in women who have undergone stroke.
   b. *Routes/dosages/frequencies:* 20 minutes twice a day of aromatherapy acupressure using lavender, rosemary, and peppermint.

c. *Cautions:* Test sensitivity to essential oils.

d. *Assessments:* Assess pain level prior to and after aromatherapy acupressure.

e. *Tips on use:* Go to http://www.positivehealth.com/article-list.php?subject id=18

f. *Other considerations:* None.

g. *References/other sources:*

Shin, B. C., & Lee, M. S. (2007). Effects of aromatherapy acupressure on hemiplegic shoulder pain and motor power in stroke patients: A pilot study. *Journal of Alternative and Complementary Medicine, 13*(2), 347–351.

Appendix

COMPLEMENTARY AND HOLISTIC TRAINING PROGRAMS

The training programs listed below are taught by either board-certified advanced holistic practitioners and/or are certified by the American Holistic Nurses Association Certification Board. More information about continuing education units for participating in these programs as well as other programs that may only be offered once is available at http://www.ahna.org

Anti-Aging Holistic Certificate Program, holisticnurse@earthlink.net, http://www.carolynchambersclark.com

AsOneHolisticCoaching Training Program, contact Linda@asonecoaching.com or http://www.asonecoaching.com

Assertiveness Certification Program, holisticnurse@earthlink.net or http://www.carolynchambersclark.com

Certificate Program in Aromatherapy for Health Professional, R.J. Buckle Associates, LLC, rjbinfo@aol.com or http://www.rjbuckle.com

Certificate Program in Integrative Imagery, Beyond Ordinary Nursing (650) 570–6157, imagine@integrativeimagery.com, or http://www.integrative imagery.com

Great River Craniosacral Therapy Institute Training Program, Great River Craniosacral Therapy Institute, (845) 358-4815, doctorwishcst@gmail.com, or http://www.drwishcraniosacral.com

Healing Touch Certification Program, Healing Touch International Inc., (303) 989–7982, htiheal@aol.com, or http://wwwhealingtouchinterna tional.com

Holistic Stress Management Instructor Certification Workshop, Paramount Wellness Institute, (303) 678–9962, brianlukes@cs.com, or http://www.brianlukeseaward.net

Integrative Healing Arts Certificate Program, the BirchTree Center for Healthcare Transformation, contact info@birchtreecenter.com or http://www.birchtreecenter.com

Self-Healing Certificate Program, holisticnurse@earthlink.net or http://www.carolynchambersclark.com

Whole Health Education Certificate, National Institute of Whole Health, (781) 237–7971 or http://www.wholehealtheducation.com

Woman's Health Complementary Skills Certification Program, holistic nurse@earthlink.net or http://www.carolynchambersclark.com

Index

Acidic dietary patterns, osteoporosis
   and, 273
Acrylamide, breast cancer and, 66
Acupressure
   anxiety and, 35
   breast cancer and, 89–90
   colon and rectal cancer and, 118
   depression and, 130
   digestion and, 143–144
   endometrial cancer and, 155–156
   fatigue and, 167–168
   gastric cancer and, 182
   heart/blood vessels and, 207
   insomnia and, 219
   kidney conditions and, 227–228
   nausea and vomiting due to
     chemotherapy and, 250
   pain and, 307–309
   pancreatic cancer and, 323–324
   pregnancy and, 356–357
   stroke and, 365–366
Acupuncture, hypertension and, 62–63
Aerobic exercise
   heart/blood vessels and, 190–191
   overweight/obesity and, 288–289
   pregnancy and, 345–346
Affirmations
   anxiety and, 28–29
   bladder infections and, 39–40
   blood pressure/hypertension and, 49–50
   breast cancer and, 77–78
   colon and rectal cancer and, 109–110
   depression and, 125
   digestion and, 139
   endometrial cancer and, 149
   falls and, 159–160
   fatigue and, 165–166
   fibroids and, 170–171
   gastric cancer and, 176
   heart/blood vessels and, 195
   incontinence and, 212
   insomnia and, 218–219

   kidney conditions and, 224–225
   lung conditions and, 244
   migraines and, 265
   osteoporosis and, 272
   ovarian cancer and, 284–285
   overweight/obesity and, 291–292
   pain and, 304
   pancreatic cancer and, 317
   PMS and, 327
   polycystic ovary syndrome and, 334
   pregnancy and, 347–348
   stroke and, 362
Aggravation and colon and rectal cancer, 106
Agricultural exposures, gastric cancer
   and, 173–174
Air pollution, pregnancy/labor/delivery
   and, 337–338
Alcohol
   blood pressure and, 45–46
   breast cancer and, 66
   endometrial cancer and, 145–146
   PMS and, 328–329
Almonds, colon and rectal cancer and, 110
Aloe vera
   digestion and, 135
   gastric cancer and, 175
   pancreatic cancer and, 322
Alpha-linolenic acid, heart/blood vessels
   and, 196
Aluminum
   Alzheimer's and, 2
   breast cancer and, 66–67
Alzheimer's, 1–22
   aluminum and, 2
   environment and, 1–6
   exercise/movement and, 6–9
   herbs/essential oils and, 7–9
   mindset and, 9–10
   nutrition and, 10–18
   stress management and, 18–19
   supplements and, 19
   touch and, 21–22

Animal fat and animal protein
   endometrial cancer and, 150
   kidney conditions and, 225
   pregnancy and, 341
Animal fat versus antioxidant foods,
   heart/blood vessels and, 196
Antidepressants, osteoporosis and,
   269–270. *See also* SSRIs
Antioxidants, heart/blood vessels and, 196
Anxiety, 23–26
   environment and, 23–24
   exercise/movement and, 24–26
   herbs/essential oils and, 26–28
   mindset and, 28–29
   nutrition and, 29–31
   stress management and, 32–34
   supplements and, 32–34
   touch and, 35–36
Apples/apple juice
   Alzheimer's and, 10–11
   hypertension and, 50–51
Aromatherapy
   breast cancer and, 84
   colon and rectal cancer and, 108
   endometrial cancer and, 148
   gastric cancer and, 175
   insomnia and, 217
   kidney conditions and, 223–224
   pain and, 309–310
   pancreatic cancer and, 315–316
   pregnancy and, 346
   stroke and, 365–366
Aspirin, heart/blood vessels and, 185–186
Astragalus, breast cancer and, 74
Atkins type-diet
   digestion and, 140
   kidney conditions and, 225
Autogenic training
   hypertension and, 59
   migraines and, 265–266

Back pain, massage and, 310
Basil, gastric cancer and, 176
B-complex vitamins
   heart/blood vessels and, 207
   lung/TB and, 249
Beef, red meat, ham, fibroids and, 171
Beet juice, hypertension and, 51
Behavioral program, overweight/obesity
   and, 289
Berries/berry juice
   Alzheimer's and, 11
   bladder infections and, 40

blood pressure/hypertension and, 50–51
   breast cancer and, 78
   colon and rectal cancer and, 100
   falls and, 160
Beta-carotene, gastric cancer and, 180
Binge-eating, overweight/obesity and,
   296–297
Bingo, Alzheimer's/memory and, 9
Biofeedback
   blood pressure/hypertension and, 63
   incontinence and, 209–210
Black cohosh
   breast cancer and, 74
   insomnia and, 217
   menopause and, 255–256
Black tea
   Alzheimer's and, 13–14
   bladder infections and, 41
   endometrial cancer and, 153
   falls and, 161
Bladder hygiene and cystitis, 37–38
Bladder infections (cystitis)
   environment and, 37–38
   exercise/movement and, 38–39
   herbs/essential oils and, 39
   mindset and, 39–40
   nutrition and, 40–42
   stress management and, 42
   supplements and, 42
   touch and, 43
Bladder irritants
   bladder infections and, 41–42
   incontinence and, 212
Bladder training, incontinence and, 211
Blood pressure (hypertension)
   environment and, 45–48
   exercise/movement and, 48–49
   herbs/essential oils and, 49
   mindset and, 49–50
   nutrition and, 50–59
   stress management and, 50–59
   supplements and, 61–62
   touch and, 62–64
Blueberries, Alzheimer's and, 11
Blue light, fatigue, and, 163
Board games, Alzheimer's and, 9
Brassica vegetables, endometrial cancer
   and, 151–152
Breast cancer
   environment and, 65–72
   exercise and, 72–74
   herbs/essential oils and, 74–77
   mindset and, 77–78

nutrition and, 78–83
stress management and, 83–86
supplements and, 86–89
touch and, 89–91
Breast feeding, pregnancy/labor/delivery
and, 338
Breathing therapy, pain and, 305
Breech presentations, 340–341
Butterbur, migraines and, 265
Butter-flavored popcorn, lung conditions
and, 244–245

Caffeine
heart/blood vessels and, 199
pregnancy, miscarriage and, 348
Calcium
absorption, oxalic acid and, 274
colon and rectal cancer and, 117–118
heart/blood vessel and, 198
hypertension and, 51
osteoporosis and, 273–274, 278–279
PMS and, 327–328
Carbohydrates
Pancreatic cancer and, 321
PMS and, 328
Carbonated beverages, kidney conditions
and, 225
Cell phones, breast cancer and, 68–69
CenteringPregnancy, adolescents and,
338–339
Cervical cancer
environment and, 93–94
exercise/movement and, 94–95
herbs/essential oils and, 95
mindset and, 96
nutrition and, 95–100
stress management, 100–101
supplements, 101–102
touch, 102–104
Chamomile
digestion and, 135
heart/blood vessels and, 193
Chaste tree, PMS and, 326–327
Chemical exposures and breast cancer,
71–72
Cherries
heart/blood vessels and, 198
overweight/obesity and, 292
pain and, 304–305
Chinese approaches, fibroids and, 172
Chinese herbs, polycystic ovary syndrome
and, 334
Chlordane, gastric cancer and, 173–174

Chocolate, osteoporosis and, 274
Cholesterol
chamomile tea lowers and, 193
coffee elevates and, 199
eggs lower and, 19
exercise increase HDL ("good") form
and, 191
fenugreek lowers and, 136
flaxseed lowers and, 259
green tea lowers and, 193
hawthorn lowers, 194
heart/blood vessels and, 196
lecithin protects against and, 19
low fat diet increases and, 197
magnesium lowers and, 201
mate tea lower and, 195
pancreatic cancer and, 321
pecans lower and, 203
psyllium lowers and, 206
sitting increases and, 191
stress elevates and, 204
sugar intake and, 15, 202
yoga reduces and, 204
Chromium, depression and, 129
Cinnamon
digestion and, 138–139
heart/blood vessels and, 198–199
overweight/obesity and, 292–293
Circadian rhythm, breast cancer and, 61
Clove, bladder infections, and, 39
Coenzyme Q10
heart/blood vessels and, 205–206
migraines and, 266
with riboflavin and niacin for breast
cancer, 86–87
Coffee
anxiety increase and, 29–30
blood pressure/hypertension increase
and, 51–52
osteoporosis and, 274–275
Cognitive-behavioral therapy
anxiety and, 29
blood pressure/hypertension reduction
and, 50
breast cancer and, 78
depression and, 125–126
digestion and, 138, 141
fatigue and, 165–166
heart/blood vessels and, 195–196
incontinence and, 213–214
menopause and, 258–259
migraines and, 266
PMS and, 329–330

Colas
  kidney conditions and, 225
  osteoporosis and, 275
Colon and rectal cancer
  environment and, 105–107
  exercise/movement and, 107–108
  herbs/essential oils and, 108–109
  mindset and, 109–110
  nutrition and, 110–117
  stress management and, 117
  supplements and, 117–118
  touch and, 118–119
Computer game, lung conditions and,
  241–242
Constipation. *See* Digestion
Cooked meat carcinogens, breast cancer
  and, 67–68
Cookware and fetus, 342–343
Copper, bladder infections and, 42
Counseling, overweight/obesity and, 291
Cow's milk, digestion and, 139
C-reactive protein, heart/blood vessels
  and, 186
Crohn's. *See* Digestion
Crossword puzzles, Alzheimer's and, 9
C-sections, 339–340
CT scans
  colon and rectal cancer and, 105–106
  endometrial cancer and, 146
  gastric cancer and, 174
  ovarian cancer and, 281–282
  pancreatic cancer and, 313–314
Curry (curcumin/tumeric)
  Alzheimer's and, 11–12
  breast cancer and, 76–76
  colon and rectal cancer and, 108–109
  digestion and, 139
  endometrial cancer and, 150
  heart/blood vessels and, 200
  lung conditions and, 245
  osteoporosis and, 275–276
  pancreatic cancer and, 316
Cycling, hypertension and, 48–49
Cystitis. *See* Bladder infections

Dairy products, overweight/obesity
  and, 293
Dancing
  Alzheimer's and, 9
  anxiety and, 24–25
DASH diet
  hypertension and, 53
  stroke and, 362–363

Denial, overweight/obesity and, 291
Depression
  environment and, 121–122
  exercise/movement and, 122–123
  herbs/essential oils and, 123–124
  mindset and, 125–126
  nutrition and, 126–128
  stress management and, 128–129
  supplements and, 129–130
  touch and, 130–131
Diarrhea. *See* Digestion
Dietary advice, overweight/obesity and,
  295–296
Dietary cholesterol, pancreative cancer
  and, 321
Dieting
  osteoporosis and, 270
  overweight/obesity and, 288–290
Digestion
  environment and, 133–134
  exercise/movement and, 134–135
  herbs/essential oils and, 135–137
  mindset and, 137–138
  nutrition and, 138–141
  stress management and, 141–142
  supplements and, 142–143
  touch and, 143
Dioxin
  breast cancer and, 68
  pregnancy and, 340
Doulas and pregnancy, 340
Dysmenorrhea, static magnet and, 311

Ear reflexology, PMS and, 331
Electromagnetic fields
  breast cancer and, 68–69
  digestion and, 134
  heart/blood vessels and, 189
Endometrial cancer
  environment and, 145–147
  exercise/movement and, 147–148
  herbs/essential oils and, 148–149
  mindset and, 149
  nutrition and, 150–153
  stress management and, 153–154
  supplements and, 154–155
  touch and, 155–156
Environment
  Alzheimer's and, 1–6
  anxiety and, 23–24
  bladder infections and, 37–38
  blood pressure and, 45–48
  breast cancer and, 65–72

cervical cancer and, 93–94
colon and rectal cancer and, 105–107
depression and, 121–122
digestion and, 133–134
endometrial cancer and, 145–147
falls and, 157–158
fatigue and, 163–164
fibroids and, 169–170
gastric cancer and, 173–174
heart and blood vessels and, 185–190
incontinence and, 209–210
insomnia and, 215–216
kidney conditions and, 221–222
liver conditions and, 229–230
lung conditions and, 241–243
menopause and, 253–254
migraines and, 263–264
osteoporosis and, 269–171
overweight/obesity and, 287–288
pain and, 299–301
pancreatic cancer and, 313–315
PMS and, 325–326
pregnancy/labor/delivery and, 337–345
stroke and, 359–360
Environmental behavioral training,
    insomnia and, 215–216
Exercise/Movement
    Alzheimer's and, 6–7
    anxiety and, 24–26
    bladder infections and, 38–39
    blood pressure and, 48–49
    breast cancer and, 72–74
    cervical cancer and, 94–95
    colon and rectal cancer and, 107–108
    depression and, 134–135
    digestion and, 134–135
    endometrial cancer and, 147–148
    falls and, 158–159
    fatigue and, 164
    fibroids and, 170
    heart/blood vessels and, 190–103
    incontinence and, 211
    insomnia and, 216–217
    kidney conditions and, 222–223
    liver conditions and, 230–231
    lung conditions and, 243–244
    menopause and, 254–255
    migraines and, 264
    osteoporosis and, 271–272
    ovarian cancer and, 283–284
    overweight/obesity and, 288
    pain and, 302–303
    pancreatic cancer and, 315

PMS and, 326
    polycystic ovary syndrome and, 333–334
    pregnancy/labor/delivery and, 345–346
    stroke and, 361
External cephalic version (ECV), 339

Faith, stroke and, 365
Falls
    affirmations and, 159–160
    environment and, 157–158
    exercise and, 158–159
    mindset and, 159–160
    nutrition and, 160–161
    prevention and, 157–158
    stretching exercises and, 158–159
    supplements and, 161–162
    yoga and, 159
Fasting, digestion and, 140
Fat (high) diet
    Alzheimer's and, 14
    overweight/obesity and, 293–294
    PMS and, 328–329
Fat and spices, reflux and, 140
Fatigue
    environment and, 163–164
    exercise/movement and, 164
    herbs/essential oils and, 164–165
    mindset and, 165–166
    nutrition and, 166–167
    touch and, 167–168
Fatty acids, depression and, 127
Fenugreek
    digestion and, 136
    heart/blood vessels and, 193–194
Fetus
    aerobic exercise, anxiety, depression
        and, 353
    caffeine and, 348
    copper and, 349–350
    folate and, 351–352
    fresh water fish and, 342
    non-stick cookware and, 342
    ocean fish and, 351
    overweight (maternal) and, 350
    power-frequency fields and, 343
    smoking and, 343–344
    SSRIs and, 344
    trans-fat, sugar and fertility, 353
    vitamin D deficiency and, 344
    whole wheat and, 351
Fiber
    endometrial cancer and, 152–153
    hypertension and, 53–54

Fiber (*continued*)
overweight/obesity and, 293–294
polycystic ovary syndrome and, 335
pregnancy and need for, 350–351
Fibroids
environment and, 169–170
exercise/movement and, 170
mindset, 170–171
nutrition and, 171–172
touch and, 172
Fish/fish oil
Alzheimer's and, 12
blood pressure and, 54
depression and, 128
falls and, 160–161
heart/blood vessels and, 196–197
pregnancy and, 351
Flavonoids, fruits and vegetables
Alzheimer's and, 12–13
stroke and, 363
Flavonols, pancreatic cancer and, 317–318
Flaxseed
breast cancer and, 78–79
colon and rectal cancer and, 110–111
menopause and, 259–260
Floating, pain and, 299–300
Fluoride in drinking water, heart/blood
vessels and, 187
Folate
Alzheimer's and, 16
bladder infections and, 42
blood pressure/hypertension and, 54–55
depression and, 126–127
endometrial cancer and, 150–151
gastric cancer and, 176–177
lung conditions and, 245
pancreatic cancer and, 318
pregnancy and, 351–352
Food/mood diary, fatigue and, 166–167
Foot acupressure, massage, Alzheimer's
and, 21–22
Foot reflexology
bladder infections and, 43
blood pressure/hypertension and, 63
breast cancer and, 90
colon and rectal cancer and, 119
depression and, 131
fatigue and, 168
gastric cancer and, 182
incontinence and, 214
kidney conditions and, 228
lung cancer and, 250–251
ovarian cancer and, 285–286

pancreatic cancer and, 324–325
PMS and, 331
Fresh water fish, mercury and PCBs, 342
Fried potatoes, white bread, polycystic
ovary syndrome and, 335
Fructose, overweight/obesity and, 294
Fruits, osteoporosis and, 277–278
Fruits and vegetables
Alzheimer's and, 12–13
anxiety and, 30
blood pressure and, 53–54
breast cancer and, 80
colon and rectal cancer and, 113
depression and, 130
endometrial cancer and, 152
falls and, 160
fatigue and, 166
gastric cancer and, 177–178
heart/blood vessels and, 196
liver conditions and, 233–234
lung conditions and, 246
osteoporosis and, 273
pancreatic cancer and, 321
pregnancy and, 352
stroke and, 363

Gardening, endometrial cancer and, 147
Garlic
Alzheimer's and, 13
bladder infections and, 41
blood pressure/hypertension and, 56
colon and rectal cancer and, 111–112
endometrial cancer and, 151–152
fatigue and, 164–165
gastric cancer and, 179
heart/blood vessels and, 200–201
kidney conditions and, 225
stroke and, 362
Gasoline, pregnancy and, 341
Gastric cancer
environment and, 173–174
herbs/essential oils and, 175–176
mindset and, 176
nutrition and, 176–180
propargite and, 173–174
supplements and, 180–181
touch and, 182–184
Ginger, digestion and, 136
Gingko biloba
Alzheimer's and, 7–8
anxiety and, 26–27
colon and rectal cancer and, 118
depression and, 123–124

endometrial cancer and, 154
gastric cancer and, 180–181
kidney conditions and, 226–227
liver conditions and, 249
Ginseng, fatigue and, 165
Grapeseed extract, breast cancer and, 87
Green tea
  Alzheimer's and, 13–14
  blood pressure/hypertension and, 56
  breast cancer and, 79–80
  colon and rectal cancer and, 112
  endometrial cancer and, 153
  falls and, 161
  gastric cancer and, 178
  heart/blood vessels and, 194
  kidney conditions and, 225
  lung conditions and, 246–247
  pancreatic cancer and, 318–319
  stroke and, 262–364
Guided imagery, pain and, 305, 310

Hair dyes, ovarian cancer and, 282
Hand aromatherapy and massage,
  Alzheimer's and, 21–22
Hand reflexology, PMS, and, 331
Hand washing, digestion and, 133–134
Hawthorn, heart/blood vessels and,
  194–195
Headache diary, migraines and, 263
Healing touch, pain and, 310
Heart/blood vessels
  environment and, 185–190
  exercise/movement and, 190–193
  herbs/essential oils and, 193–194
  mindset and, 195–196
  nutrition and, 196–203
  stress management and, 204–205
  supplements and, 205–207
  touch and, 207
Heartburn. *See* Digestion
Herbs/essential oils
  Alzheimer's and, 7–9
  anxiety and, 26–28
  bladder infections and, 39
  blood pressure and, 49
  breast cancer and, 74–79
  cervical cancer and, 95
  colon and rectal cancer and, 108–109
  depression and, 123–124
  digestion and, 135–137
  endometrial cancer and, 148
  fatigue and, 164–165
  gastric cancer and, 175–176

heart/blood vessels and, 193–195
insomnia and, 217–218
kidney conditions and, 223–224
liver conditions and, 231–233
menopause and, 255–256
migraines and, 265
pain and, 303–304
PMS and, 326–327
polycystic ovary syndrome and,
  346–347
pregnancy/labor/delivery and, 346–347
stroke and, 362
Hexavalent chromium, gastric cancer
  and, 174
Homeocysteine, vitamin B12, osteoporosis
  and, 276–277
Hormone therapy, heart/blood vessels
  and, 187–188
Housework
  anxiety and, 25
  endometrial cancer and, 147
Hydrotherapy, pain and, 302
Hypnosis
  digestion and, 138
  osteoporosis and, 272–273
  pain and, 305–306
  pregnancy and, 353–354
Hysterectomy, incontinence and, 210

IBS/IBD. *See* Digestion
Imagery, Alzheimer's and, 18
Inactivity, colon and rectal cancer and,
  107–108
Incontinence
  environment and, 209–210
  exercise/movement and, 211
  mindset and, 212
  nutrition and, 212–213
  stress management and, 213–214
  touch and, 214
Inositol, polycystic ovary syndromes and,
  335–336
Insomnia
  environment and, 215–216
  exercise/movement and, 216–217
  herbs/essential oils and, 217–218
  mindset and, 218–219
  touch and, 219
Iron
  bladder infections and, 42
  heart/blood vessels and, 196

Journaling, breast cancer and, 84–85

Kegels/bladder training, incontinence and, 211
Kidney conditions
    environment and, 221–222
    exercise/movement and, 222–223
    herbs/essential oils and, 223–224
    mindset and, 224–225
    nutrition and, 225–226
    stress management and, 226
    supplements and, 226–227
    touch and, 227–228
Kneeling during labor, 342

Labor, kneeling during and, 342
Laughter, heart/blood vessels and, 204
Lavender essential oils
    anxiety and, 27
    insomnia and, 217
Lecithin
    Alzheimer's and, 19
    memory and, 19
Lemon balm
    Alzheimer's and, 8–9
    anxiety and, 27
Licorice
    breast cancer and, 76–77
    colon and rectal cancer and, 109
    endometrial cancer and, 148
Liver conditions
    environment and, 229–230
    exercise/movement and, 230–231
    herbs/essential oils and, 231–233
    nutrition and, 233–237
    stress management and, 237
    supplements and, 237–238
    touch and, 238–240
Low back pain, massage and, 310
Low carbohydrate diets, digestion and, 140
Lung conditions
    environment and, 241–243
    exercise/movement and, 243–244
    mindset and, 244
    nutrition and, 244–248
    stress management and, 248
    supplements and, 248
    touch and, 250–251
Lysine
    lowers cholesterol, 307
    pain and, 306–307

Magnesium
    blood pressure/hypertension and, 56–57
    heart/blood vessels and, 201–202

osteoporosis and, 277
    overweight/obesity and, 294–295
Maitake mushrooms
    breast cancer and, 87–99
    gastric cancer and, 179
    lung cancer and, 247
Mammograms, breast cancer and, 72
Massage
    anxiety and, 35–36
    blood pressure/hypertension and, 63–64
    breast cancer and, 91
    depression and, 130
    fatigue and, 167–168
    menopause and, 261
    migraines and, 267
    pain and, 310–311
Mastectomy, preventive, breast cancer and, 69
Mate tea, heart/blood vessels and, 195
Meat
    fibroids and, 171
    pancreatic cancer and, 321
Meditation
    Alzheimer's and, 18
    hypertension and, 59–60
Mediterranean diet
    Alzheimer's and, 17
    breast cancer and, 80–81
    colon and rectal cancer and, 112–113
    kidney conditions and, 225
Memory
    environment and, 1–6
    exercise/movement and, 6–9
    herbs/essential oils and, 7–9
    medication/memory loss diary and, 2
    mindset and, 9–10
    nutrition and, 10–18
    stress management and, 18–19
    supplements and, 19
    touch and, 21–22
Menopause
    environment and, 253–254
    exercise/movement and, 254–255
    herbs/essential oils and, 255–256
    mindset and, 256
    nutrition and, 256–258
    stress management and, 258–259
    supplements and, 259–261
    touch and, 261
Menthol, bladder infections and, 39
Mercury, air pollution, heart/blood vessels and, 188
Methylmercury, PCBs, and pregnancy, 342

Migraines
    environment and, 263–264
    exercise/movement and, 264
    herbs/essential oils and, 265
    mindset and, 265
    stress management and, 265–266
    supplements and, 266
    touch and, 267
Milk, digestion and, 139
Milk thistle
    breast cancer and, 88
    digestion and, 136–137
    endometrial cancer and, 149
    kidney conditions and, 224
    lung conditions and, 243–244
    ovarian cancer and, 284
    pancreatic cancer and, 316–317
Mindfullness-based stress reduction
    breast cancer and, 85
    colon and rectal cancer and, 117
    pain and, 306
Mindset
    Alzheimer's and, 9–10
    anxiety and, 28–29
    bladder infections and, 39–40
    blood pressure and, 49–50
    breast cancer and, 77–78
    cervical cancer and, 16
    colon and rectal cancer and, 109–110
    depression and, 125–126
    digestion and, 137–138
    endometrial cancer and, 149
    falls and, 159–160
    fatigue and, 165–166
    fibroids and, 170–171
    heart/blood vessels and, 195–106
    incontinence and, 212–213
    insomnia and, 218–219
    kidney conditions and, 224–225
    lung conditions and, 244
    menopause and, 256
    migraines and, 265
    osteoporosis and, 272
    ovarian cancer and, 284–285
    overweight/obesity and, 292–292
    pain and, 304
    pancreatic cancer and, 317
    PMS and, 327
    polycystic ovary syndrome and,
        334–335
    pregnancy/labor/delivery and, 347–348
    stroke and, 362
Mirror treatment, pain and, 300
Molasses, depression and, 128

Multivitamins
    Alzheimer's and, 20
    memory and, 20
    pregnancy and, 354
Music
    anxiety and, 24–25
    insomnia and, 216–217
    pain and, 300–301, 310
    stroke and, 359–360
Musical instruments, Alzheimer's and, 9

Neighborhood conditions, breast cancer
        and, 69–70
Nutrition
    Alzheimer's and, 10–18
    anxiety and, 29–31
    bladder infections and, 40–42
    blood pressure and, 50–59
    breast cancer and, 78–83
    cervical cancer and, 96–100
    colon and rectal cancer and, 110–117
    depression and, 126–128
    digestion and, 138–141
    endometrial cancer and, 150–153
    falls and, 160–161
    fatigue and, 166–167
    fibroids and, 171–172
    gastric cancer and, 176–180
    heart/blood vessels and, 196–203
    incontinence and, 213–214
    kidney conditions and, 225–226
    liver conditions and, 233–237
    lung conditions and, 244–248
    menopause and, 256–258
    osteoporosis and, 273–278
    ovarian cancer and, 285
    overweight/obesity and, 292–296
    pain and, 304–305
    pancreatic cancer and, 317–321
    PMS and, 327–329
    polycystic ovary syndrome and, 335
    pregnancy/labor/delivery and, 348–353
    stroke and, 362–365

Obesity, PMS and, 329
Occupational therapy, stroke and, 361
Olive oil, heart/blood vessels and, 203
Omega-3 fatty acids
    depression and, 127
    falls and, 160
    osteoporosis and, 277–278
    pancreatic cancer and, 319
    polycystic ovary syndrome and, 335
    pregnancy and, 351

Onion
Alzheimer's and, 14
blood pressure/hypertension and, 50–51
gastric cancer and, 179
Organochlorides, pancreatic cancer
and, 314
Osteoporosis
environment and, 269–271
exercise/movement and, 271–272
mindset and, 272
nutrition and, 273–278
supplements and, 278–279
Outdoors, incontinence and, 210
Ovarian cancer
environment and, 282–283
exercise/movement and, 281–283
mindset and, 284–285
nutrition and, 285
touch and, 285–296
Overweight/obesity
digestion and, 141
endometrial cancer and, 146
environment and, 287–288
exercise/movement and, 288
mindset and, 291–292
nutrition and, 292–296
PMS and, 329
pregnancy and, 320
stress management and, 296–298
stroke and, 364
supplements and, 297–298
Oxalic acid, calcium absorption and, 274

Pain
environment and, 299–301
exercise/movement and, 302–303
herbs/essential oils and, 303–304
mindset and, 304
nutrition and, 304–305
stress management and, 305–306
supplements and, 306–307
touch and, 307–311
Pancreatic cancer
environment and, 313–315
exercise/movement and, 315
herbs/essential oil and, 315–317
mindset and, 317
nutrition and, 317–321
stress management and, 321–322
supplements and, 322–323
touch and, 323–324
Parental identity and pregnancy, 348
Pecans, heart/blood vessels and, 203

Peppermint
anxiety and, 27–28
bladder infections and, 39
digestion and, 137
pain and, 303–304, 307
Perineal talc
fibroids and, 169–170
ovarian cancer and, 282
Pesticides
breast cancer and, 70
pregnancy and, 341
Physical activity/inactivity
incontinence and, 211
lung cancer and, 243
pancreatic cancer and, 315
stroke and, 361
PMS
environment and, 325–326
exercise/movement and, 326
herbs/essential oils and, 326–327
mindset and, 327
nutrition and, 327–329
obesity and, 329
protein and, 328–329
stress management and, 329–330
supplements and, 330–331
touch and, 331
Polycystic ovary syndrome
exercise/movement and, 333–334
herbs/essential oils and, 334
mindset and, 334–335
nutrition and, 335
supplements and, 335–336
Pomegranate juice/oil/extract
colon and rectal cancer and, 114
heart/blood vessels and, 201–202
hypertension and, 57
lung conditions and, 248–249
menopause and, 260
overweight/obesity and, 297
Postoperative pain, massage and, 310
Potassium
blood pressure/hypertension and, 61
incontinence and, 212
Power lines, breast cancer and, 68–69
Prayer, depression and, 126
Pregnancy/labor/delivery
adolescence and, 338–339
environment and, 337–345
exercise/movement and, 345–346
herbs/essentials oils and, 346–347
methylmercury, PCBs and, 342
mindset and, 347–348

nutrition and, 348–353
stress management and, 353–354
supplements ands, 354–356
touch and, 356–357
Prempro, menopause and, 253
Preventive mastectomy, breast
cancer and, 69
Probiotics
bladder infections and, 40–41
breast cancer and, 82
colon and rectal cancer and, 114–115
digestion and, 142–143
pregnancy and, 354
Processed meat, gastric cancer and, 179
Propargite, gastric cancer and, 173–174
Protein
incontinence and, 212
kidney conditions and, 225
PMS and, 328–329
Psyllium, heart/blood vessels and, 206
Pycnogenol
Alzheimer's and, 19
blood pressure/hypertension and, 61–62
breast cancer and, 88
colon and rectal cancer and, 118
digestion and, 143
endometrial cancer and, 154
gastric cancer and, 180–181
heart/blood vessels and, 206
kidney conditions and, 226–227
liver cancer and, 249
memory and, 19
menopause and, 260–261
pancreatic cancer and, 322
PMS and, 330
Pregnancy and, 355

Qi gong, PMS and, 326
Quercetin, stroke and, 363

Reading, Alzheimer's and, 9–10
Red meat, processed meat and/or ham
fibroids and, 171
gastric cancer and, 179
heart/blood vessels and, 196–197
lung cancer and, 248
menopause and, 256–257
Red wine, polycystic ovary syndrome
and, 335
Relaxation therapy/breathing
bladder infections and, 42
depression and, 128–129
pain and, 305

Resistance training
heart/blood vessels and, 191–192
menopause and, 255
Rocking chair
Alzheimer's and, 6–7
anxiety and, 25
Room mold, lung conditions and, 242
Rosemary
anxiety and, 27
bladder infections and, 39
breast cancer and, 77
Running
breast cancer and, 72–73
hypertension and, 48

Sage
anxiety and, 28
depression and, 124
Salt
hypertension and, 57–58
stroke and, 364
Seaweed alginate, pectin, overweight/
obesity and, 295
Selenium
Alzheimer's and, 19
bladder infections and, 42
breast cancer and, 88–89
colon and rectal cancer and, 115
gastric cancer and, 180
TB and, 249
Sesame oil
hypertension and, 58
overweight/obesity and, 295
Sexual assault, breast cancer and, 70–71
Shift work, breast cancer and, 67
Sitz baths, pain and, 301
Smoking
anxiety and, 24
colon and rectal cancer and, 106
osteoporosis and, 271
PMS and, 325–326
pregnancy and, 343
Snoezelen, multi-sensory intervention,
Alzheimer's and, 6
Social support
heart/blood vessels and, 189
overweight/obesity and, 288–289
stroke and, 360
Sodas, Alzheimer's and, 14–15
Soy/soy nuts
blood pressure/hypertension and, 58
breast cancer and, 82–83
colon and rectal cancer and, 115

Soy/soy nuts (*continued*)
  endometrial cancer and, 152–153
  fibroids and, 171–172
  menopause and, 257
  osteoporosis and, 277–278
  PMS and, 329
Spearmint, menopause and, 256
Sports participation, heart/blood vessels
    and, 192
SSRIs (e.g., Paxil) and pregnancy, 344
Starchy diet, pancreatic cancer and, 320
Static magnets and pain, 311
St. John's wort and depression, 124
Stress management
  Alzheimer's and, 18–19
  anxiety and, 32–34
  blood pressure and, 59–60
  breast cancer and, 83–86
  cervical cancer and, 100–101
  colon and rectal cancer and, 117
  depression and, 128–129
  digestion and, 141–142
  endometrial cancer and, 153–154
  heart/blood vessels and, 204–205
  kidney conditions and, 226
  liver conditions and, 237
  lung conditions and, 248
  menopause and, 258–259
  migraines and, 265–266
  overweight/obesity and, 296–297
  pain and, 305–306
  pancreatic cancer and, 321–322
  PMS and, 329–330
  pregnancy/labor/delivery and, 353–354
  stroke and, 365
Sugar, refined carbohydrates, and/or
    animal products
  Alzheimer's and, 17
  colon and rectal cancer and, 116
  fatigue and, 167
  heart/blood vessels and, 202
Sugar and sugary foods
  pancreatic cancer and, 320
  PMS and, 328–329
Sulfur foods
  Alzheimer's and, 14
  depression and, 128
  endometrial cancer and, 153
Supplements
  Alzheimer's and, 19
  anxiety and, 34
  bladder infections and, 42
  blood pressure and, 61–62
  breast cancer and, 86–89

  cervical cancer and, 101–102
  colon and rectal cancer and, 117
  depression and, 129–130
  digestion and, 142–143
  endometrial cancer and, 154–155
  falls and, 161–162
  gastric cancer and, 180–181
  heart/blood vessels and, 205–207
  kidney conditions and, 226–227
  liver conditions and, 237–238
  lung conditions and, 248
  menopause and, 259–261
  migraines and, 266
  osteoporosis and, 278–279
  overweight/obesity and, 297–298
  pain and, 306–307
  pancreatic cancer and, 322–323
  PMS and, 330–331
  polycystic ovarian syndrome and, 335–336
  pregnancy/labor/delivery and, 354–357
Survivor strategies, breast cancer and,
    73–74
Swimming and hypertension, 48–49

Tai chi
  blood pressure/hypertension and, 48
  heart/blood vessels and, 192
  pain and, 302–303
Talc, fibroids and, 169–170
Talking and Alzheimer's, 10
Targeted dietary advice, overweight/
    obesity and, 295–296
Therapeutic touch (TT)
  Alzheimer's and, 22
  anxiety and, 36
  colon and rectal cancer and, 119
  endometrial cancer and, 156
  gastric cancer and, 183
  lung cancer and, 251
Thyrotropin and heart/blood vessels, 190
Tobacco smoke and PMS, 325–326
Tomatoes and hypertension, 59
Touch
  Alzheimer's and, 21–22
  anxiety and, 35–36
  bladder infections and, 43
  blood pressure and, 62–64
  breast cancer and, 89–91
  cervical cancer and, 118–119
  colon and rectal cancer and, 118–119
  depression and, 130–131
  digestion and, 143
  endometrial cancer and, 155–156
  fatigue and, 167–168

gastric cancer and, 182–183
heart/blood vessels and, 207
incontinence and, 214
insomnia and, 219
kidney conditions and, 227–228
liver conditions and, 238–240
lung conditions and, 250–251
menopause and, 261
migraines and, 267
ovarian cancer and, 285–286
pain and, 307–311
pancreatic cancer and, 323–324
PMS and, 331
pregnancy/labor/delivery and, 356–357
stroke and, 365–366
Trans fat
  heart/blood vessels and, 202–203
  pregnancy and, 352–253
Trifluin and gastric cancer, 173–174
Triggering foods and bladder infections,
  41–42
24-D, chlordane, propargite, trifluin and
  gastric cancer, 173–174

Vegetables and gastric cancer, 177–178
Vegetarian diets and overweight/obesity,
  296
Vinegar and overweight/obesity,
  297–298
Vitamin A
  bladder infections and, 42
  breast cancer and, 89
  endometrial cancer and, 154–155
  gastric cancer and, 181
  lung cancer and, 249
  pancreatic cancer and, 322–323
Vitamin B1 (thiamine)
  Alzheimer's and, 15
  breast cancer and, 89
Vitamin B3 (niacin)
  Alzheimer's and, 15
  breast cancer and, 89
  incontinence and, 212
Vitamin B6
  bladder infections and, 42
  breast cancer and, 89
  depression and, 129–130
  incontinence and, 212
  PMS and, 330
  pregnancy and, 355–356
Vitamin B12 and folate
  Alzheimer's and, 16
  bladder infections and, 42
  breast cancer and, 89

Vitamin B12 and osteoporosis, 276–277
Vitamin C and E
  Alzheimer's and, 20–21
  bladder infections and, 42
  blood pressure and, 62
  breast cancer and, 89
  colon and rectal cancer and, 116–117
  endometrial cancer and, 154–155
  gastric cancer and, 181
  pancreatic cancer and, 322–323
  TB and, 249
Vitamin C and stroke, 365
Vitamin D
  bladder infections and, 42
  blood pressure/hypertension and, 47
  breast cancer and, 71, 89
  colon and rectal cancer and, 106–107
  depression and, 121–122
  endometrial cancer and, 146–147
  falls and, 161–162
  heart/blood vessels and, 189–190
  incontinence and, 212
  kidney conditions and, 221–222
  lung conditions and, 242–243
  osteoporosis and, 270–271
  ovarian cancer and, 282–283
  pain and, 301
  pancreatic cancer and, 314–315
  PMS and, 327–328
  pregnancy/labor/delivery and,
    344–345
Vitamin E
  gastric cancer and, 180
  heart/blood vessels and, 207
  PMS and, 330–331
  polycystic ovary syndrome and, 335
Vitamin K
  menopause and, 257–258
  osteoporosis and, 278

Walking
  Alzheimer's and, 7
  anxiety and, 25–26
  blood pressure/hypertension and,
    48–49
  breast cancer and, 72–73
  endometrial cancer and, 147
  menopause and, 254–255
Walnuts
  depression and, 128
  heart/blood vessels and, 203
Water
  blood pressure and, 47–48
  colon and rectal cancer and, 107

Water (*continued*)
  digestion and, 141
  gastric cancer and, 174
  heart/blood vessels and, 186–187
  overweight/obesity and, 298
  stroke and, 360
Watercress
  ovarian cancer and, 285
  pancreatic cancer and, 320–321
Weighted exercise and osteoporosis,
  271–272
Western diet and pancreatic cancer, 321
Whole grains
  anxiety and, 31
  blood pressure and, 53
  breast cancer and, 79
  cervical cancer and, 98, 100
  colon and rectal cancer and, 113, 117
  endometrial cancer, 152, 155
  gastric cancer and, 177–178
  lung cancer and, 246

Workplace
  aggravation and colon and rectal cancer,
    106
  chemical exposures and breast cancer,
    71–72

X-rays
  breast cancer and, 72
  pregnancy and, 340

Yoga
  anxiety and, 26
  bladder infections and, 38–39
  blood pressure/hypertension and, 60
  breast cancer and, 85–86
  heart/blood vessels and, 192–193
  migraines and, 264
  pain and, 303
  pregnancy and, 346

Zinc and bladder infections, 42